Diabetic
Cooking

Publications International, Ltd.

Favorite Brand Name Recipes at www.fbnr.com

Pictured on the front cover: Fresh Vegetable Lasagna *(page 244).*

Pictured on the back cover *(clockwise from left):* Scallop and Spinach Salad *(page 142),* Low Fat Lemon Soufflé Cheesecake *(page 328)* and Grilled Chicken & Fresh Salsa Wrap *(page 67).*

ISBN: 0-7853-7996-7

Library of Congress Control Number: 2002116494

Manufactured in China.

8 7 6 5 4 3 2 1

Nutritional Analysis: The nutritional information that appears with each recipe was submitted in part by the participating companies and associations. Every effort has been made to check the accuracy of these numbers. However, because numerous variables account for a wide range of values for certain foods, nutritive analyses in this book should be considered approximate.

Microwave Cooking: Microwave ovens vary in wattage. Use the cooking times as guidelines and check for doneness before adding more time.

Preparation/Cooking Times: Preparation times are based on the approximate amount of time required to assemble the recipe before cooking, baking, chilling or serving. These times include preparation steps such as measuring, chopping and mixing. The fact that some preparations and cooking can be done simultaneously is taken into account. Preparation of optional ingredients and serving suggestions is not included.

Contents

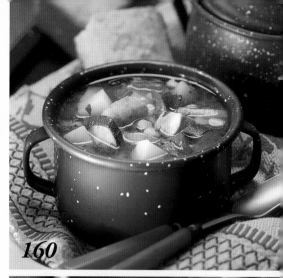

160

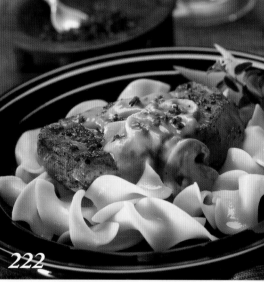

222

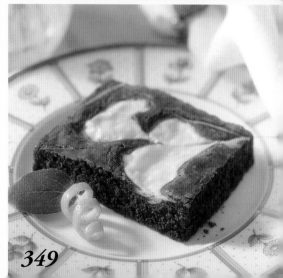

349

Introduction

Whether you or someone close to you has only recently been diagnosed with diabetes or has been living with it for years, don't be discouraged. We now know more about diabetes than ever before, and research is constantly providing us with information on new and better ways of managing it. Today people with diabetes are living long, happy and healthy lives.

No Foods are Forbidden

In the past, people with diabetes were told to monitor the amount of sugar in every food they ate. While it used to be thought that simple sugar, such as the type in cake and cookies, caused a larger rise in blood glucose than other types of carbohydrates, research has proven otherwise. Today the focus has shifted away from sugar to focus on the total amount of carbohydrates consumed throughout the day. Better known as "Carbohydrate Counting," this system is much more flexible than the older, more rigid Exchange System.

Instead of telling patients what foods to avoid, health professionals are now instructing them on healthy eating and foods to choose. Registered dietitians and certified diabetes educators everywhere are working with patients, instructing them on ways to include a wide variety of foods—even sugary ones in moderation—in their meal plans. Because this system, "Carbohydrate Counting," is the one being taught by so many health professionals today, the amount of sugar is not included with the nutritional analyses for the recipes in this book. You will, however, find the total amount of carbohydrates and the exchange information given with each recipe.

If you haven't already, ask your medical doctor or endocrinologist to refer you to a registered dietitian or a certified diabetes educator. Either of these professionals will talk with you and help you better understand your diabetes and instruct you on ways to control it. They will likely be able to calculate the number of servings of carbohydrates you need each day and can work with you to devise a meal plan that best fits your lifestyle.

It's All About Balance

Goals for healthful eating are based on total foods consumed throughout the day or over a period of time, instead of only on individual foods. A food might be high in carbohydrates, but if other foods eaten throughout the day are adjusted to meet a person's total suggested carbohydrate intake, the single high-carbohydrate food will not likely pose a problem. Because of this, a range of healthful recipes are included within this book. Some of the recipes are higher in sodium; some are higher in fat; and some are higher in carbohydrates or cholesterol. Moderation, portion sizes and planning are the keys to success with any healthful eating plan.

A diagnosis of diabetes brings about a whole new way of living. This collection of scrumptiously satisfying recipes is intended to help make this transition as smooth as possible. Let it be your guide to providing delicious and nutritious meals each and every day of the week!

Within This Book...

Daybreak Delights

Purported to be the most important meal of the day, breakfast is even more crucial for someone with diabetes. If you find yourself in a toast or cereal rut, this chapter's for you. It offers a variety of delicious new breakfast creations that'll have you looking forward to mornings.

Snacking Sensations

Health professionals often recommend people with diabetes eat several smaller meals and snacks throughout the day to help keep blood glucose levels more even. This chapter is filled with a mix of salty, crunchy, savory and sweet quick-fixing snack recipes sure to make snacktime easier and more enjoyable than ever.

Sandwich Splendor

Steer clear of tempting and often unhealthy take-out. Pull out your brown bag and start packing! This chapter's jam-packed with a plethora of delicious and exciting new sandwiches and wraps—both hot and cold—you can create right in your own kitchen.

Satisfying Salads

Salad for lunch, salad for dinner, salad anytime! You'll find a medley of over 30 mouthwatering salad recipes—many without a hint of lettuce—in this chapter.

Simmering Soups

Clear soups, hearty stews, meaty chilis and creamy chowders are just a sampling of the home-style goodness you'll find inside this chapter. Served alone or alongside a sandwich or salad, these piping-hot creations will please your palate and warm your belly.

Sizzling Skillets

Pull out your skillets! This chapter's filled with healthy meals you can prepare right on your stovetop. Super quick and easy to make, these hot skillet meals are perfect for times when you don't feel like spending hours in the kitchen, but still want delicious and nutritious fare.

One-Dish Wonders

Turkey Breast with Barley-Cranberry Stuffing, Cannelloni with Tomato-Eggplant Sauce and Chicken Pot Pie are just a sampling of the tasty, wholesome, good-for-you meals you'll find within this chapter. And the best part? They're all served up in a single dish, which means less cleanup for you!

Especially Eastern

Often low in fat and filled with fresh vegetables, foods from the East are some of the healthiest. Enjoy the splendor of this chapter's stir-fries, rice and noodle dishes, and fresh seafood dinners.

World Fare

This chapter is proof that healthy dishes can be found the world over. Inside you'll find a compilation of some of the finest dishes from such countries as Mexico, Italy and Spain, to name a few.

Pieced Perfection

A whole chapter devoted to cakes and pies? You bet! Lusciously moist cakes and cupcakes, deliciously rich cheesecakes and decadently creamy pies all take center stage here.

Sumptuous Sweets

Some of the most delectable sweet treats imaginable are included within this chapter. And since sweets are no longer forbidden, you can enjoy these decadent pleasures—without the guilt.

Regarding the Nutritional Analyses

The nutritional information that appears with each recipe in this book was calculated by an independent nutrition consulting firm, and The Dietary Exchanges are based on the Exchange Lists for Meal Planning developed by The American Diabetes Association, Inc., and the American Dietetic Association. The following also apply:

- The analysis of each recipe includes all the ingredients that are listed in that recipe, except ingredients labeled as "optional" or "for garnish." If a range is given for an ingredient, the first amount was used to calculate the nutritional information. If an ingredient is presented with an option (e.g., 2 cups hot cooked rice or noodles), the first item listed was used in the nutritional calculations.

- In photographs, extra foods shown on the same serving plate with the food of interest and offered as "serve with" suggestions at the end of the recipe are not included in the nutritional analyses unless they are included in the ingredient list.

- To be consistent with ingredients used in the nutritional analyses, meats should be trimmed of all visible fat.

- The analyses for recipes calling for cooked rice or noodles were based on the preparation of these ingredients without added salt or fat.

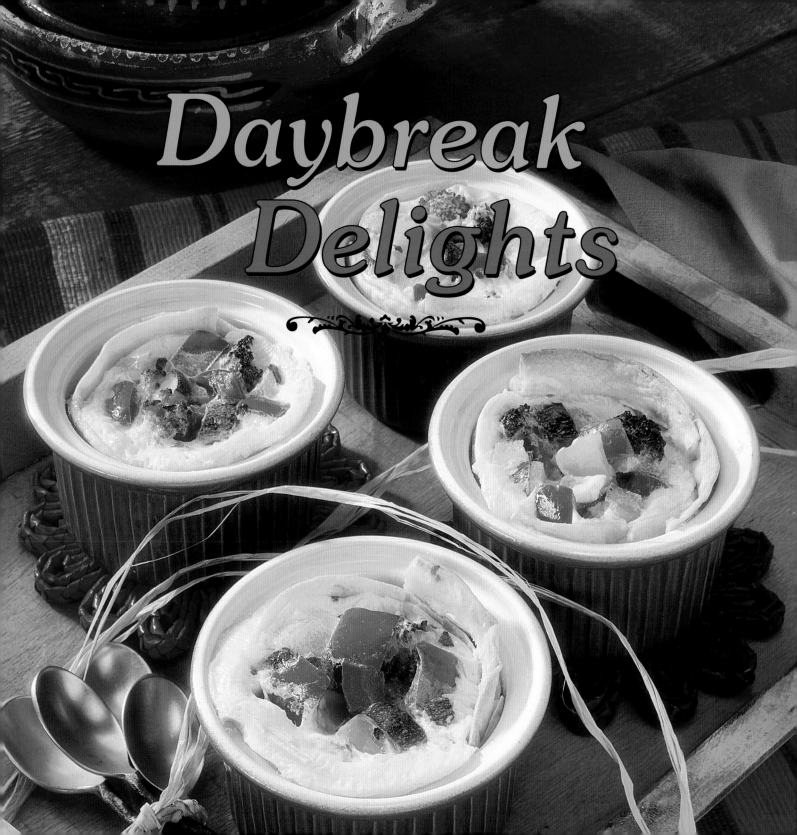

Daybreak Delights

Mini Vegetable Quiches

2 cups cut-up vegetables (bell peppers, broccoli, zucchini and/or carrots)
2 tablespoons chopped green onions
2 tablespoons FLEISCHMANN'S® Original Margarine
4 (8-inch) flour tortillas, each cut into 8 triangles
1 cup EGG BEATERS® Healthy Real Egg Product
1 cup fat-free (skim) milk
½ teaspoon dried basil leaves

In medium nonstick skillet, over medium-high heat, sauté vegetables and green onions in margarine until tender.

Arrange 4 tortilla pieces in each of 8 (6-ounce) greased custard cups or ramekins, placing points of tortilla pieces at center of bottom of each cup and pressing lightly to form shape of cup. Divide vegetable mixture evenly among cups. In small bowl, combine Egg Beaters®, milk and basil. Pour evenly over vegetable mixture. Place cups on baking sheet. Bake at 375°F for 20 to 25 minutes or until puffed and knife inserted into centers comes out clean. Let stand 5 minutes before serving.

Makes 8 servings

Nutrients per Serving (1 quiche):
Calories: 115, Calories from Fat: 30%, Total Fat: 4g, Saturated Fat: 1g, Cholesterol: 1mg, Sodium: 184mg, Carbohydrate: 14g, Dietary Fiber: 1g, Protein: 6g

Dietary Exchanges: ½ Starch, 2 Vegetable, ½ Fat

Mini Vegetable Quiches

Apricot-Almond Coffee Ring

1 cup dried apricots, sliced
1 cup water
3½ teaspoons EQUAL® FOR RECIPES *or* 12 packets EQUAL® sweetener *or* ½ cup
    EQUAL® SPOONFUL™
⅛ teaspoon ground mace
1 loaf (16 ounces) frozen Italian bread dough, thawed
⅓ cup sliced or slivered almonds, divided
  Skim milk
1 teaspoon EQUAL® FOR RECIPES *or* 3 packets EQUAL® sweetener *or*
    2 tablespoons EQUAL® SPOONFUL™

• Heat apricots, water, 3½ teaspoons Equal® For Recipes or 12 packets Equal® sweetener or ½ cup Equal® Spoonful™ and mace to boiling in small saucepan; reduce heat and simmer, covered, until apricots are tender and water is absorbed, about 10 minutes. Simmer, uncovered, until no water remains, 2 to 3 minutes. Cool.

• Roll dough on floured surface into 14×8-inch rectangle. Spread apricot mixture on dough to within 1 inch of edges; sprinkle with ¼ cup almonds. Roll dough up jelly-roll style, beginning with long edge; pinch edge of dough to seal. Place dough, seam side down, on greased cookie sheet, forming circle; pinch ends to seal. Using scissors, cut dough from outside edge almost to center, making cuts 1 inch apart. Turn each section, cut side up, so filling shows. Let rise, covered, in warm place until dough is double in size, about 1 hour.

• Brush top of dough lightly with milk; sprinkle with remaining almonds and 1 teaspoon Equal® for Recipes or 3 packets Equal® sweetener or 2 tablespoons Equal® Spoonful™. Bake coffee cake in preheated 375°F oven until golden, 25 to 30 minutes. Cool on wire rack.   *Makes about 12 servings*

Nutrients per Serving (¹⁄₁₂ of total recipe):
Calories: 158, Calories from Fat: 20%, Total Fat: 3g, Saturated Fat: <1g, Cholesterol: 2mg, Sodium: 184mg, Carbohydrate: 25g, Dietary Fiber: 2g, Protein: 5g

Dietary Exchanges: 1 Starch, 1 Fruit, ½ Fat

Apricot-Almond Coffee Ring

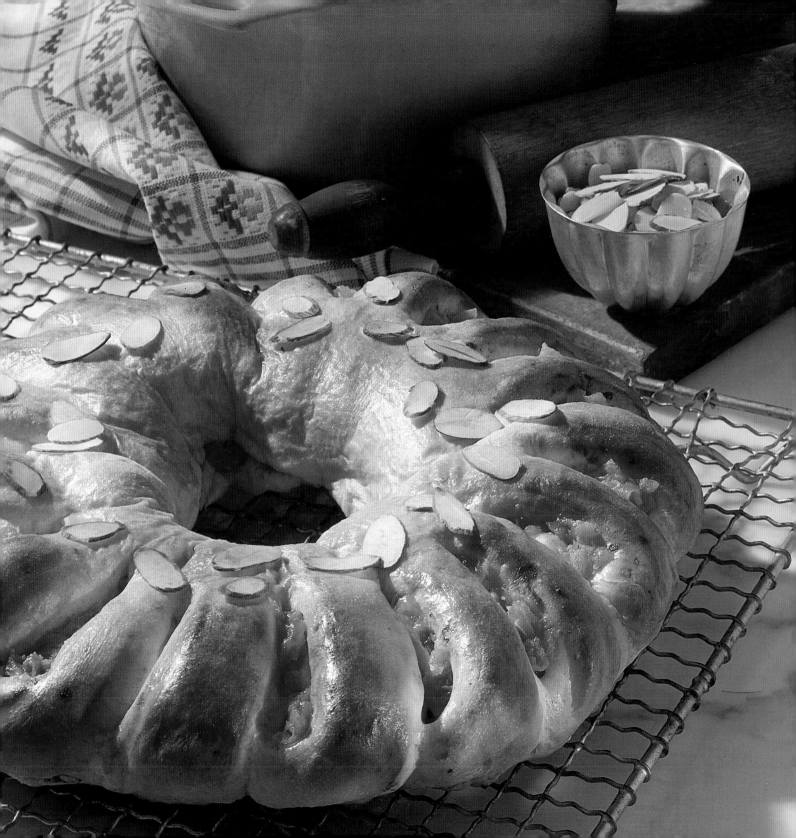

Farmstand **Frittata**

Nonstick cooking spray
½ cup chopped onion
1 medium red bell pepper, seeded and cut into thin strips
1 cup broccoli florets, blanched and drained
1 cup cooked quartered, unpeeled red potatoes
6 egg whites
1 cup cholesterol-free egg substitute
1 tablespoon chopped fresh parsley
½ teaspoon salt
¼ teaspoon black pepper
½ cup (2 ounces) shredded reduced-fat Cheddar cheese

1. Spray large nonstick ovenproof skillet with cooking spray; heat over medium heat until hot. Add onion and bell pepper; cook and stir 3 minutes or until crisp-tender.

2. Add broccoli and potatoes; cook and stir 1 to 2 minutes or until heated through.

3. Whisk together egg whites, egg substitute, parsley, salt and black pepper in medium bowl.

4. Spread vegetables into even layer in skillet. Pour egg white mixture over vegetables; cover and cook over medium heat 10 to 12 minutes or until egg mixture is set.

5. Meanwhile, preheat broiler. Top frittata with cheese. Broil 4 inches from heat 1 minute or until cheese is bubbly and golden brown. Cut into wedges. Garnish as desired. *Makes 4 servings*

Nutrients per Serving (¼ of total recipe):
Calories: 163, Calories from Fat: 12%, Total Fat: 2g, Saturated Fat: 1g, Cholesterol: 8mg, Sodium: 686mg, Carbohydrate: 19g, Dietary Fiber: 2g, Protein: 17g

Dietary Exchanges: 1 Starch, 2 Lean Meat

Farmstand Frittata

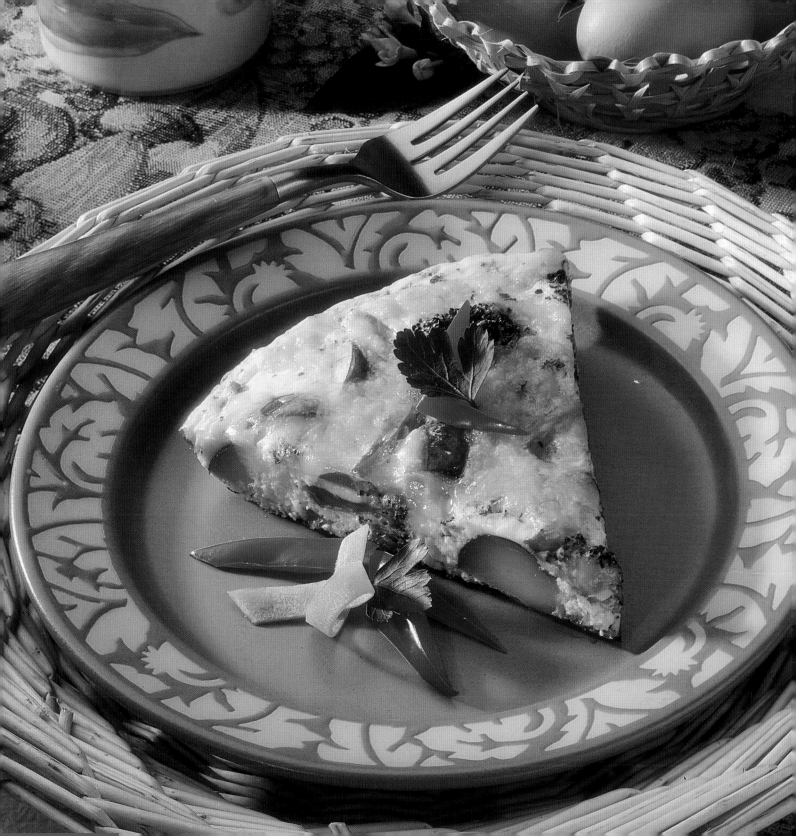

Cinnamon French Toast

1 cup EGG BEATERS® Healthy Real Egg Product
⅓ cup skim milk
1 teaspoon ground cinnamon
1 teaspoon vanilla extract
10 (1-inch-thick) slices French bread
2 tablespoons FLEISCHMANN'S® Original Margarine, divided
   Additional FLEISCHMANN'S® Original Margarine, optional
   Maple-flavored syrup, optional

In small bowl, combine Egg Beaters®, milk, cinnamon and vanilla. Pour half of egg mixture into 13×9×2-inch baking pan. Arrange bread slices in pan; pour remaining egg mixture evenly over bread slices. Let stand for 15 to 20 minutes to absorb egg mixture.

In large nonstick griddle or skillet, over medium heat, melt 1 tablespoon margarine. Cook half the bread slices for 3 minutes on each side or until golden. Cook remaining bread slices, using remaining 1 tablespoon margarine as needed. Serve topped with additional margarine and syrup if desired.

Makes 5 servings

Prep Time: 25 minutes
Cook Time: 15 minutes

Nutrients per Serving (2 slices without additional spread or syrup):
Calories: 334, Calories from Fat: 20%, Total Fat: 8g, Saturated Fat: 2g, Cholesterol: <1mg, Sodium: 682mg, Carbohydrate: 54g, Dietary Fiber: 2g, Protein: 13g

Dietary Exchanges: 4 Starch, 1 Fat

Vegetable Soufflé in **Pepper Cups**

1 cup chopped broccoli
½ cup shredded carrot
¼ cup chopped onion
1 teaspoon dried basil leaves, crushed
½ teaspoon ground black pepper
2 teaspoons FLEISCHMANN'S® Original Margarine
2 tablespoons all-purpose flour
1 cup skim milk
1 cup EGG BEATERS® Healthy Real Egg Product
3 large red, green or yellow bell peppers, halved lengthwise

In nonstick skillet over medium-high heat, cook and stir broccoli, carrot, onion, basil and black pepper in margarine until vegetables are tender. Stir in flour until smooth. Gradually add milk, stirring constantly until thickened. Remove from heat; set aside.

In medium bowl, with electric mixer at high speed, beat Egg Beaters® until foamy, about 3 minutes. Gently fold into broccoli mixture; spoon into bell pepper halves. Place in 13×9-inch baking pan. Bake at 375°F for 30 to 35 minutes or until knife inserted into centers comes out clean. Garnish as desired and serve immediately.   *Makes 6 servings*

Nutrients per Serving (1 filled pepper half):
Calories: 75, Calories from Fat: 16%, Total Fat: 1g, Saturated Fat: <1g, Cholesterol: 1mg, Sodium: 107mg, Carbohydrate: 10g, Dietary Fiber: 2g, Protein: 7g

Dietary Exchanges: 2 Vegetable, ½ Fat

French Breakfast Crêpes

1 cup all-purpose flour
1 cup fat-free (skim) milk
⅔ cup EGG BEATERS® Healthy Real Egg Product
1 tablespoon FLEISCHMANN'S® Original Margarine, melted

In medium bowl, combine flour, milk, Egg Beaters® and margarine; let stand 30 minutes.

Heat lightly greased 8-inch nonstick skillet or crêpe pan over medium-high heat. Pour in scant ¼ cup batter, tilting pan to cover bottom. Cook for 1 to 2 minutes; turn and cook for 30 seconds to 1 minute more. Place crêpe on waxed paper. Stir batter and repeat to make 10 crêpes. Fill with desired fillings, or use in recipes calling for prepared crêpes. *Makes 10 crêpes*

Strawberry Yogurt Crêpes: In medium bowl, combine 1 pint low-fat vanilla yogurt and 2 tablespoons orange-flavored liqueur or orange juice; reserve ½ cup. Stir 2 cups sliced strawberries into remaining yogurt mixture. Spoon ¼ cup strawberry mixture down center of each prepared crêpe; roll up. Top with reserved yogurt mixture.

Blueberry Crêpes: In medium saucepan, combine 2 cups fresh or frozen blueberries, ⅓ cup water, 2 teaspoons lemon juice and 2 teaspoons cornstarch. Cook over medium-high heat, stirring frequently until mixture thickens and begins to boil. Reduce heat; simmer 1 minute. Chill. Spoon 2 tablespoons low-fat vanilla yogurt down center of each prepared crêpe; roll up. Top with blueberry sauce.

Prep Time: 10 minutes
Cook Time: 40 minutes

Nutrients per Serving (per crêpe without filling and topping):
Calories: 73, Calories from Fat: 16%, Total Fat: 1g, Saturated Fat: <1g, Cholesterol: <1mg, Sodium: 55mg, Carbohydrate: 11g, Dietary Fiber: <1g, Protein: 4g

Dietary Exchanges: 1 Starch

Strawberry Yogurt Crêpe

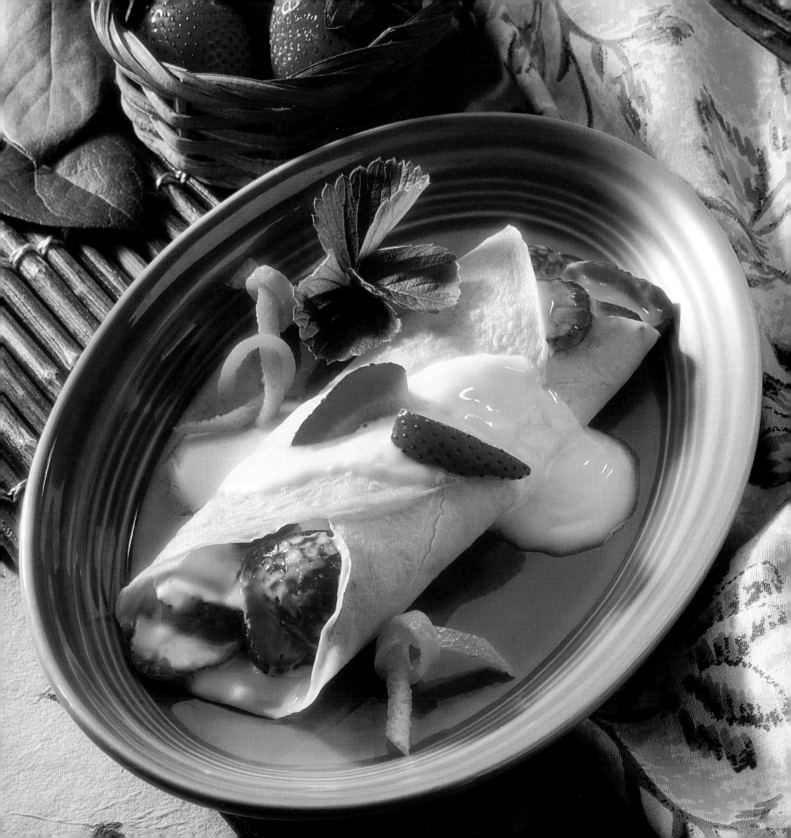

Spinach Feta Frittata

1½ cups cholesterol-free egg substitute

⅓ cup evaporated fat-free milk

1 package (10 ounces) frozen chopped spinach, thawed and squeezed dry

½ cup finely chopped green onions

1½ teaspoons dried oregano or basil leaves

¼ teaspoon salt

⅛ teaspoon black pepper

2 cups cooked spaghetti noodles (4 ounces uncooked)

4 ounces crumbled sun-dried tomato and basil or plain feta

Nonstick cooking spray

Diced red bell pepper (optional)

1. Preheat broiler.

2. Combine egg substitute and milk in medium bowl; whisk together until well blended. Stir in spinach, green onions, oregano, salt and black pepper. Stir in noodles and feta.

3. Spray 10-inch cast iron or ovenproof skillet with cooking spray. Heat over medium heat. Add egg mixture and cook 5 minutes or until nearly cooked through, stirring occasionally.

4. Place skillet under broiler 3 to 5 minutes or until just beginning to lightly brown and set. Remove from broiler. Cut into 4 wedges. Top each wedge with diced bell pepper, if desired.

Makes 4 servings

Nutrients per Serving (1 wedge):
Calories: 254, Calories from Fat: 25%, Total Fat: 7g, Saturated Fat: 5g, Cholesterol: 21mg, Sodium: 762mg, Carbohydrate: 26g, Dietary Fiber: 4g, Protein: 20g

Dietary Exchanges: ½ Starch, 2 Vegetable, 3 Lean Meat

Spinach Feta Frittata

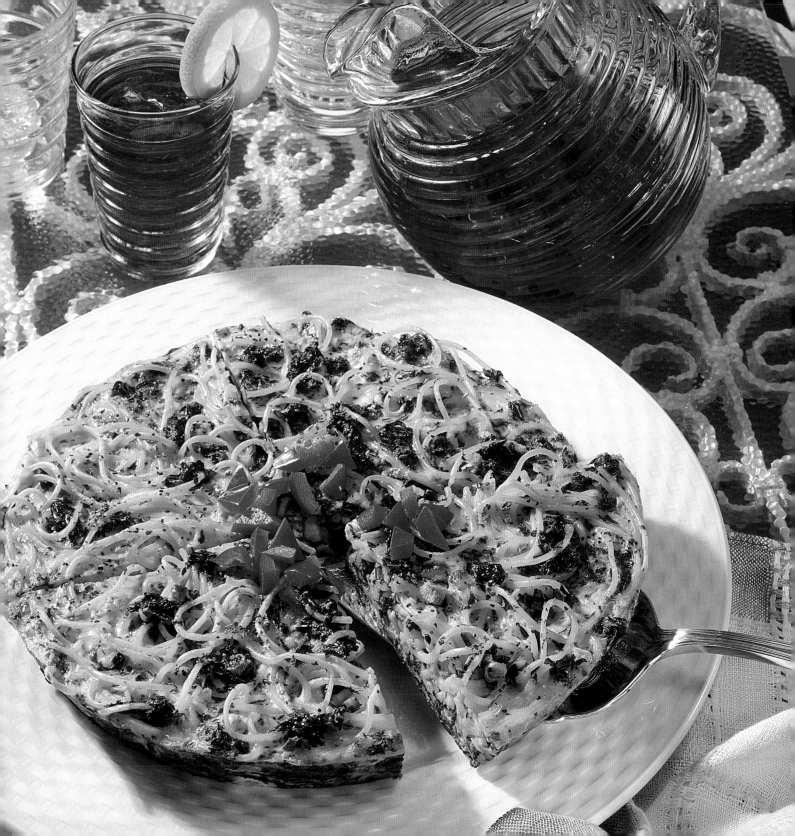

Orange **Muffins**

    2 cups all-purpose flour
    2 teaspoons baking powder
    ½ teaspoon baking soda
    ¼ teaspoon salt
    1 tablespoon grated orange peel
    1 egg, beaten
    ¾ cup orange juice
    ¼ cup butter or margarine, melted
    2 tablespoons milk
    1 teaspoon vanilla
       Whipped butter (optional)
       No-sugar-added orange marmalade fruit spread (optional)

Preheat oven to 400°F. Grease twelve medium-size muffin cups or line with paper liners; set aside. Combine dry ingredients and orange peel in medium bowl. Add beaten egg, orange juice, butter, milk and vanilla to dry ingredients; mix just until moistened. Spoon batter into prepared muffin cups, filling each cup ½ full. Bake 18 to 20 minutes or until golden brown. Let cool in pan on wire rack 5 minutes. Remove from pan; cool. Serve warm or at room temperature. Spread with whipped butter and marmalade, if desired. *Makes 12 muffins*

Nutrients per Serving (1 muffin):
Calories: 128, Calories from Fat: 34%, Total Fat: 5g, Saturated Fat: 3g, Cholesterol: 29mg, Sodium: 231mg, Carbohydrate: 18g, Dietary Fiber: 1g, Protein: 3g

Dietary Exchanges: 1 Starch, 1 Fat

Mushroom-Herb Omelet

1 cup EGG BEATERS® Healthy Real Egg Product
1 tablespoon chopped fresh parsley
1 teaspoon finely chopped oregano, basil or thyme (*or* ¼ teaspoon dried)
2 cups sliced fresh mushrooms
2 teaspoons FLEISCHMANN'S® Original Margarine, divided

In small bowl, combine Egg Beaters®, parsley and oregano, basil or thyme; set aside.

In 8-inch nonstick skillet, over medium heat, sauté mushrooms in 1 teaspoon margarine until tender; set aside. In same skillet, over medium heat, melt ½ teaspoon margarine. Pour half the egg mixture into skillet. Cook, lifting edges to allow uncooked portion to flow underneath. When almost set, spoon half of mushrooms over half of omelet. Fold other half over mushrooms; slide onto serving plate. Repeat with remaining margarine, egg mixture and mushrooms. *Makes 2 servings*

Prep Time: 10 minutes
Cook Time: 20 minutes

Nutrients per Serving (1 omelet):
Calories: 114, Calories from Fat: 27%, Total Fat: 3g, Saturated Fat: 1g, Cholesterol: 0mg, Sodium: 239mg, Carbohydrate: 7g, Dietary Fiber: 1g, Protein: 14g

Dietary Exchanges: 1 Vegetable, 2 Lean Meat

Apricot Walnut Swirl Coffeecake

2⅓ cups reduced-fat baking mix (Bisquick®)
3½ teaspoons EQUAL® FOR RECIPES *or* 12 packets EQUAL® sweetener *or* ½ cup
    EQUAL® SPOONFUL™
⅔ cup skim milk
⅓ cup fat-free sour cream
1 egg
2 tablespoons melted margarine
   Apricot Walnut Filling (page 24)
⅓ cup light apricot preserves sweetened with NutraSweet® brand sweetener or
    apricot spreadable fruit

- Combine baking mix and Equal®; mix in milk, sour cream, egg and margarine. Spread ⅓ of batter in greased and floured 6-cup Bundt pan; spoon half the filling over batter. Repeat layers, ending with batter.

- Bake in preheated 375°F oven until coffeecake is browned on top and toothpick inserted in center comes out clean, about 25 minutes. Cool in pan 5 minutes; invert onto rack and cool 5 to 10 minutes.

- Spoon apricot preserves over top of coffeecake; serve warm. *Makes 12 servings*

continued on page 24

Apricot Walnut Swirl Coffeecake

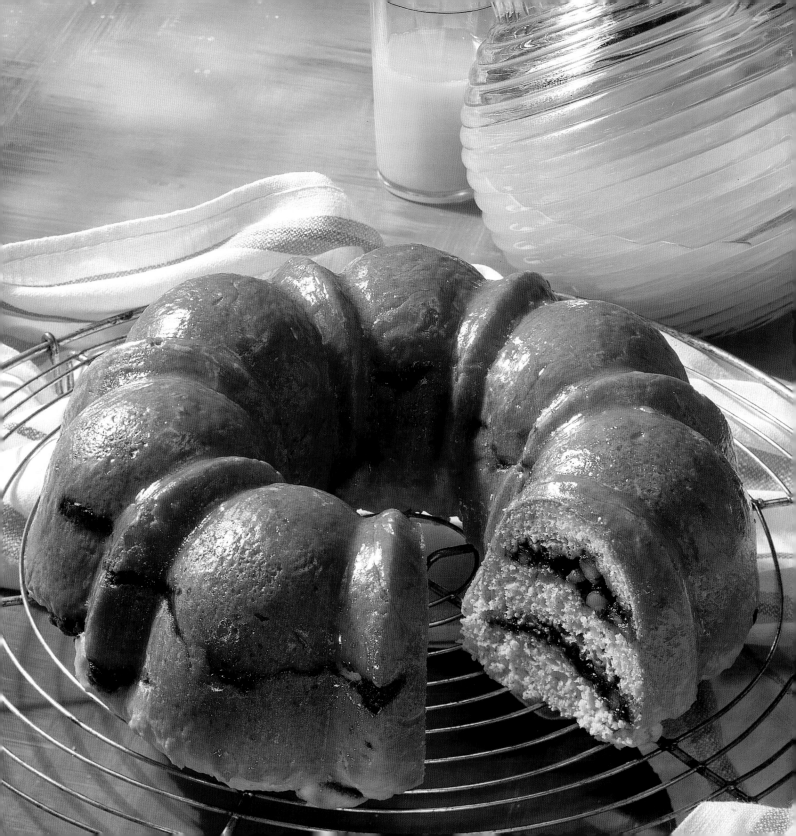

Apricot Walnut Swirl Coffeecake, continued

Apricot Walnut Filling

½ cup light apricot preserves sweetened with NutraSweet® brand sweetener or apricot spreadable fruit

5½ teaspoons EQUAL® FOR RECIPES *or* 18 packets EQUAL® sweetener *or* ¾ cup EQUAL® SPOONFUL™

4 teaspoons ground cinnamon

½ cup chopped walnuts

• Mix all ingredients in small bowl.

Makes 12 servings

Nutrients per Serving (¹⁄₁₂ of total coffeecake):
Calories: 189, Calories from Fat: 34%, Total Fat: 7g, Saturated Fat: 1g, Cholesterol: 18mg, Sodium: 332mg, Carbohydrate: 28g, Dietary Fiber: 1g, Protein: 4g

Dietary Exchanges: 2 Starch, 1 Fat

Triple Fruit Smoothie

1 (8-fluid-ounce) can chilled Vanilla GLUCERNA® Shake

½ cup frozen whole raspberries, unsweetened

½ cup frozen whole strawberries, unsweetened

½ banana, sliced

1 to 2 packets artificial sweetener, if desired

In blender, combine all ingredients. Blend until smooth. Pour into glasses and serve.

Makes 2 servings

Nutrients per Serving (1 cup):
Calories: 162, Calories from Fat: 31%, Total Fat: 6g, Saturated Fat: 1g, Cholesterol: 1mg, Sodium: 107mg, Carbohydrate: 24g, Dietary Fiber: 3g, Protein: 6g

Dietary Exchanges: ½ Fruit, 1 Milk, 1 Fat

Mexican Strata Olé

4 (6-inch) corn tortillas, halved, divided
1 cup chopped onion
½ cup chopped green bell pepper
1 clove garlic, crushed
1 teaspoon dried oregano leaves
½ teaspoon ground cumin
1 teaspoon FLEISCHMANN'S® Original Margarine
1 cup dried kidney beans, cooked in unsalted water according to package
  directions
½ cup (2 ounces) shredded reduced-fat Cheddar cheese
1½ cups fat-free (skim) milk
1 cup EGG BEATERS® Healthy Real Egg Product
1 cup thick and chunky salsa

Arrange half the tortilla pieces in bottom of greased 12×8×2-inch baking dish; set aside.

In large nonstick skillet, over medium-high heat, sauté onion, bell pepper, garlic, oregano and cumin in margarine until tender; stir in beans. Spoon half the mixture over tortillas; repeat layers once. Sprinkle with cheese.

In medium bowl, combine milk and Egg Beaters®; pour evenly over cheese. Bake at 350°F for 40 minutes or until puffed and golden brown. Let stand 10 minutes before serving. Serve topped with salsa.   *Makes 8 servings*

Nutrients per Serving (⅛ of total recipe):
Calories: 185, Calories from Fat: 13%, Total Fat: 3g, Saturated Fat: 1g, Cholesterol: 6mg, Sodium: 397mg, Carbohydrate: 27g, Dietary Fiber: 7g, Protein: 13g

Dietary Exchanges: 2 Starch, 1 Lean Meat

Chile Scramble

2 tablespoons minced onion
1 teaspoon FLEISCHMANN'S® Original Margarine
1 cup EGG BEATERS® Healthy Real Egg Product
1 (4-ounce) can diced green chiles, drained
¼ cup whole kernel corn
2 tablespoons diced pimientos

In 10-inch nonstick skillet, over medium-high heat, sauté onion in margarine for 2 to 3 minutes or until onion is translucent. Pour Egg Beaters® into skillet; cook, stirring occasionally, until mixture is set. Stir in chiles, corn and pimientos; cook 1 minute more or until heated through.   *Makes 2 servings*

Prep Time: 5 minutes
Cook Time: 10 minutes

Nutrients per Serving (½ of total recipe):
Calories: 122, Calories from Fat: 12%, Total Fat: 2g, Saturated Fat: <1g, Cholesterol: 0mg, Sodium: 427mg, Carbohydrate: 13g, Dietary Fiber: 3g, Protein: 13g

Dietary Exchanges: 1 Vegetable, 2 Lean Meat

recipe tip ....
Low in fat and cholesterol, Chile Scramble is also sure to please the palate of any egg lover.

Chile Scramble

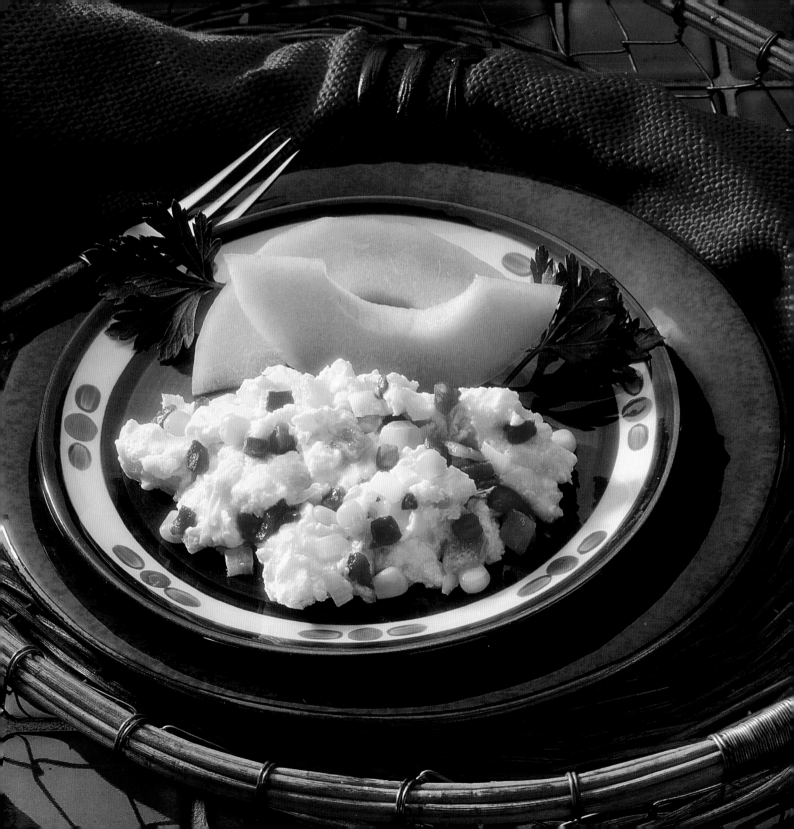

Sweet and Russet Potato Latkes

2 cups shredded russet potatoes
1 cup shredded sweet potato
1 cup shredded apple
¾ cup cholesterol-free egg substitute
⅓ cup all-purpose flour
1 teaspoon sugar
¼ teaspoon baking powder
¼ teaspoon salt
⅛ teaspoon ground nutmeg
   Nonstick cooking spray
1 cup unsweetened cinnamon applesauce

1. Combine potatoes and apple in medium bowl. Combine egg substitute, flour, sugar, baking powder, salt and nutmeg in small bowl; add to potato mixture.

2. Spray large nonstick skillet with cooking spray; heat over medium-low heat until hot. Spoon 1 rounded tablespoonful potato mixture into skillet to form pancake about ¼ inch thick and 3 inches in diameter.* Cook 3 minutes or until browned. Turn latkes and cook second side 3 minutes or until browned. Repeat with remaining batter. Keep cooked latkes warm in preheated 250°F oven.

3. Top each latke with 1 tablespoon applesauce. Garnish, if desired.   *Makes 8 servings*

Three to four latkes can be cooked at one time.

Nutrients per Serving (2 latkes):
Calories: 107, Calories from Fat: 2%, Total Fat: <1g, Saturated Fat: <1g, Cholesterol: 0mg, Sodium: 119mg, Carbohydrate: 23g, Dietary Fiber: 2g, Protein: 4g

Dietary Exchanges: 1 Starch, ½ Fruit

Sweet and Russet Potato Latkes

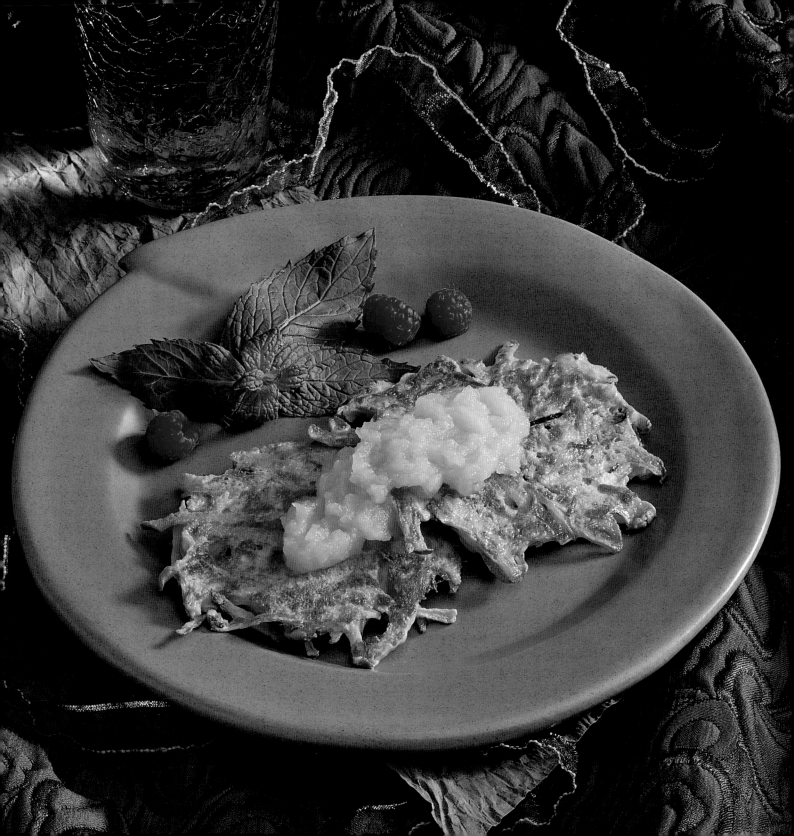

Vegetable Omelet

Ratatouille (page 32)
Nonstick Cooking Spray
5 whole eggs
6 egg whites *or* ¾ cup cholesterol-free egg substitute
¼ cup fat-free (skim) milk
½ teaspoon salt
⅛ teaspoon black pepper
4 to 6 slices Italian bread
2 cloves garlic, halved

1. Prepare Ratatouille; keep warm.

2. Spray 12-inch skillet with cooking spray; heat over medium heat. Beat whole eggs, egg whites, milk, salt and pepper in large bowl until foamy. Pour egg mixture into skillet; cook over medium-high heat 2 to 3 minutes or until bottom of omelet is set. Reduce heat to medium-low. Cover; cook 8 minutes or until top of omelet is set. Remove from heat.

3. Spoon half of Ratatouille down center of omelet. Carefully fold omelet in half; slide onto serving plate. Spoon remaining Ratatouille over top.

4. Toast bread slices; rub both sides of warm toast with cut garlic cloves. Serve with omelet. Serve with fresh fruit, if desired. *Makes 4 to 6 servings*

continued on page 32

Vegetable Omelet

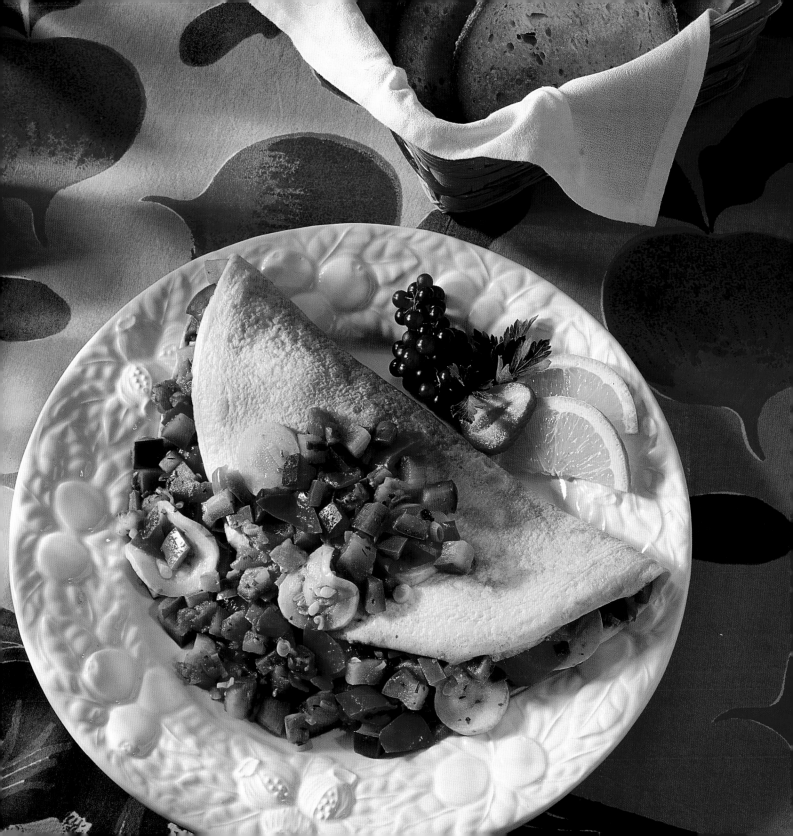

Daybreak Delights

Ratatouille

> Nonstick cooking spray
> 1 cup chopped onion
> ½ cup chopped green bell pepper
> 2 cloves garlic, minced
> 4 cups cubed unpeeled eggplant
> 1 medium yellow summer squash, sliced
> 1 cup chopped fresh tomatoes
> ¼ cup finely chopped fresh basil *or* 1½ teaspoons dried basil leaves
> 1 tablespoon finely chopped fresh oregano *or* 1 teaspoon dried oregano leaves
> 2 teaspoons finely chopped fresh thyme *or* ½ teaspoon dried thyme leaves

Spray large skillet with cooking spray; heat over medium heat. Add onion, bell pepper and garlic; cook and stir 5 minutes or until tender. Add eggplant, summer squash, tomatoes, basil, oregano and thyme. Cover; cook over medium heat 8 to 10 minutes or until vegetables are tender. Uncover; cook 2 to 3 minutes or until all liquid is absorbed.　　　　　*Makes about 4 cups*

Nutrients per Serving (⅙ of omelet with Ratatouille plus toast slice):
Calories: 274, Calories from Fat: 26%, Total Fat: 8g, Saturated Fat: 2g, Cholesterol: 266mg, Sodium: 620mg, Carbohydrate: 32g, Dietary Fiber: 2g, Protein: 19g

Dietary Exchanges: 1½ Starch, 1½ Vegetable, 2 Lean Meat, ½ Fat

recipe tip ....
When purchasing an eggplant, look for one that is plump, glossy and heavy. Avoid any with scarred, bruised or dull surfaces.

Spinach-Cheddar Squares

1½ cups EGG BEATERS® Healthy Real Egg Product
¾ cup fat-free (skim) milk
1 tablespoon dried onion flakes
1 tablespoon grated Parmesan cheese
¼ teaspoon garlic powder
⅛ teaspoon ground black pepper
¼ cup plain dry bread crumbs
¾ cup shredded fat-free Cheddar cheese, divided
1 (10-ounce) package frozen chopped spinach, thawed and well drained
¼ cup diced pimentos

In medium bowl, combine Egg Beaters®, milk, onion flakes, Parmesan cheese, garlic powder and pepper; set aside.

Sprinkle bread crumbs evenly onto bottom of lightly greased 8×8×2-inch baking dish. Top with ½ cup Cheddar cheese and spinach. Pour egg mixture evenly over spinach; top with remaining Cheddar cheese and pimentos.

Bake at 350°F for 35 to 40 minutes or until knife inserted in center comes out clean. Let stand 10 minutes before serving.

Makes 16 servings

Prep Time: 15 minutes
Cook Time: 40 minutes

Nutrients per Serving (1 square):
Calories: 37, Calories from Fat: 6%, Total Fat: <1g, Saturated Fat: <1g, Cholesterol: <1mg, Sodium: 116mg, Carbohydrate: 4g, Dietary Fiber: 1g, Protein: 5g

Dietary Exchanges: 1 Lean Meat

Breakfast Quesadilla

1 frozen BOCA® Breakfast Patty *or* **2 frozen BOCA Breakfast Links**
1 TACO BELL® HOME ORIGINALS®* Flour Tortilla
1 tablespoon PHILADELPHIA® Light Cream Cheese Spread
　TACO BELL® HOME ORIGINALS® Thick 'N Chunky Salsa (optional)
*TACO BELL and HOME ORIGINALS are registered trademarks owned and licensed by Taco Bell Corp.

HEAT breakfast patty or links as directed on package.

SPREAD flour tortilla with cream cheese. Top with chopped patty or links; fold tortilla in half.

HEAT tortilla in nonstick or lightly oiled skillet on medium heat about 2 minutes on each side. Serve with salsa, if desired.　　　　　　　　　　　　　　　　*Makes 1 serving*

Prep Time: 5 minutes
Cook Time: 4 minutes

Nutrients per Serving (1 quesadilla):
Calories: 220, Calories from Fat: 37%, Total Fat: 9g, Saturated Fat: 3g, Cholesterol: 10mg, Sodium: 560mg, Carbohydrate: 22g, Dietary Fiber: 4g, Protein: 12g

Dietary Exchanges: 1½ Starch, 1 Lean Meat, 1 Fat

recipe tip ....
For a zesty twist, spoon a small amount of salsa onto the tortilla mixture before folding.

Breakfast Quesadilla

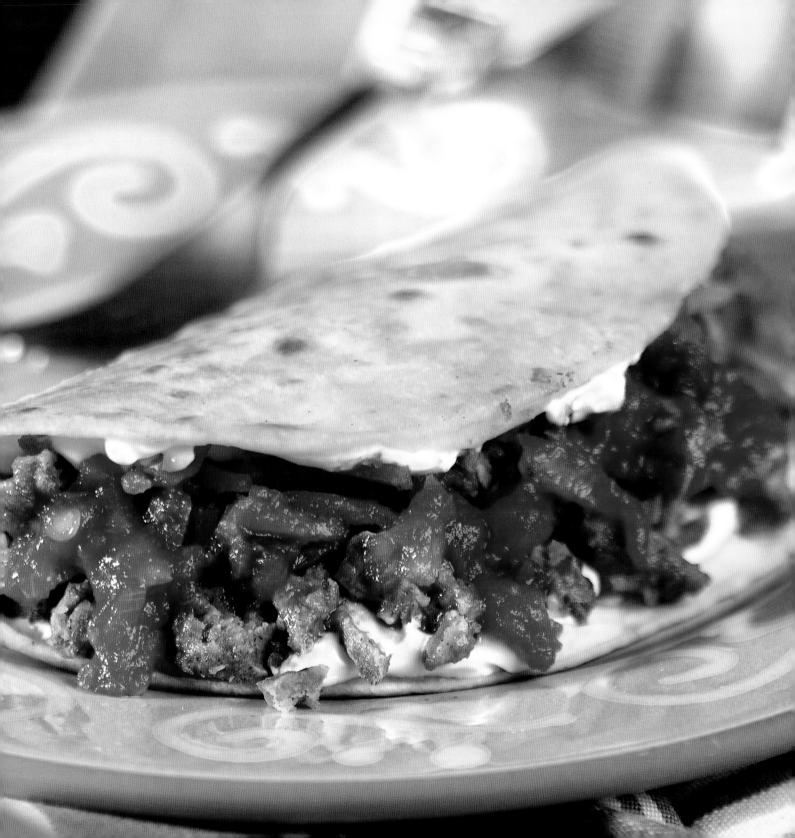

Silver Dollar Pancakes with Mixed Berry Topping

1¼ cups all-purpose flour
2 tablespoons sugar
2 teaspoons baking soda
1½ cups buttermilk
½ cup EGG BEATERS® Healthy Real Egg Product
3 tablespoons FLEISCHMANN'S® Original Margarine, melted, divided
Mixed Berry Topping (recipe follows)

In large bowl, combine flour, sugar and baking soda. Stir in buttermilk, Egg Beaters® and 2 tablespoons margarine just until blended.

Brush large nonstick griddle or skillet with some of remaining margarine; heat over medium-high heat. Using 1 heaping tablespoon batter for each pancake, spoon batter onto griddle. Cook until bubbly; turn and cook until lightly browned. Repeat with remaining batter, using remaining margarine as needed to make 28 pancakes. Serve hot with Mixed Berry Topping.

Makes 28 (2-inch) pancakes

Mixed Berry Topping: In medium saucepan, over medium-low heat, combine 1 (12-ounce) package frozen mixed berries,* thawed, ¼ cup honey and ½ teaspoon grated gingerroot (or ⅛ teaspoon ground ginger). Cook and stir just until hot and well blended. Serve over pancakes.

Three cups mixed fresh berries may be substituted.

Prep Time: 20 minutes
Cook Time: 20 minutes

Nutrients per Serving (4 pancakes plus ¼ cup topping):
Calories: 220, Calories from Fat: 23%, Total Fat: 6g, Saturated Fat: 1g, Cholesterol: 2mg, Sodium: 502mg, Carbohydrate: 37g, Dietary Fiber: 1g, Protein: 6g

Dietary Exchanges: 2 Starch, ½ Fruit, 1 Fat

*Silver Dollar Pancakes with Mixed
Berry Topping*

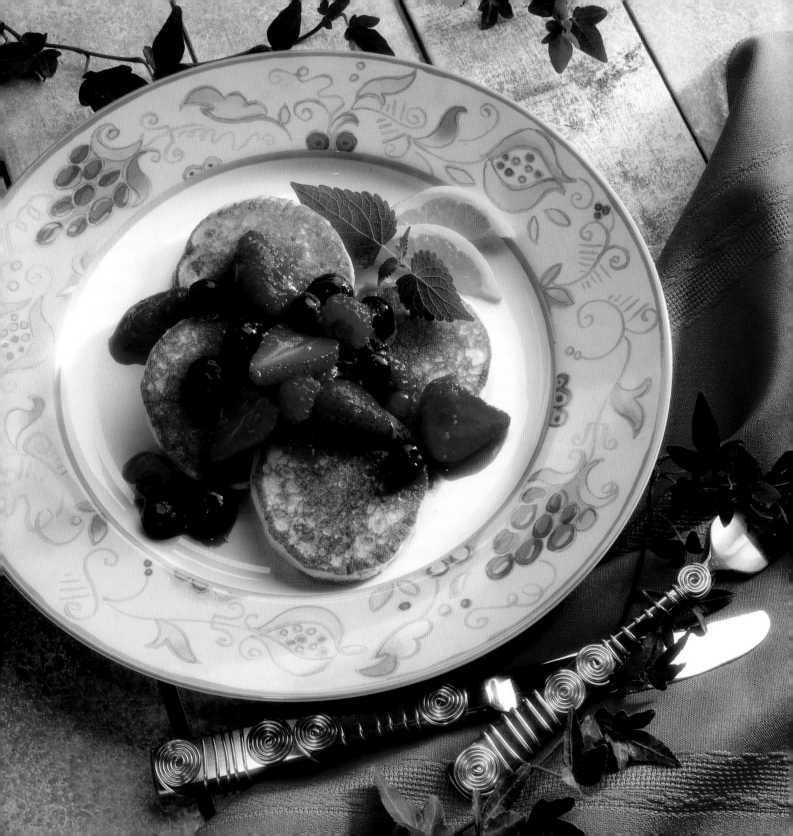

Roasted Pepper **and Sourdough Brunch Casserole**

3 cups sourdough bread cubes

1 jar (12 ounces) roasted pepper strips, drained

4 ounces (1 cup) shredded reduced-fat sharp Cheddar cheese

4 ounces (1 cup) shredded reduced-fat Monterey Jack cheese

1 cup nonfat cottage cheese

12 ounces cholesterol-free egg substitute

1 cup fat-free (skim) milk

¼ cup chopped fresh cilantro

¼ teaspoon black pepper

1. Spray 11×9-inch baking pan with nonstick cooking spray. Place bread cubes in pan. Arrange roasted peppers evenly over bread cubes. Sprinkle Cheddar and Monterey Jack cheeses over peppers.

2. Place cottage cheese in food processor or blender; process until smooth. Add egg substitute; process 10 seconds. Combine cottage cheese mixture and milk in small bowl; pour over ingredients in baking pan. Sprinkle with cilantro and black pepper. Cover with plastic wrap; refrigerate 4 to 12 hours.

3. Preheat oven to 375°F. Bake, uncovered, 40 minutes or until hot and bubbly and golden brown on top. *Makes 8 servings*

Nutrients per Serving (⅛ of total recipe):
Calories: 179, Calories from Fat: 28%, Total Fat: 6g, Saturated Fat: 3g, Cholesterol: 22mg, Sodium: 704mg, Carbohydrate: 13g, Dietary Fiber: 1g, Protein: 19g

Dietary Exchanges: 1 Starch, 2 Lean Meat

*Roasted Pepper and Sourdough
Brunch Casserole*

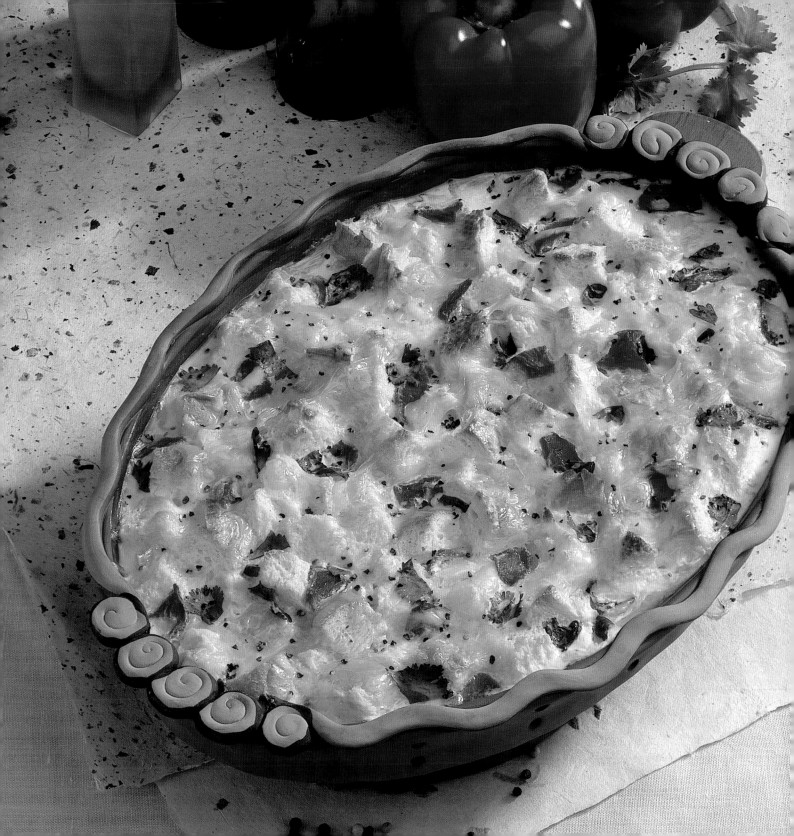

Apricot Oatmeal Muffins

1 cup QUAKER® Oats (quick or old fashioned, uncooked)

1 cup low-fat buttermilk

¼ cup egg substitute or 2 egg whites

2 tablespoons margarine, melted

1 cup all-purpose flour

⅓ cup finely chopped dried apricots

¼ cup chopped nuts (optional)

3 tablespoons granulated sugar *or* 1¾ teaspoons EQUAL® MEASURE™
     (7 packets) *or* 2 tablespoons fructose

1 teaspoon baking powder

½ teaspoon baking soda

¼ teaspoon salt (optional)

Heat oven to 400°F. Lightly spray 12 medium muffin cups with vegetable oil cooking spray. Combine oats and buttermilk; let stand 10 minutes. Add egg substitute and margarine; mix well. In large bowl, combine remaining ingredients; mix well. Add wet ingredients to dry ingredients; mix just until moistened. Fill muffin cups almost full. Bake 20 to 25 minutes or until golden brown. Let muffins stand a few minutes; remove from pan.   *Makes 1 dozen*

Hint: Toast nuts for extra flavor. Spread evenly in small baking pan. Bake in 400°F oven 5 to 7 minutes or until light golden brown. Or, spread nuts on plate. Microwave on HIGH 1 minute; stir. Continue microwaving, checking every 30 seconds, until nuts are crunchy.

Nutrients per Serving (1 muffin without nuts, made with granulated sugar):
Calories: 110, Calories from Fat: 25%, Total Fat: 3g, Saturated Fat: 1g, Cholesterol: 0mg, Sodium: 125mg, Carbohydrate: 19g, Dietary Fiber: 1g, Protein: 4g

Dietary Exchanges: 1 Starch, ½ Fat

Spinach **Cheese Roulade**

4 teaspoons FLEISCHMANN'S® Original Margarine, divided
2 tablespoons all-purpose flour
1 cup skim milk
2 cups EGG BEATERS® Healthy Real Egg Product
1 medium onion, chopped
1 (10-ounce) package fresh spinach, coarsely chopped
½ cup low-fat cottage cheese (1% milkfat)
1 (8-ounce) can no-salt-added tomato sauce
½ teaspoon dried basil leaves
½ teaspoon garlic powder

In small saucepan, over medium heat, melt 3 teaspoons margarine; blend in flour. Cook, stirring until smooth and bubbly; remove from heat. Gradually blend in milk; return to heat. Heat to a boil, stirring constantly until thickened; cool slightly. Stir in Egg Beaters®. Spread mixture in bottom of 15½×10½×1-inch baking pan that has been greased, lined with foil and greased again. Bake at 350°F for 20 minutes or until set.

In medium skillet, sauté onion in remaining margarine until tender. Add spinach and cook until wilted, about 3 minutes; stir in cottage cheese. Keep warm.

Invert egg mixture onto large piece of foil. Spread with spinach mixture; roll up from short end. In small saucepan, combine tomato sauce, basil and garlic; heat until warm. To serve, slice roll into 8 pieces; top with warm sauce. *Makes 8 servings*

Prep Time: 30 minutes
Cook Time: 25 minutes

Nutrients per Serving (⅛ of total recipe):
Calories: 92, Calories from Fat: 22%, Total Fat: 2g, Saturated Fat: 1g, Cholesterol: 1mg, Sodium: 233mg, Carbohydrate: 7g, Dietary Fiber: 3g, Protein: 10g

Dietary Exchanges: 1½ Vegetable, 1 Lean Meat

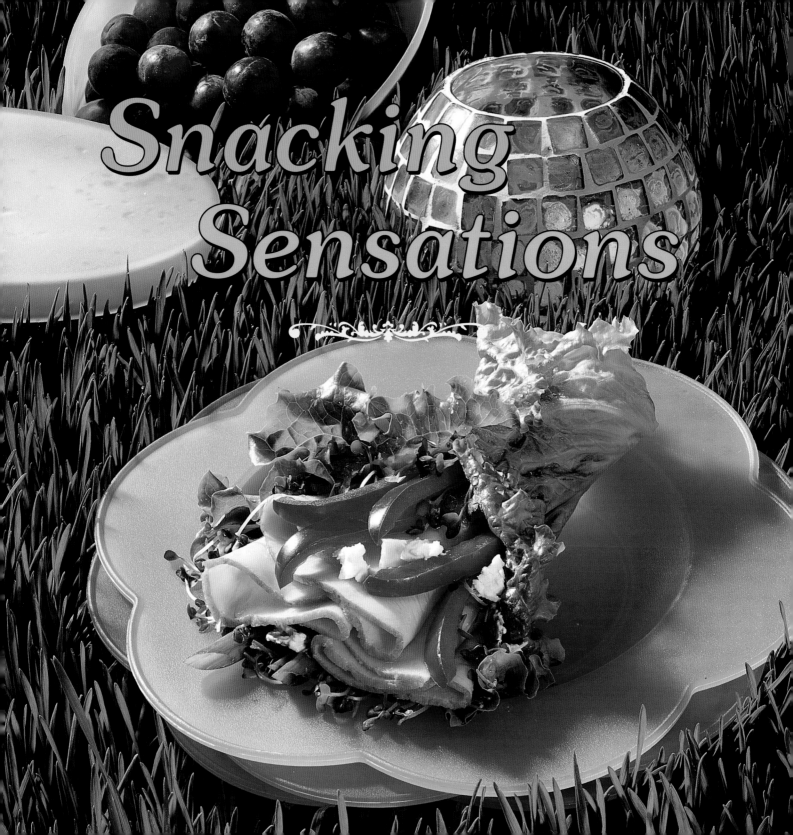

Snacking Sensations

Curly Lettuce Wrappers

    4 green leaf lettuce leaves
    ¼ cup low-fat sour cream
    4 turkey bacon slices, crisp-cooked and crumbled
    ½ cup (2 ounces) crumbled feta or blue cheese
    8 ounces thinly sliced deli turkey breast
    4 whole green onions
    ½ medium red or green bell pepper, thinly sliced
    1 cup broccoli sprouts

1. Rinse lettuce leaves and pat dry.

2. Combine sour cream and bacon in small bowl. Spread ¼ of sour cream mixture evenly over center third of one lettuce leaf. Sprinkle 2 tablespoons cheese over sour cream. Top with 2 ounces turkey.

3. Cut off green portion of each green onion, reserving white onion bottoms for later use. Place green portion of 1 onion, ¼ of bell pepper slices and ¼ cup sprouts on top of turkey.

4. Fold right edge of lettuce over filling; fold bottom edge up over filling. Loosely roll up from folded right edge, leaving left edge of wrap open. Repeat with remaining ingredients.   *Makes 4 servings*

Nutrients per Serving (1 Lettuce Wrapper):
Calories: 155, Calories from Fat: 41%, Total Fat: 7g, Saturated Fat: 4g, Cholesterol: 75mg, Sodium: 987mg, Carbohydrate: 6g, Dietary Fiber: <1g, Protein: 17g

Dietary Exchanges: 1 Vegetable, 2 Lean Meat, ½ Fat

Curly Lettuce Wrapper

Southwest Snack Mix

4 cups corn cereal squares

2 cups unsalted pretzels

½ cup unsalted pumpkin or squash seeds

1½ teaspoons chili powder

1 teaspoon minced fresh cilantro or parsley

½ teaspoon garlic powder

½ teaspoon onion powder

1 egg white

2 tablespoons olive oil

2 tablespoons lime juice

1. Preheat oven to 300°F. Spray large nonstick baking sheet with nonstick cooking spray.

2. Combine cereal, pretzels and pumpkin seeds in large bowl. Combine chili powder, cilantro, garlic powder and onion powder in small bowl.

3. Whisk together egg white, oil and lime juice in separate small bowl. Pour over cereal mixture; toss to coat evenly. Add seasoning mixture; mix lightly to coat evenly. Transfer to prepared baking sheet.

4. Bake 45 minutes, stirring every 15 minutes; cool. Store in airtight container.

Makes about 12 servings

Variation: Substitute ½ cup unsalted peanuts for pumpkin seeds.

Nutrients per Serving (½ cup):
Calories: 93, Calories from Fat: 28%, Total Fat: 3g, Saturated Fat: <1g, Cholesterol: 0mg, Sodium: 114mg, Carbohydrate: 15g, Dietary Fiber: 1g, Protein: 2g

Dietary Exchanges: 1 Starch, ½ Fat

Southwest Snack Mix

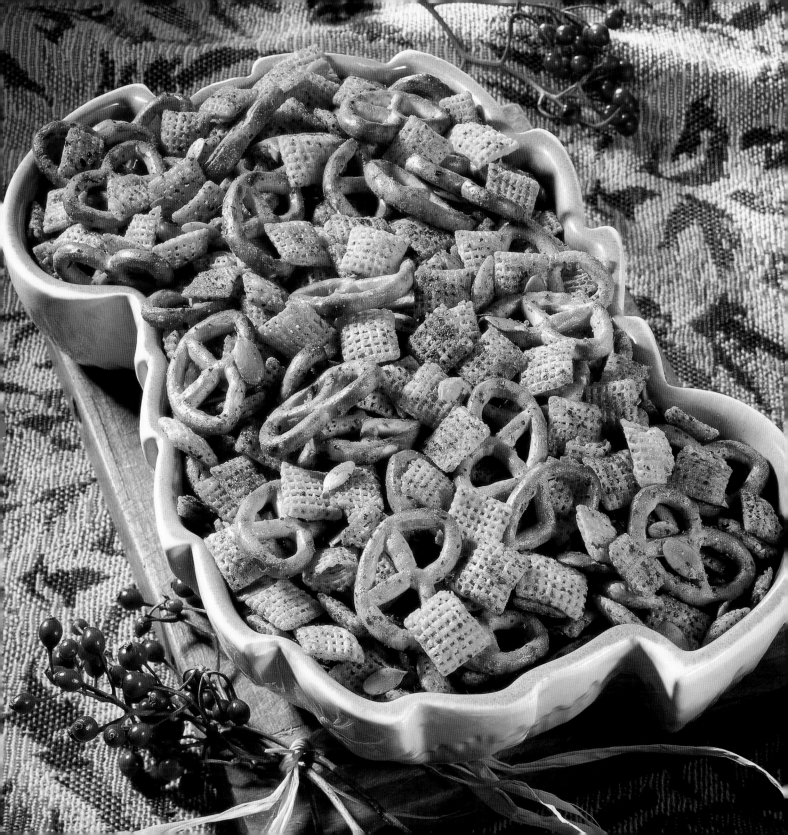

Chili-Cheese Quesadillas with Salsa Cruda

2 tablespoons part-skim ricotta cheese

6 (6-inch) corn tortillas

½ cup (2 ounces) shredded reduced-fat Monterey Jack cheese

2 tablespoons diced mild green chilies

Salsa Cruda (page 48)

1. To make 1 quesadilla, spread 2 teaspoons ricotta over tortilla. Sprinkle with heaping tablespoonful Monterey Jack cheese and 2 teaspoons diced chilies. Top with 1 tortilla. Repeat to make 2 more quesadillas.

2. Spray small nonstick skillet with nonstick cooking spray. Heat over medium-high heat. Add 1 quesadilla; cook 2 minutes or until bottom is golden. Turn quesadilla over; cook 2 minutes. Remove from heat. Cut into 4 wedges. Repeat with remaining quesadillas. Serve warm with Salsa Cruda.

Makes 4 servings

continued on page 48

recipe tip ....

Serve up these tasty quesadilla bites before your next Mexican dinner, or bring them to the annual neighborhood barbecue. Let the fiesta begin!

Chili-Cheese Quesadillas with Salsa Cruda

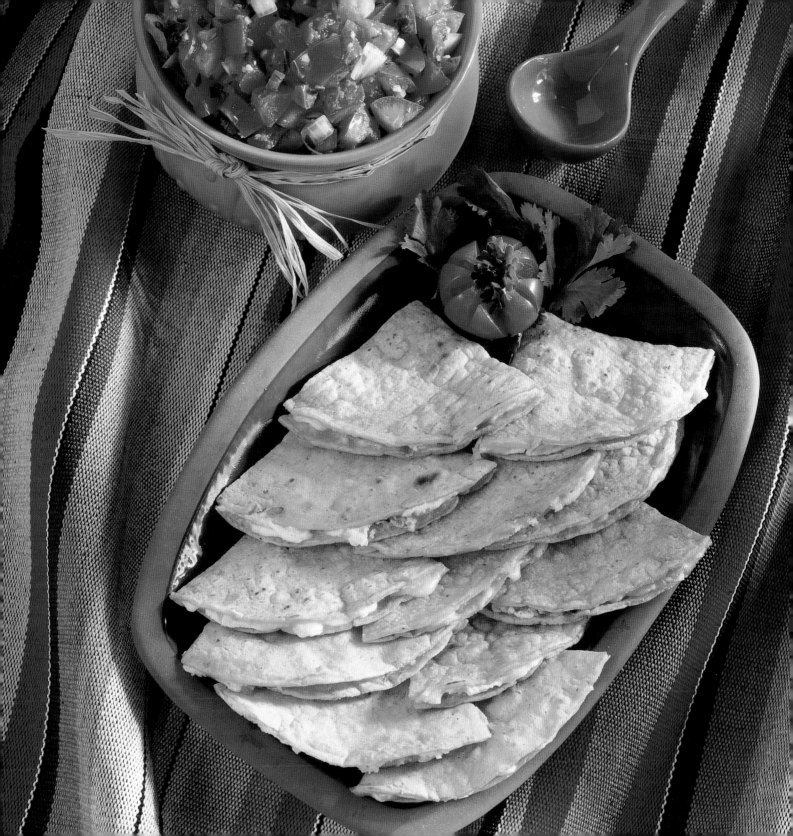

Chili-Cheese Quesadillas with Salsa Cruda, continued

Salsa Cruda

1 cup chopped tomato

2 tablespoons minced onion

2 tablespoons minced fresh cilantro (optional)

2 tablespoons lime juice

½ jalapeño pepper,* seeded and minced

1 clove garlic, minced

*Jalapeño peppers can sting and irritate the skin; wear rubber gloves when handling peppers and do not touch eyes. Wash hands after handling peppers.

Combine tomato, onion, cilantro, lime juice, jalapeño and garlic in small bowl. Stir to combine.

Makes 4 servings

Nutrients per Serving (3 quesadilla wedges plus Salsa Cruda):
Calories: 150, Calories from Fat: 35%, Total Fat: 6g, Saturated Fat: 2g, Cholesterol: 33mg, Sodium: 411mg, Carbohydrate: 18g, Dietary Fiber: 2g, Protein: 6g

Dietary Exchanges: 1 Starch, 1½ Fat

recipe tip ⋯⋯⋯⋯⋯⋯⋯⋯⋯⋯⋯⋯⋯⋯⋯⋯⋯⋯⋯⋯⋯

Tomatoes should never be refrigerated before being cut. Cold temperatures cause the flesh to become mealy and the tomatoes to lose their flavor. Instead, store them at room temperature. Ripening can be hastened by placing the tomatoes in a paper bag.

Ham and Cheese Corn Muffins

1 package (about 8 ounces) corn muffin mix
½ cup chopped deli ham
½ cup (2 ounces) shredded Swiss cheese
⅓ cup reduced-fat (2%) milk
1 egg
1 tablespoon Dijon mustard

1. Preheat oven to 400°F. Combine muffin mix, ham and cheese in medium bowl.

2. Combine milk, egg and mustard in 1-cup glass measure. Stir milk mixture into dry ingredients; mix just until moistened.

3. Fill 9 paper cup-lined 2¾-inch muffin cups two-thirds full with batter.

4. Bake 18 to 20 minutes or until light golden brown. Remove muffin pan to cooling rack. Let stand 5 minutes. Serve warm.

Makes 9 muffins

Serving Suggestion: For added flavor, serve Ham and Cheese Corn Muffins with honey-flavored butter. To prepare, stir together equal amounts of honey and softened butter.

Prep and Cook Time: 30 minutes

Nutrients per Serving (1 muffin without honey-flavored butter):
Calories: 150, Calories from Fat: 35%, Total Fat: 6g, Saturated Fat: 2g, Cholesterol: 33mg, Sodium: 411mg, Carbohydrate: 18g, Dietary Fiber: 2g, Protein: 6g

Dietary Exchanges: 1 Starch, 1½ Fat

Smoked Salmon Appetizers

¼ cup reduced-fat or fat-free cream cheese, softened

1 tablespoon chopped fresh dill *or* 1 teaspoon dried dill weed

⅛ teaspoon ground red pepper

4 ounces thinly sliced smoked salmon or lox

24 melba toast rounds or other low-fat crackers

1. Combine cream cheese, dill and pepper in small bowl; stir to blend. Spread evenly over each slice of salmon. Roll up salmon slices jelly-roll fashion. Place on plate; cover with plastic wrap. Chill at least 1 hour or up to 4 hours before serving.

2. Using a sharp knife, cut salmon rolls crosswise into ¾-inch pieces. Place pieces cut-side-down on serving plate. Garnish each salmon roll with dill sprig, if desired. Serve cold or at room temperature with melba rounds.

Makes about 2 dozen appetizers

Nutrients per Serving (1 appetizer):
Calories: 80, Calories from Fat: 21%, Total Fat: 2g, Saturated Fat: 1g, Cholesterol: 6mg, Sodium: 241mg, Carbohydrate: 10g, Dietary Fiber: 1g, Protein: 6g

Dietary Exchanges: ½ Starch, ½ Lean Meat

recipe tip

A member of the parsley family, dill weed is the dried soft feathery leaves of the dill plant. Its distinctive flavor can easily dominate a dish, so you may want to use it sparingly at first.

Smoked Salmon Appetizers

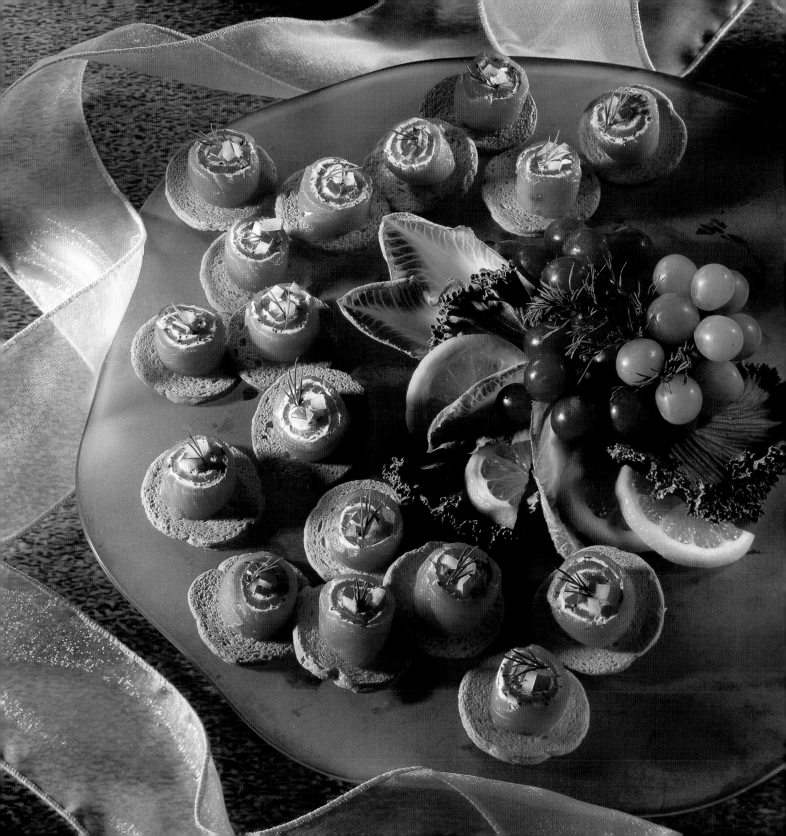

Harvest-Time Popcorn

2 tablespoons vegetable oil

1 cup popcorn kernels

2 cans (1¾ ounces each) shoestring potatoes (3 cups)

1 cup salted mixed nuts or peanuts

¼ cup margarine, melted

1 teaspoon dried dill weed

1 teaspoon Worcestershire sauce

½ teaspoon lemon-pepper seasoning

¼ teaspoon garlic powder

¼ teaspoon onion salt

1. Heat oil in 4-quart saucepan over high heat until hot. Add popcorn kernels. Cover pan; shake continuously over heat until popping stops. Popcorn should measure 2 quarts (8 cups). Do not add butter or salt.

2. Preheat oven to 325°F. Combine popcorn, shoestring potatoes and nuts in large roasting pan. Set aside.

3. Combine margarine, dill, Worcestershire, lemon-pepper seasoning, garlic powder and onion salt in small bowl. Pour evenly over popcorn mixture, stirring until evenly coated.

4. Bake 8 to 10 minutes, stirring once. Remove from oven; let stand at room temperature until cool. Store in airtight containers. *Makes 2½ quarts (10 cups)*

Nutrients per Serving (2 cups popcorn):
Calories: 339, Calories from Fat: 75%, Total Fat: 29g, Saturated Fat: 5g, Cholesterol: 0mg, Sodium: 297mg, Carbohydrate: 15g, Dietary Fiber: 4g, Protein: 7g

Dietary Exchanges: 1 Starch, 6 Fat

Harvest-Time Popcorn

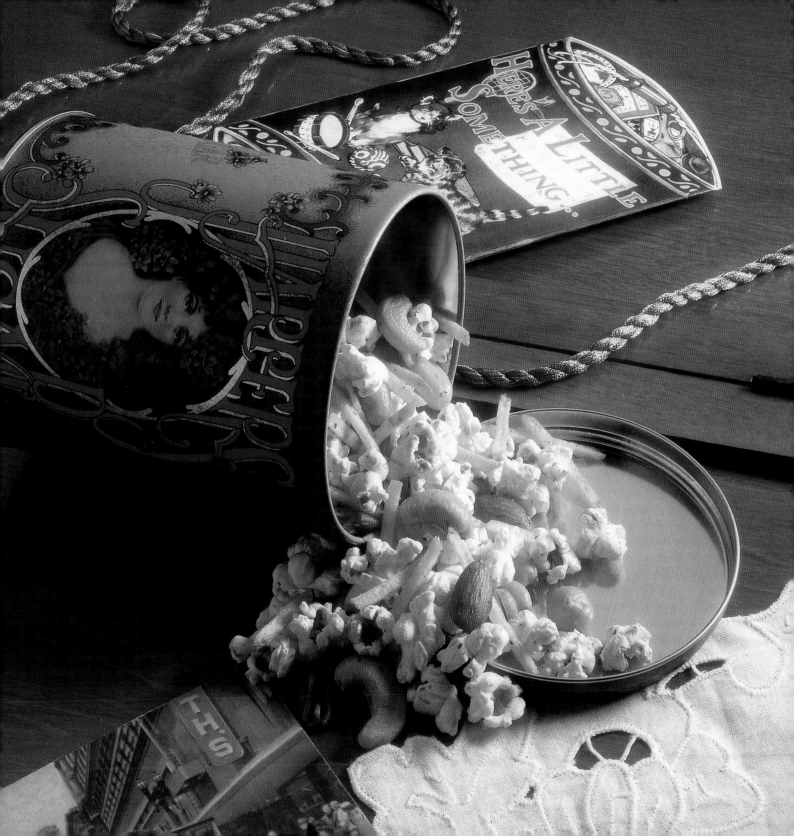

Pita Pizzas

Nonstick cooking spray
½ pound boneless skinless chicken breasts, cut into ½-inch cubes
½ cup thinly sliced red bell pepper
½ cup thinly sliced mushrooms
½ cup thinly sliced red onion (about 1 small)
2 cloves garlic, minced
1 teaspoon dried basil leaves
½ teaspoon dried oregano leaves
1 cup torn fresh spinach leaves
6 mini whole wheat pita bread rounds
½ cup (2 ounces) shredded part-skim mozzarella cheese
1 tablespoon grated Parmesan cheese

1. Preheat oven to 375°F. Spray medium nonstick skillet with cooking spray; heat over medium heat until hot. Add chicken; cook and stir 6 minutes or until browned and no longer pink in center. Remove chicken from skillet.

2. Spray same nonstick skillet again with cooking spray; add bell pepper, mushrooms, onion, garlic, basil and oregano. Cook and stir over medium heat 5 to 7 minutes or until vegetables are crisp-tender. Return chicken to skillet; stir well.

3. Place spinach on top of pita bread rounds. Divide chicken and vegetable mixture evenly over top of spinach. Sprinkle evenly with mozzarella and Parmesan cheese. Bake, uncovered, 7 to 10 minutes or until cheese is melted. *Makes 6 servings*

Nutrients per Serving (1 pita pizza):
Calories: 158, Calories from Fat: 17%, Total Fat: 3g, Saturated Fat: 2g, Cholesterol: 125mg, Sodium: 198mg, Carbohydrate: 19g, Dietary Fiber: 4g, Protein: 14g

Dietary Exchanges: 1 Starch, ½ Vegetable, 1½ Lean Meat

Cheesy Spinach Dip

    1 cup reduced-fat sour cream

    1 cup 1% low-fat cottage cheese

    1 box (10 ounces) frozen chopped spinach, thawed and squeezed dry

    1 can (8 ounces) sliced water chestnuts, drained and chopped

    1 package (1.4 ounces) instant vegetable soup mix

    ¼ cup (1 ounce) grated Parmesan cheese

    2 tablespoons milk (plus additional milk, if necessary)

    1½ teaspoons dried chives

    Cut-up raw vegetables and crackers

Combine sour cream, cottage cheese, spinach, water chestnuts, instant soup mix, Parmesan cheese, milk and chives in large bowl; mix well. Cover and refrigerate at least 2 hours or overnight. Stir well before serving. Add more milk if dip is too thick. Serve with raw vegetables and crackers.

Makes about 3½ cups

Nutrients per Serving (2 tablespoons):
Calories: 34, Calories from Fat: 32%, Total Fat: 1g, Saturated Fat: 1g, Cholesterol: 4mg, Sodium: 187mg, Carbohydrate: 3g, Dietary Fiber: 1g, Protein: 3g

Dietary Exchanges: ½ Starch

recipe tip

Easy to prepare, this healthy, low-fat spinach dip is the perfect appetizer to serve to family and friends. Or, store it in the refrigerator for a quick snack during the week.

Smoked Chicken Bagel Snacks

⅓ cup fat-free cream cheese, softened

2 teaspoons spicy brown mustard

¼ cup chopped roasted red peppers

1 green onion with top, sliced

5 mini-bagels, split

3 ounces smoked chicken or turkey, cut into 10 very thin slices

¼ medium cucumber, cut into 10 thin slices

1. Combine cream cheese and mustard in small bowl; mix well. Stir in peppers and green onion.

2. Spread cream cheese mixture evenly onto cut sides of bagels. Cover bottom halves of bagels with chicken, folding chicken to fit onto bagels; top with cucumber slices and tops of bagels.

Makes 5 servings

Nutrients per Serving (1 bagel snack):
Calories: 139, Calories from Fat: 7%, Total Fat: 1g, Saturated Fat: <1g, Cholesterol: 12mg, Sodium: 502mg, Carbohydrate: 21g, Dietary Fiber: <1g, Protein: 10g

Dietary Exchanges: 1 Starch, 1 Lean Meat

Smoked Chicken Bagel Snacks

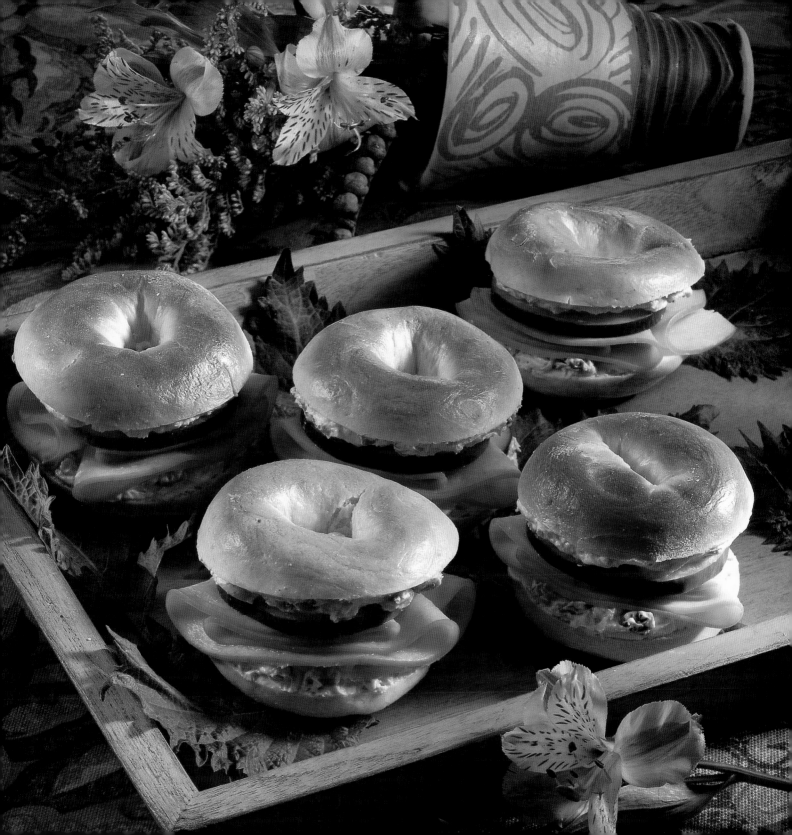

Fresh Fruit with Creamy Lime Dipping Sauce

2 tablespoons lime juice

1 small jicama, peeled and cut into ½-inch-thick strips 3 to 4 inches long

2 pounds watermelon, rind removed and fruit cut into ½-inch-thick wedges 2 to
 3 inches wide

½ small pineapple, peeled, halved lengthwise and cut crosswise into wedges

1 ripe papaya, peeled, seeded and sliced crosswise

Creamy Lime Dipping Sauce (recipe follows)

Combine lime juice and jicama in large bowl; toss. Drain. Arrange jicama, watermelon, pineapple and papaya on large platter. Serve with Creamy Lime Dipping Sauce. Garnish as desired.

Makes 12 servings

Creamy Lime Dipping Sauce

1 carton (6 ounces) nonfat vanilla yogurt

2 tablespoons minced fresh cilantro

2 tablespoons lime juice

1 tablespoon minced jalapeño pepper*

*Jalapeños can irritate skin. Wear rubber gloves when handling; do not touch eyes. Wash hands following.

Combine all ingredients in small bowl; mix well to combine.

Makes about 1 cup

Nutrients per Serving (¹⁄₁₂ of total recipe):
Calories: 65, Calories from Fat: 5%, Total Fat: <1g, Saturated Fat: 0g, Cholesterol: <1mg, Sodium: 23mg, Carbohydrate: 15g, Dietary Fiber: 1g, Protein: 1g

Dietary Exchanges: 1 Fruit

***Fresh Fruit with Creamy Lime
Dipping Sauce***

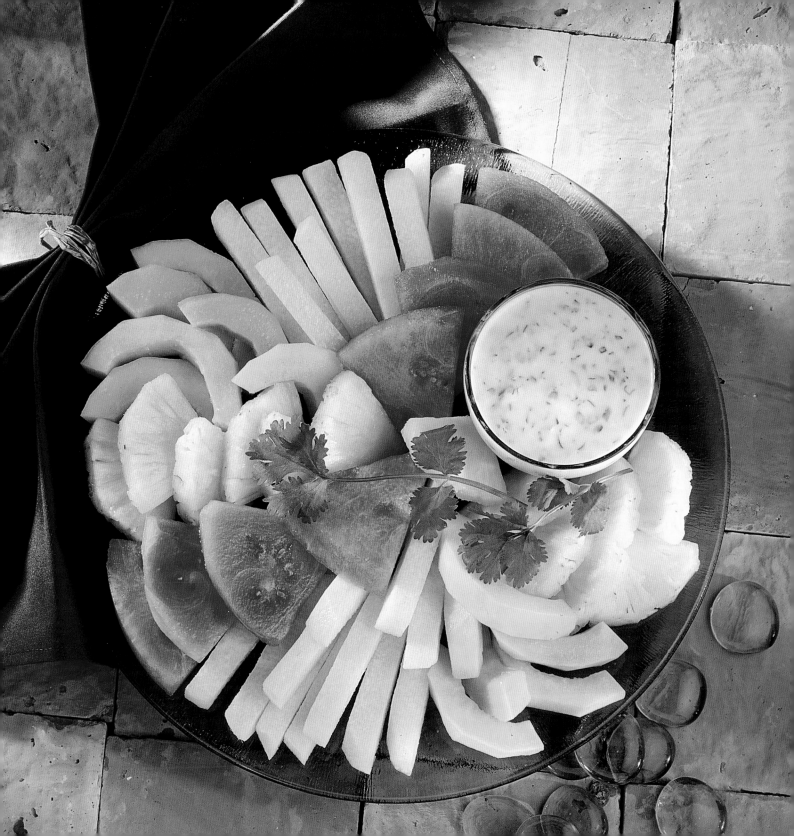

Peanut Butter-Pineapple Celery Sticks

½ cup 1% low-fat cottage cheese
½ cup reduced-fat peanut butter
½ cup crushed pineapple in juice, drained
12 (3-inch-long) celery sticks

1. Combine cottage cheese and peanut butter in food processor. Blend until smooth. Stir in pineapple.

2. Stuff celery sticks with peanut butter-pineapple mixture.   *Makes 6 servings*

Nutrients per Serving (2 celery sticks plus ⅙ of peanut butter-pineapple filling):
Calories: 165, Calories from Fat: 43%, Total Fat: 8g, Saturated Fat: 2g, Cholesterol: 1mg, Sodium: 313mg, Carbohydrate: 17g, Dietary Fiber: 3g, Protein: 8g

Dietary Exchanges: 1 Fruit, 1 Lean Meat, 1 Fat

recipe tip

The peanut butter-pineapple mixture in this recipe tastes great on apples, too.

Savory Zucchini Stix

Nonstick olive oil cooking spray
3 tablespoons seasoned dry bread crumbs
2 tablespoons grated Parmesan cheese
1 egg white
1 teaspoon reduced-fat (2%) milk
2 small zucchini (about 4 ounces each), cut lengthwise into quarters
⅓ cup spaghetti sauce, warmed

1. Preheat oven to 400°F. Spray baking sheet with cooking spray; set aside.

2. Combine bread crumbs and Parmesan cheese in shallow dish. Combine egg white and milk in another shallow dish; beat with fork until well blended.

3. Dip each zucchini wedge first into crumb mixture, then into egg white mixture, letting excess drip back into dish. Roll again in crumb mixture to coat.

4. Place zucchini sticks on prepared baking sheet; coat well with cooking spray. Bake 15 to 18 minutes or until golden brown. Serve with spaghetti sauce. *Makes 4 servings*

Nutrients per Serving (2 Stixs plus about 1 tablespoon spaghetti sauce):
Calories: 69, Calories from Fat: 26%, Total Fat: 2g, Saturated Fat: 1g, Cholesterol: 6mg, Sodium: 329mg, Carbohydrate: 9g, Dietary Fiber: 1g, Protein: 4g

Dietary Exchanges: 2 Vegetable, ½ Fat

Bruschetta

Nonstick cooking spray
1 cup thinly sliced onion
½ cup chopped seeded tomato
2 tablespoons capers
¼ teaspoon black pepper
3 cloves garlic, finely chopped
1 teaspoon olive oil
4 slices French bread
½ cup (2 ounces) shredded reduced-fat Monterey Jack cheese

1. Spray large nonstick skillet with cooking spray. Heat over medium heat until hot. Add onion. Cook and stir 5 minutes. Stir in tomato, capers and pepper. Cook 3 minutes.

2. Preheat broiler. Combine garlic and oil in small bowl; brush bread slices with mixture. Top with onion mixture; sprinkle with cheese.

3. Place bread slices on baking sheet. Broil 3 minutes or until cheese melts.   *Makes 4 servings*

Nutrients per Serving (1 Bruschetta slice):
Calories: 90, Calories from Fat: 20%, Total Fat: 2g, Saturated Fat: <1g, Cholesterol: 0mg, Sodium: 194mg, Carbohydrate: 17g, Dietary Fiber: <1g, Protein: 3g

Dietary Exchanges: 1 Starch

Bruschetta

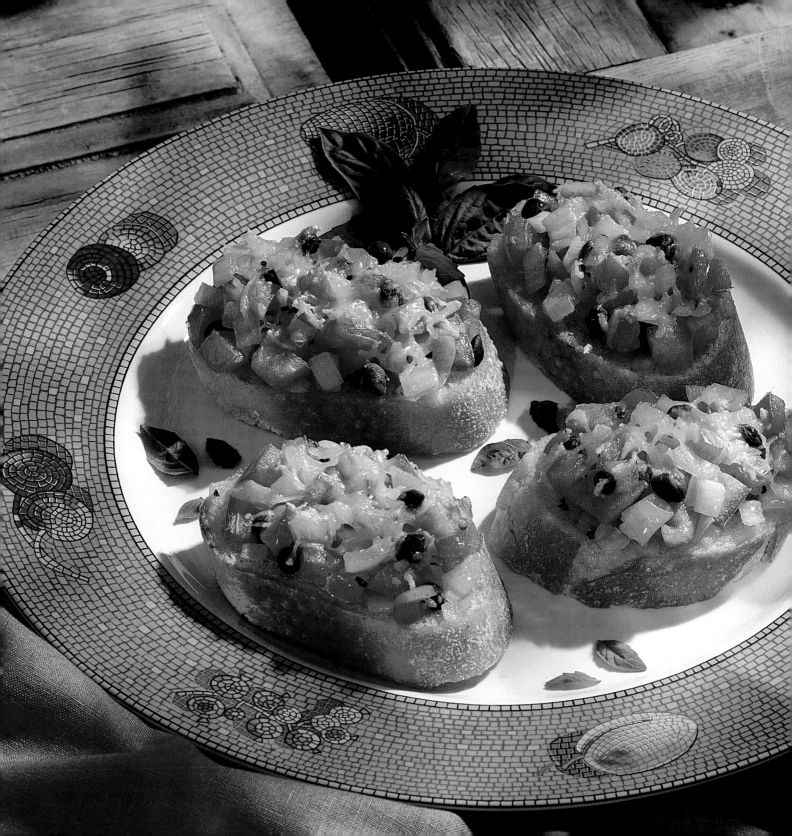

Hot Spiced Tea

1 tub CRYSTAL LIGHT® Iced Tea Mix or CRYSTAL LIGHT® Peach Flavor Iced Tea Mix or CRYSTAL LIGHT® Raspberry Flavor Iced Tea Mix
1 tub CRYSTAL LIGHT® Lemonade Flavor Low Calorie Soft Drink Mix
1 teaspoon ground cinnamon
⅛ to ¼ teaspoon ground cloves

MIX drink mixes and spices. Store in tightly covered jar.   *Makes about 8 teaspoons or 16 servings*

To Make 1 Quart: Measure 3 level teaspoons mix into heatproof pitcher or bowl. Add 1 quart boiling water; stir to dissolve mix.

For Single Serving: Measure ½ level teaspoon mix into cup. Add ¾ cup (6 ounces) boiling water; stir to dissolve mix.

Prep: 10 minutes

Nutrients per Serving (½ teaspoon mix):
Calories: 5, Calories from Fat: 0%, Total Fat: 0g, Saturated Fat: 0g, Cholesterol: 0mg, Sodium: 5mg, Carbohydrate: 0g, Dietary Fiber: 0g, Protein: 0g

Dietary Exchanges: Free

recipe tip ....
Hot Spiced Tea is a wonderful beverage to serve for holiday parties.

"Light" Fresh Lemonade

Juice of 6 SUNKIST® lemons (1 cup)
Low calorie sugar substitute to equal ¾ cup sugar
¼ cup sugar
4 cups cold water
1 fresh SUNKIST® lemon, unpeeled, cut into cartwheel slices
Ice cubes

In large pitcher, combine lemon juice, sugar substitute and sugar; stir to dissolve sugar. Add cold water, lemon cartwheel slices and ice; stir well.   *Makes about 6 servings*

Nutrients per Serving (1 cup):
Calories: 53, Calories from Fat: 0%, Total Fat: 0g, Saturated Fat: 0g, Cholesterol: 0mg, Sodium: 3mg, Carbohydrate: 15g, Dietary Fiber: <1g, Protein: <1g

Dietary Exchanges: 1 Fruit

Iced Apple Tea

1 tub CRYSTAL LIGHT® Iced Tea Low Calorie Soft Drink Mix
6 cups cold water
2 cups cold apple juice
Ice cubes

PLACE drink mix in large pitcher. Add water and juice; stir to dissolve. Serve over ice.

Makes 8 servings

Nutrients per Serving (1 cup):
Calories: 30, Calories from Fat: 0%, Total Fat: 0g, Saturated Fat: 0g, Cholesterol: 0mg, Sodium: 10mg, Carbohydrate: 8g, Dietary Fiber: 0g, Protein: 0g

Dietary Exchanges: ½ Fruit

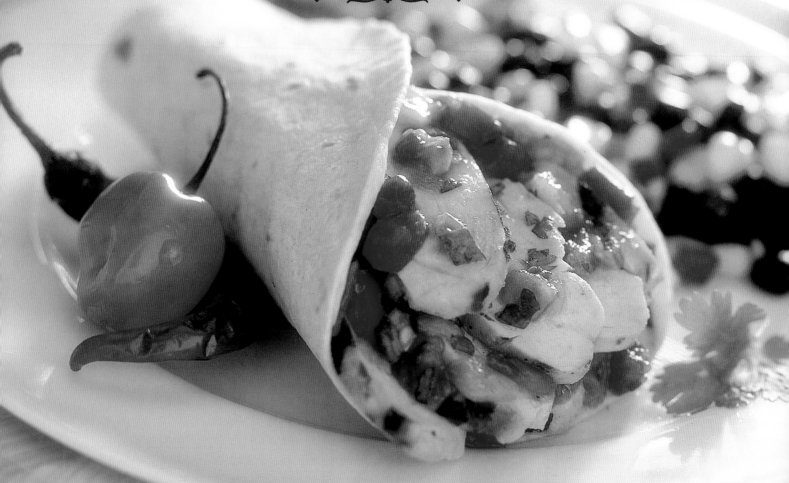

Sandwich
Splendor

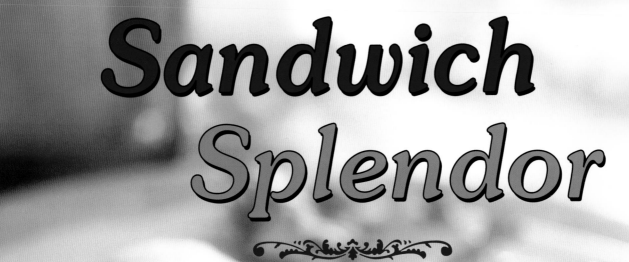

Grilled Chicken & Fresh Salsa Wraps

1 bottle (12 ounces) LAWRY'S® Herb & Garlic Marinade with Lemon Juice,
   divided
4 boneless, skinless chicken breast halves (about 1 pound)
1 large tomato, chopped
1 can (4 ounces) diced mild green chiles, drained (optional)
¼ cup thinly sliced green onions
1 tablespoon red wine vinegar
1 tablespoon chopped fresh cilantro
½ teaspoon LAWRY'S® Garlic Salt
4 to 8 flour tortillas, warmed

In large resealable plastic food storage bag, combine 1 cup Herb & Garlic Marinade and chicken; seal bag. Marinate in refrigerator at least 30 minutes. In medium bowl, combine tomato, chiles, if desired, green onions, additional ¼ cup Herb & Garlic Marinade, vinegar, cilantro and Garlic Salt; mix well. Cover and refrigerate 30 minutes or until chilled. Remove chicken from marinade; discard used marinade. Grill or broil chicken until no longer pink, about 10 to 15 minutes, turning halfway through grilling time. Cut chicken into strips. Place chicken on tortillas; spoon salsa on top and wrap to enclose. Serve immediately. *Makes 4 servings*

Hint: This is an excellent recipe for picnics or outdoor dining. Assemble wraps when ready to serve.

Nutrients per Serving (¼ of total recipe):
Calories: 294, Calories from Fat: 18%, Total Fat: 6g, Saturated Fat: 1g, Cholesterol: 69mg, Sodium: 1283mg, Carbohydrate: 26g, Dietary Fiber: 2g, Protein: 29g

Dietary Exchanges: 1 Starch, 2 Vegetable, 3 Lean Meat

Grilled Chicken & Fresh Salsa Wrap

Garden Tuna Salad

1 can (6 ounces) tuna packed in water, drained
1 medium carrot, chopped
1 rib celery, chopped
½ cup reduced-fat Monterey Jack cheese cubes (¼ inch)
¼ cup frozen green peas, thawed and drained
¼ teaspoon dried parsley flakes
⅓ cup reduced-fat Italian salad dressing
 Lettuce
 Tomato slices
2 pita bread rounds, cut into halves

1. Place tuna in large bowl; break into chunks. Add carrot, celery, cheese, peas and parsley; toss to blend.

2. Pour dressing over tuna mixture; toss lightly to coat.

3. Place one piece lettuce and tomato slices into each pita half. Divide tuna salad evenly among pita halves.   *Makes 4 servings*

Prep Time: 15 minutes

Nutrients per Serving (¼ of total recipe):
Calories: 213, Calories from Fat: 23%, Total Fat: 6g, Saturated Fat: 2g, Cholesterol: 24mg, Sodium: 605mg, Carbohydrate: 22g, Dietary Fiber: 4g, Protein: 19g

Dietary Exchanges: 1 Starch, 2 Lean Meat

Garden Tuna Salad

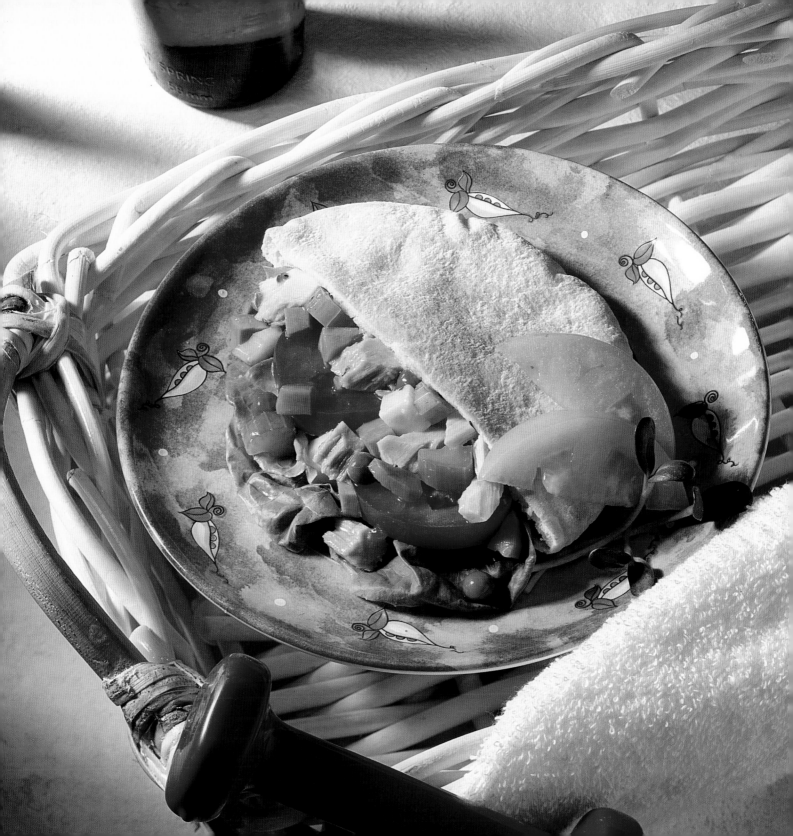

Dad's Turkey Dagwood

Mock Guacamole (page 72)
16 slices low-calorie whole wheat bread
2 tomatoes, sliced
8 cups shredded iceberg lettuce
2 packages (6 ounces) smoked turkey breast slices
8 slices (1 ounce each) reduced-fat Cheddar cheese
8 tablespoons sweet hot mustard

Prepare Mock Guacamole. Spread 3 tablespoons Mock Guacamole onto each of 8 bread slices. Arrange 2 tomato slices, 1 cup lettuce, 2 slices turkey and 1 slice cheese over Mock Guacamole on each bread slice. Spread 1 tablespoon mustard over each remaining slice of bread and place on top of each to form sandwich. Cut each sandwich in half, if desired. *Makes 8 servings*

*Favorite recipe from **National Turkey Federation***

continued on page 72

recipe tip

The smoked turkey breasts in this recipe tend to be higher in sodium content. You can lower the amount of sodium by substituting lightly salted turkey breast meat you've cooked yourself for the precooked packaged poultry.

Dad's Turkey Dagwood

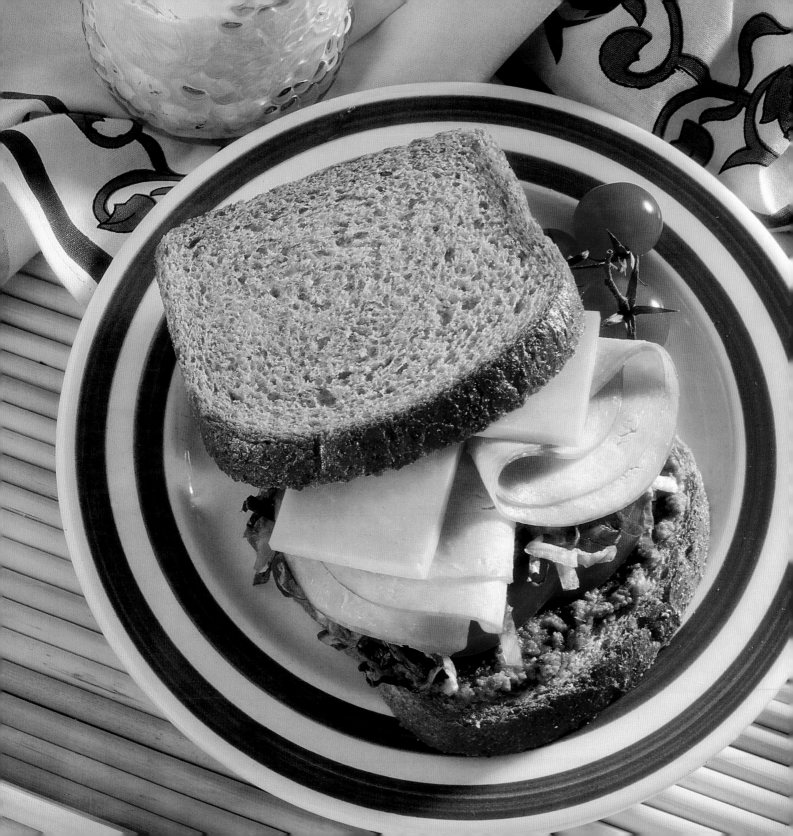

Dad's Turkey Dagwood, continued

Mock Guacamole

2 large cloves garlic
2 cups frozen peas, cooked and drained
½ cup fresh cilantro leaves
¼ cup chopped onion
1 tablespoon lemon juice
¼ teaspoon black pepper
⅛ teaspoon hot pepper sauce

Drop garlic cloves through feed tube of food processor fitted with metal blade while motor is running; process 10 seconds. Add peas, cilantro, onion, lemon juice, black pepper and hot pepper sauce; process until smooth. Refrigerate at least 1 hour.

Makes 8 servings

Favorite recipe from **National Turkey Federation**

Nutrients per Serving (1 sandwich):
Calories: 320, Calories from Fat: 22%, Total Fat: 8g, Saturated Fat: 4g, Cholesterol: 39mg, Sodium: 971mg, Carbohydrate: 42g, Dietary Fiber: 10g, Protein: 23g

Dietary Exchanges: 3 Starch, 2 Lean Meat

recipe tip

Made with peas, Mock Guacamole contains less fat than traditional guacamole, which is made from avocados.

Sloppy Joes **on Whole Wheat Buns**

1 tablespoon CRISCO® Oil*
½ cup chopped onion
½ cup chopped celery
½ cup chopped green bell pepper
½ cup shredded carrots
1¼ pounds ground beef round
½ cup ketchup
½ cup water
1 teaspoon chili powder
½ teaspoon salt
¼ teaspoon pepper
Dash of hot pepper sauce
8 whole wheat light sandwich buns

Use your favorite Crisco Oil product.

1. Heat oil in large skillet on medium heat. Add onion, celery, green pepper and carrots. Cook and stir until tender.

2. Add meat. Cook until browned, stirring occasionally. Drain. Stir in ketchup, water, chili powder, salt, pepper and hot pepper sauce. Reduce heat to low.

3. Simmer 15 minutes or until thick. Spoon evenly into buns.   *Makes 8 servings*

Nutrients per Serving (1 sandwich):
Calories: 233, Calories from Fat: 35%, Total Fat: 9g, Saturated Fat: 3g, Cholesterol: 42mg, Sodium: 510mg, Carbohydrate: 21g, Dietary Fiber: 3g, Protein: 18g

Dietary Exchanges: 1½ Starch, 2 Lean Meat, ½ Fat

Tangy Italian Chicken Sandwiches

2 cups (8 ounces) chopped cooked chicken or turkey breast

⅓ cup drained bottled hot or mild pickled vegetables (jardinière)

2 ounces reduced-fat provolone cheese slices, diced

¼ cup chopped fresh parsley

3 tablespoons reduced-fat Italian salad dressing

¼ teaspoon dried oregano leaves

4 pita bread rounds

8 leaves romaine or red leaf lettuce

1. Combine chicken, vegetables, cheese, parsley, dressing and oregano in medium bowl; mix well.

2. Cut pitas in half. Line each half with lettuce leaf. Distribute chicken mixture evenly among pockets.

Makes 4 servings

Prep Time: 15 minutes

Nutrients per Serving (2 filled pita halves):
Calories: 330, Calories from Fat: 20%, Total Fat: 7g, Saturated Fat: 3g, Cholesterol: 53mg, Sodium: 610mg, Carbohydrate: 39g, Dietary Fiber: 6g, Protein: 28g

Dietary Exchanges: 2½ Starch, 2 Lean Meat, ½ Fat

recipe tip

Pita, also known as pocket bread, is a round, flat Middle Eastern bread made from white or whole wheat flour. Usually about six to seven inches in diameter, the bread splits horizontally to form a pocket, which can be filled with a variety of ingredients to make a sandwich.

Tangy Italian Chicken Sandwiches

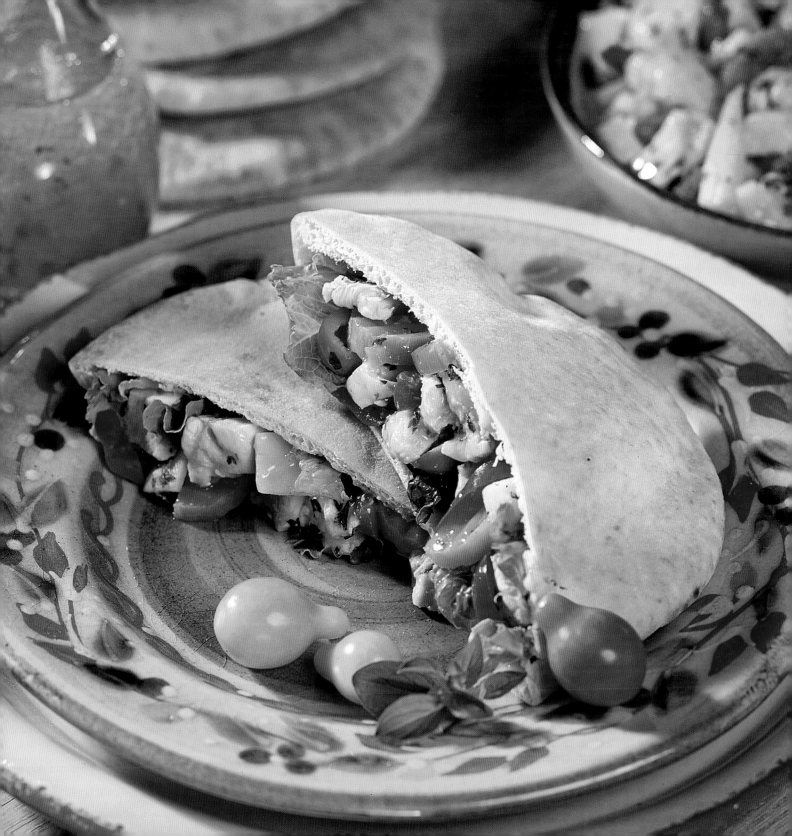

BBQ Beef **Sandwiches**

1 (2½- to 3-pound) lean boneless chuck roast

¼ cup ketchup

2 tablespoons brown sugar

2 tablespoons red wine vinegar

1 tablespoon Dijon mustard

1 tablespoon Worcestershire sauce

1 clove garlic, crushed

¼ teaspoon salt

¼ teaspoon liquid smoke flavoring

⅛ teaspoon black pepper

10 to 12 French rolls or sandwich buns

Slow Cooker Directions

1. Place beef in slow cooker. Combine remaining ingredients except rolls in medium bowl; pour over meat. Cover and cook on LOW 8 to 9 hours.

2. Remove beef from slow cooker; shred with 2 forks. Combine beef with 1 cup sauce from slow cooker. Evenly spoon meat and sauce mixture onto warmed, open-face rolls.

Makes 10 to 12 servings

Favorite recipe from **Susan Revely, Ashland, KY**

Nutrients per Serving: (1 sandwich)
Calories: 361, Calories from Fat: 45%, Total Fat: 18g, Saturated Fat: 7g, Cholesterol: 74mg, Sodium: 460mg, Carbohydrate: 24g, Dietary Fiber: 1g, Protein: 25g

Dietary Exchanges: 1½ Starch, 3 Lean Meat, 2 Fat

BBQ Beef Sandwich

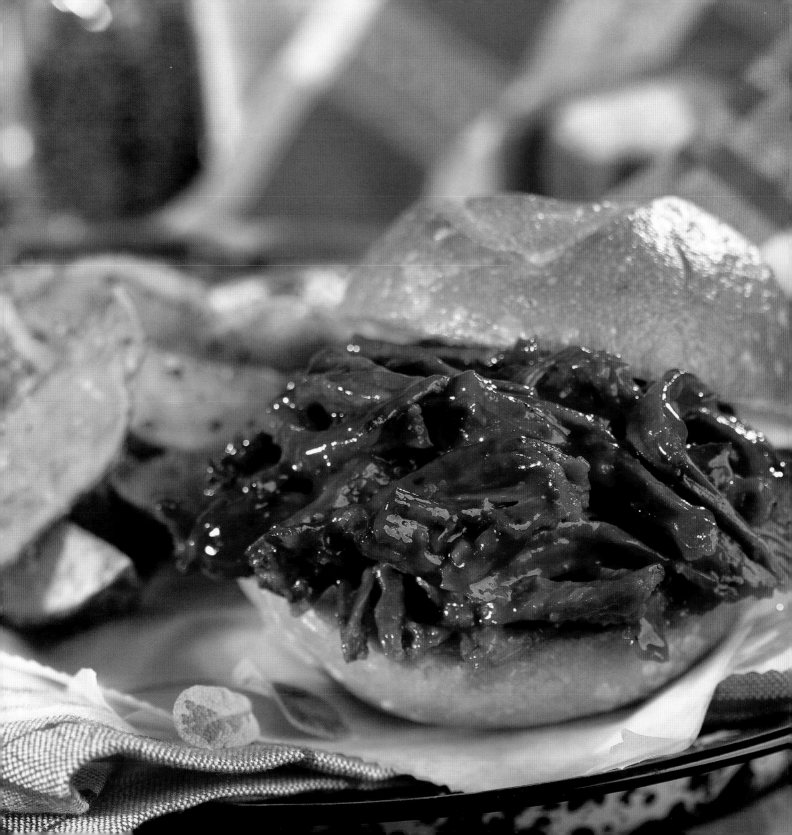

Cajun Catfish Sandwiches

Aioli Tartar Sauce (recipe follows)
4½ teaspoons paprika
1 tablespoon dried oregano leaves
1½ teaspoons salt
¾ teaspoon granulated garlic
½ teaspoon white pepper
½ teaspoon black pepper
½ teaspoon cayenne pepper
4 small catfish fillets (1¼ pounds)
Lemon juice
4 sourdough rolls, split
4 cups finely shredded cabbage
Lemon wedges

Prepare Aioli Tartar Sauce; set aside. Combine paprika, oregano, salt, garlic and peppers until blended. Brush catfish with lemon juice; sprinkle evenly with seasoning mix to coat. Lightly oil grid to prevent sticking. Grill over medium-hot KINGSFORD® Briquets, allowing 10 minutes cooking time for each inch of thickness, turning once. Spread Aioli Tartar Sauce onto insides of rolls. Top each roll with catfish fillet and 1 cup cabbage. Serve with lemon wedges. *Makes 4 sandwiches*

Aioli Tartar Sauce: Prepare Grilled Garlic (recipe page 79). Combine ½ cup mayonnaise, 12 mashed cloves Grilled Garlic, 2 teaspoons each lemon juice and chopped parsley, and 1 teaspoon chopped, drained capers; blend well.

Grilled Garlic

1 or 2 heads garlic
Olive oil

Peel outermost papery skin from garlic heads. Brush heads with oil. Grill heads at edge of grid on covered grill over medium-hot KINGSFORD® Briquets 30 to 45 minutes or until cloves are soft and buttery. Remove from grill; cool slightly. Gently squeeze softened garlic head from root end so that cloves slip out of skins into small bowl. Use immediately or cover and refrigerate up to 1 week.

Nutrients per Serving (1 sandwich with about 2 tablespoons Aioli Tartar Sauce):
Calories: 483, Calories from Fat: 52%, Total Fat: 28g, Saturated Fat: 5g, Cholesterol: 98mg, Sodium: 1,358mg, Carbohydrate: 30g, Dietary Fiber: 4g, Protein: 29g

Dietary Exchanges: 2 Starch, 4 Lean Meat, 3 Fat

recipe tip ....

While garlic's health benefits are still unclear, research seems to be giving the "thumbs-up" to this powerful bulb. In the meantime, take advantage of its super flavor-enhancing qualities.

Mediterranean **Sandwiches**

Nonstick cooking spray
1¼ pounds chicken tenders, cut crosswise in half
1 large tomato, cut into bite-size pieces
½ small cucumber, seeded and sliced
½ cup sweet onion slices (about 1 small)
2 tablespoons cider vinegar
1 tablespoon olive oil or vegetable oil
3 teaspoons minced fresh oregano *or* ½ teaspoon dried oregano leaves
2 teaspoons minced fresh mint *or* ½ teaspoon dried mint leaves
¼ teaspoon salt
12 lettuce leaves (optional)
6 whole wheat pita bread rounds, cut crosswise in half

1. Spray large nonstick skillet with cooking spray; heat over medium heat until hot. Add chicken; cook and stir 7 to 10 minutes or until browned and no longer pink in center. Cool slightly.

2. Combine chicken, tomato, cucumber and onion in medium bowl. Drizzle with vinegar and oil; toss to coat. Sprinkle with oregano, mint and salt; toss to combine.

3. Place 1 lettuce leaf in each pita bread half, if desired. Divide chicken mixture evenly between pita bread halves.

Makes 6 servings

Nutrients per Serving (2 filled pita bread halves):
Calories: 242, Calories from Fat: 21%, Total Fat: 6g, Saturated Fat: 1g, Cholesterol: 50mg, Sodium: 353mg, Carbohydrate: 24g, Dietary Fiber: 2g, Protein: 23g

Dietary Exchanges: 1½ Starch, 2½ Lean Meat

Mediterranean Sandwiches

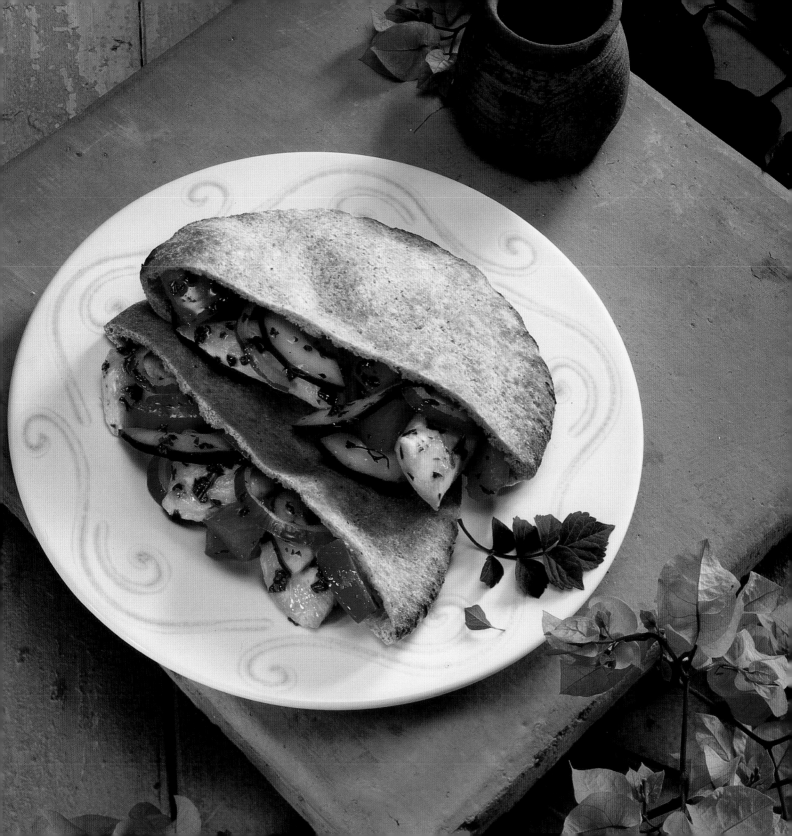

California-Style Tuna Melts

4 slices bread, cut in half, *or* 8 thin slices French bread *or* 4 (8-inch) flour tortillas,
    cut into halves
¼ cup reduced-calorie mayonnaise or salad dressing
8 thin slices tomato
1 (7-ounce) pouch of STARKIST® Premium Albacore or Chunk Light Tuna
½ cup chopped red onion
    Alfalfa sprouts
1 cup shredded low-fat Cheddar cheese
½ ripe avocado, peeled, pitted and thinly sliced

Microwave Directions
Toast bread, if desired. Arrange bread on flat microwavable plate or tray. Spread with mayonnaise.
Place 1 tomato slice on each bread half. Top with tuna, onion and alfalfa sprouts, dividing evenly.
Sprinkle cheese over top. Cover with waxed paper. Microwave on HIGH (100% power) for 2 to
4 minutes or until sandwiches are heated through and cheese is melted, rotating dish once during
cooking. Serve topped with avocado slices. Garnish as desired.   *Makes 8 Melts (4 servings)*

Nutrients per Serving (2 Melts):
Calories: 274, Calories from Fat: 52%, Total Fat: 16g, Saturated Fat: 6g, Cholesterol: 32mg,
Sodium: 533mg, Carbohydrate: 19g, Dietary Fiber: 2g, Protein: 14g

Dietary Exchanges: 1 Starch, 2 Lean Meat, 2 Fat

California-Style Tuna Melts

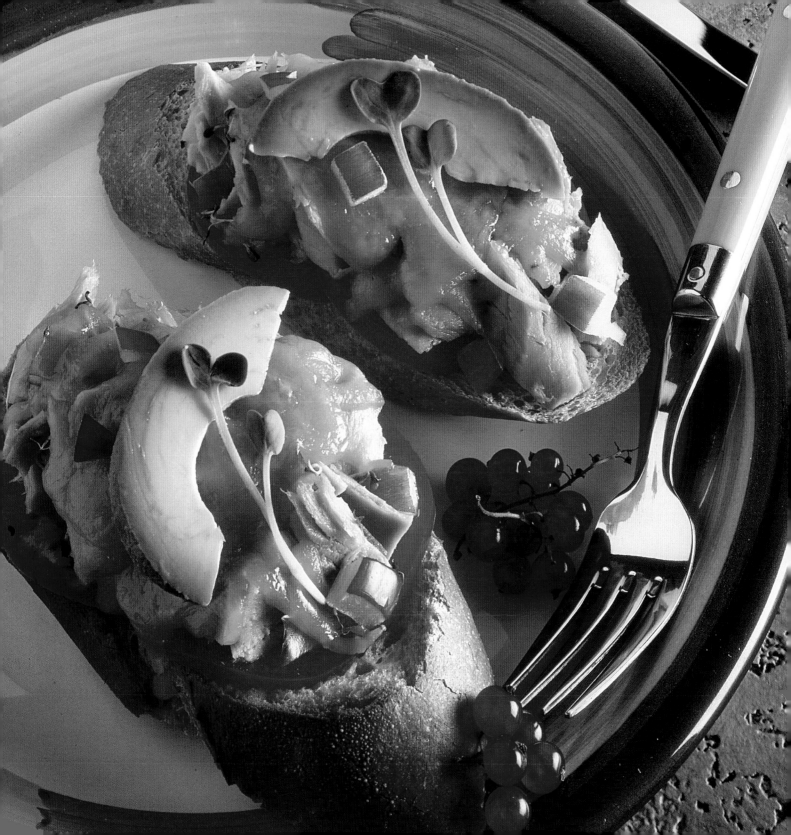

Mediterranean **Vegetable Sandwiches**

1 small eggplant, peeled, halved and cut into ¼-inch-thick slices
  Salt
1 small zucchini, halved and cut lengthwise into ¼-inch-thick slices
1 green or red bell pepper, sliced
3 tablespoons balsamic vinegar
½ teaspoon salt
½ teaspoon garlic powder
2 French bread rolls, halved

1. Place eggplant in nonaluminum colander; lightly sprinkle eggplant with salt. Let stand 30 minutes to drain. Rinse eggplant; pat dry with paper towels.

2. Preheat broiler. Spray rack of broiler pan with nonstick cooking spray. Place vegetables on rack. Broil 4 inches from heat 8 to 10 minutes or until vegetables are browned, turning once.

3. Combine vinegar, ½ teaspoon salt and garlic powder in medium bowl until well blended. Add vegetables; toss to coat. Divide vegetable mixture evenly among rolls. Serve immediately.

Makes 2 servings

Nutrients per Serving (1 sandwich):
Calories: 178, Calories from Fat: 10%, Total Fat: 2g, Saturated Fat: <1g, Cholesterol: 0mg, Sodium: 775mg, Carbohydrate: 36g, Dietary Fiber: 1g, Protein: 5g

Dietary Exchanges: 1½ Starch, 3 Vegetable

Mediterranean Vegetable Sandwich

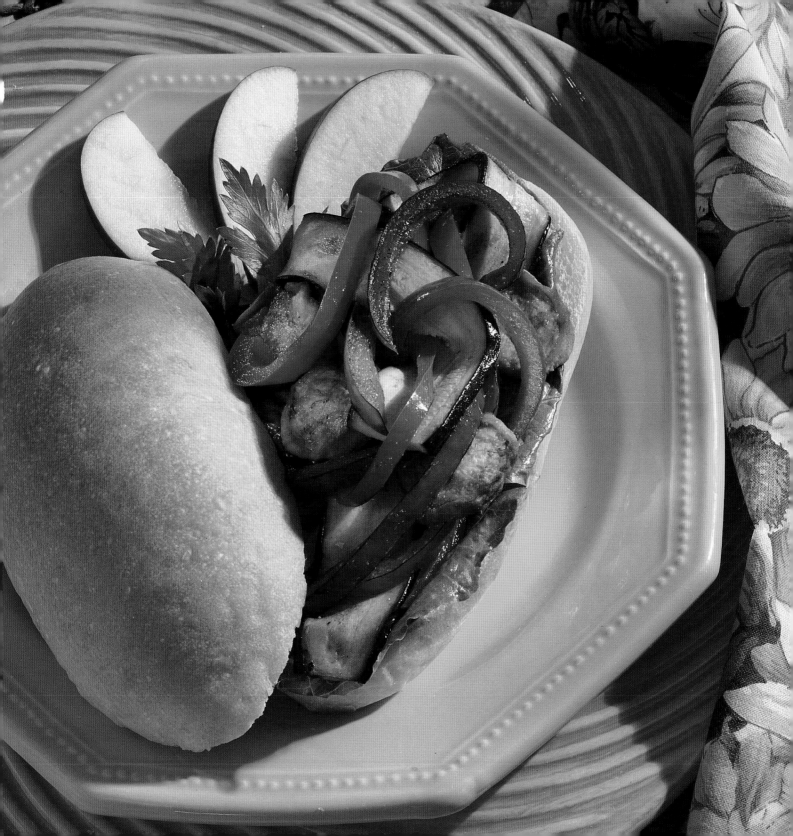

Grilled Turkey Ham Quesadillas

Nonstick cooking spray

¼ **cup salsa**

4 **(7-inch) flour tortillas**

½ **cup shredded reduced-sodium reduced-fat Monterey Jack cheese**

¼ **cup finely chopped turkey ham**

1 **can (4 ounces) diced green chilies, drained**

Additional salsa (optional)

Nonfat sour cream (optional)

1. To prevent sticking, spray grid with cooking spray. Prepare coals for grilling.

2. Spread 1 tablespoon salsa onto each tortilla. Sprinkle cheese, turkey ham and chilies equally over half of each tortilla; fold over uncovered half to make "sandwich"; spray tops and bottoms of tortilla "sandwiches" with cooking spray.

3. Grill quesadillas on uncovered grill over medium coals 1½ minutes per side or until cheese is melted and tortillas are golden brown, turning once. Quarter each quesadilla and serve with additional salsa and nonfat sour cream, if desired.   *Makes 4 servings*

Nutrients per Serving (4 quarters):
Calories: 132, Calories from Fat: 27%, Total Fat: 4g, Saturated Fat: 2g, Cholesterol: 10mg, Sodium: 390mg, Carbohydrate: 16g, Dietary Fiber: 1g, Protein: 8g

Dietary Exchanges: 1 Starch, 1 Lean Meat

Italian Meatball Subs

Nonstick cooking spray
½ cup chopped onion
3 teaspoons finely chopped garlic, divided
1 can (14½ ounces) Italian-style crushed tomatoes
2 bay leaves
2½ teaspoons dried basil leaves, divided
2 teaspoons dried oregano leaves, divided
¾ teaspoon black pepper, divided
¼ teaspoon red pepper flakes
½ pound lean ground beef
⅓ cup chopped green onions
⅓ cup plain dry bread crumbs
¼ cup chopped fresh parsley
1 egg white
½ teaspoon *each* dried marjoram leaves and ground mustard
4 French bread rolls, warmed, halved

1. Spray large nonstick saucepan with cooking spray. Heat over medium heat until hot. Add ½ cup onion and 2 teaspoons garlic. Cook and stir 5 minutes or until onion is tender. Add tomatoes, bay leaves, 2 teaspoons basil, 1 teaspoon oregano, ½ teaspoon black pepper and red pepper; cover. Simmer 30 minutes, stirring occasionally. Remove and discard bay leaves. Set sauce aside.

2. Combine beef, green onions, bread crumbs, parsley, egg white, 2 tablespoons water, remaining 1 teaspoon garlic, ½ teaspoon basil, 1 teaspoon oregano, ¼ teaspoon black pepper, marjoram and mustard in medium bowl until well blended. Shape into 16 small meatballs. Spray large nonstick skillet with cooking spray. Add meatballs. Cook 5 minutes or until meatballs are no longer pink in centers; turn occasionally. Add meatballs to tomato sauce. Cook 5 minutes; stir occasionally. Place 4 meatballs in each roll. Top meatballs with sauce. Serve immediately. *Makes 4 servings*

Nutrients per Serving (1 sub sandwich):
Calories: 282, Calories from Fat: 30%, Total Fat: 9g, Saturated Fat: 3g, Cholesterol: 35mg, Sodium: 497mg, Carbohydrate: 32g, Dietary Fiber: 1g, Protein: 18g

Dietary Exchanges: 2 Starch, 1 Vegetable, 2 Lean Meat

Tarragon Chicken Salad Sandwiches

1¼ pounds boneless skinless chicken breasts, cooked
1 cup thinly sliced celery
1 cup seedless red or green grapes, cut into halves
½ cup raisins
½ cup plain nonfat yogurt
¼ cup reduced-fat mayonnaise or salad dressing
2 tablespoons finely chopped shallots or onion
2 tablespoons minced fresh tarragon *or* 1 teaspoon dried tarragon leaves
½ teaspoon salt
⅛ teaspoon white pepper
6 lettuce leaves
6 whole wheat buns, split

1. Cut chicken into scant ½-inch pieces. Combine chicken, celery, grapes and raisins in large bowl. Combine yogurt, mayonnaise, shallots, tarragon, salt and pepper in small bowl. Spoon over chicken mixture; mix lightly.

2. Place 1 lettuce leaf in each bun. Divide chicken mixture evenly among buns.   *Makes 6 servings*

Nutrients per Serving (1 sandwich):
Calories: 353, Calories from Fat: 18%, Total Fat: 7g, Saturated Fat: 1g, Cholesterol: 76mg, Sodium: 509mg, Carbohydrate: 41g, Dietary Fiber: 4g, Protein: 34g

Dietary Exchanges: 1½ Starch, ½ Fruit, 4 Lean Meat

Tarragon Chicken Salad Sandwich

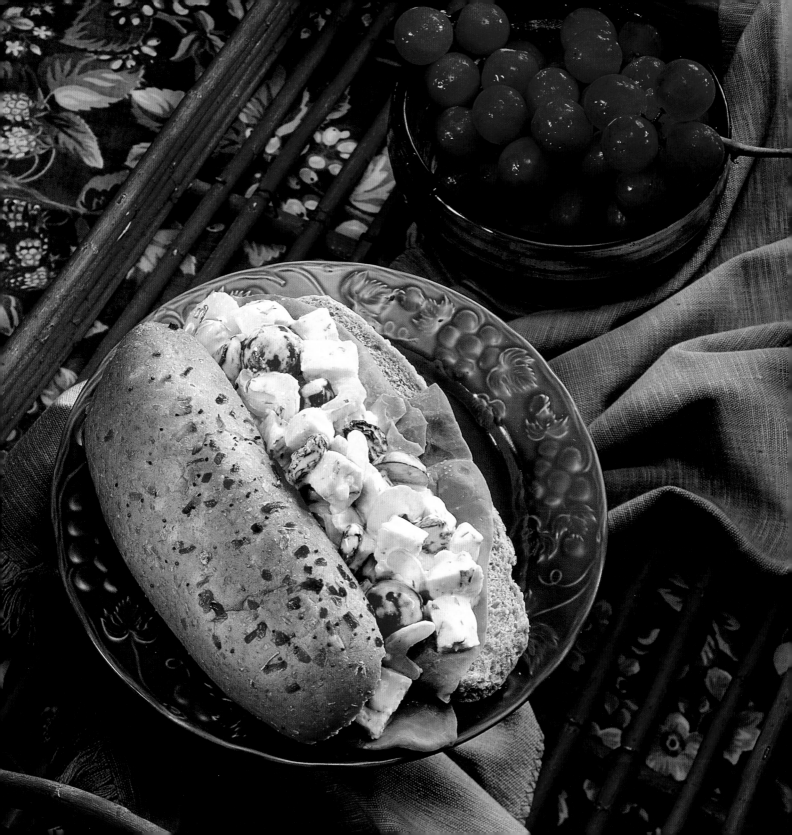

Pita **Burgers**

1 package (about 1¼ pounds) PERDUE® Fresh Ground Chicken or Turkey

2 garlic cloves, minced

2 teaspoons paprika

1 teaspoon salt

1 teaspoon ground cumin

1 teaspoon ground allspice

¼ teaspoon ground red pepper

6 pita breads, opened and lightly grilled

   Yogurt Sauce (recipe follows)

3 plum tomatoes, thinly sliced

1 small cucumber, thinly sliced

1. Prepare lightly greased grill for cooking. In medium bowl, combine ground turkey, garlic and seasonings. Form mixture into 6 burgers. Grill, uncovered, 5 to 6 inches over medium-hot coals 4 to 5 minutes on each side or until burgers are cooked through and spring back when touched.

2. Serve burgers in pita pockets, topped with yogurt sauce, tomatoes and cucumbers.

Makes 4 to 6 servings

Yogurt Sauce: Combine 1 cup plain yogurt, 1 tablespoon minced fresh parsley, 2 teaspoons minced fresh cilantro, and 1½ teaspoons minced fresh mint *or* ½ teaspoon dried mint in small bowl. Season with salt and ground pepper to taste.

Nutrients per Serving (1 burger):
Calories: 355, Calories from Fat: 24%, Total Fat: 9g, Saturated Fat: 1g, Cholesterol: 2mg, Sodium: 793mg, Carbohydrate: 42g, Dietary Fiber: 3g, Protein: 25g

Dietary Exchanges: 2 Starch, 2 Vegetable, 3 Lean Meat

Quick Pork Fajitas

1 pork tenderloin, about 1 pound, thinly sliced
2 to 3 tablespoons fajita seasoning or marinade
½ onion, sliced
½ green pepper, sliced
4 to 6 flour tortillas, warmed

In a shallow bowl, toss pork pieces with fajita seasoning. In large non-stick skillet over medium-high heat, stir-fry pork pieces with onion and green pepper until all is just tender. Wrap portions in flour tortillas with salsa, if desired. *Makes 4 servings*

Favorite recipe from **National Pork Board**

Nutrients per Serving (1 fajita):
Calories: 259, Calories from Fat: 22%, Total Fat: 6g, Saturated Fat: 2g, Cholesterol: 73mg, Sodium: 510mg, Carbohydrate: 22g, Dietary Fiber: 2g, Protein: 27g

Dietary Exchanges: 1½ Starch, 3 Lean Meat

recipe tip

Placing a pork tenderloin in the freezer for about 20 minutes makes slicing easier.

Grilled Vegetable Muffuletta

10 cloves garlic, peeled

Nonstick cooking spray

1 tablespoon balsamic vinegar

1 tablespoon fresh lemon juice

1 tablespoon olive oil

¼ teaspoon black pepper

1 medium eggplant, cut crosswise into eight ¼-inch-thick slices

2 small yellow squash, cut lengthwise into thin slices

1 small red onion, thinly sliced

1 large red bell pepper, seeded and quartered

1 loaf round whole wheat sourdough bread (1 pound)

2 slices (1 ounce each) reduced-fat Swiss cheese

8 washed spinach leaves

1. Preheat oven to 350°F. Place garlic in ovenproof dish. Spray with cooking spray. Cover with foil; bake 30 to 35 minutes or until garlic is soft and golden brown.

2. Place garlic, vinegar, lemon juice, olive oil and black pepper in food processor; process until smooth. Set aside.

3. Prepare grill for direct grilling. Brush eggplant, squash, onion and bell pepper with garlic mixture. Arrange vegetables on grid over medium coals. Grill 10 to 12 minutes or until vegetables are crisp-tender, turning once. Separate onion slices into rings.

4. Slice top from bread loaf. Hollow out loaf, leaving ½-inch-thick shell. Layer half of eggplant, squash, onion, bell pepper, cheese and spinach in hollowed bread, pressing gently after each layer. Repeat layers. Replace bread top; serve immediately or cover with plastic wrap and refrigerate up to 4 hours.

Makes 6 servings

Nutrients per Serving (⅙ of total recipe):
Calories: 214, Calories from Fat: 23%, Total Fat: 6g, Saturated Fat: 2g, Cholesterol: 7mg, Sodium: 262mg, Carbohydrate: 34g, Dietary Fiber: 1g, Protein: 9g

Dietary Exchanges: 1½ Starch, 2 Vegetable, 1 Fat

Grilled Vegetable Muffuletta

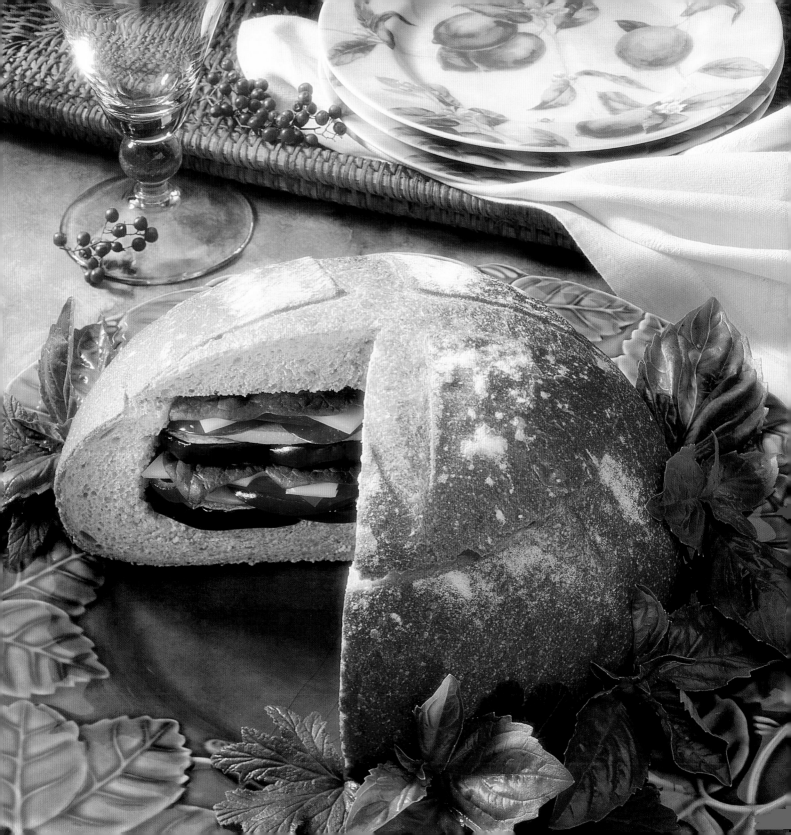

Moroccan Grilled Turkey with
Cucumber Yogurt Sauce

1 package BUTTERBALL® Fresh Boneless Turkey Breast Cutlets
⅓ cup fresh lime juice
2 cloves garlic, minced
½ teaspoon curry powder
½ teaspoon salt
¼ teaspoon ground cumin
¼ teaspoon cayenne pepper
3 large pitas, cut in half*
Cucumber Yogurt Sauce (page 96)

Pitas may be filled and folded in half.

Prepare grill for medium-direct-heat cooking. Lightly spray unheated grill rack with nonstick cooking spray. Combine lime juice, garlic, curry powder, salt, cumin and cayenne pepper in medium bowl. Dip cutlets in lime juice mixture. Place cutlets on rack over medium-hot grill. Grill 5 to 7 minutes on each side or until meat is no longer pink in center. Distribute turkey and Cucumber Yogurt Sauce evenly among pitas.

Makes 6 servings

Preparation Time: 20 Minutes

continued on page 96

Moroccan Grilled Turkey with
Cucumber Yogurt Sauce

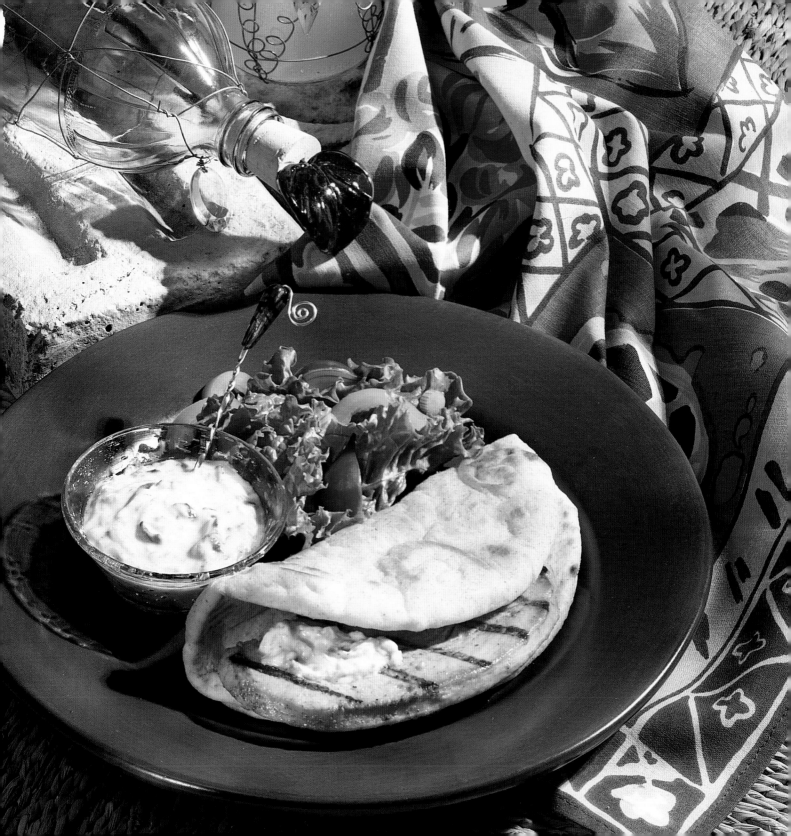

Cucumber Yogurt Sauce

---

    1 cup fat-free yogurt

    ½ cup shredded cucumber

    1 teaspoon grated lime peel

    1 teaspoon salt

    ½ teaspoon ground cumin

Combine yogurt, cucumber, lime peel, salt and cumin in medium bowl. Chill.

Nutrients per Serving (1 sandwich):
Calories: 194, Calories from Fat: 5%, Total Fat: 1g, Saturated Fat: 1g, Cholesterol: 47mg, Sodium: 648mg, Carbohydrate: 20g, Dietary Fiber: 1g, Protein: 23g

Dietary Exchanges: 2½ Starch, 2 Lean Meat

Sassy Southwestern Veggie Wraps

    ½ cup diced zucchini

    ½ cup diced red or yellow bell pepper

    ½ cup frozen corn, thawed

    1 jalapeño pepper,* seeded and chopped

    ¾ cup shredded reduced-fat Mexican cheese blend

    3 tablespoons prepared salsa or picante sauce

    2 (8-inch) fat-free flour tortillas

*Jalapeño peppers can sting and irritate the skin; wear rubber gloves when handling peppers and do not touch eyes. Wash hands after handling peppers.

---

1. Combine zucchini, bell pepper, corn and jalapeño pepper in small bowl. Stir in cheese and salsa; mix well.

2. Soften tortillas according to package directions. Spoon vegetable mixture down center of tortillas, distributing evenly; roll up burrito-style. Serve wraps cold or warm.*   *Makes 2 servings*

To warm each wrap, cover loosely with plastic wrap and microwave at HIGH 40 to 45 seconds or until cheese is melted.

Nutrients per Serving (1 wrap):
Calories: 221, Calories from Fat: 27%, Total Fat: 7g, Saturated Fat: 5g, Cholesterol: 19mg, Sodium: 664mg, Carbohydrate: 26g, Dietary Fiber: 8g, Protein: 16g

Dietary Exchanges: 1½ Starch, 1 Vegetable, 1 Lean Meat, ½ Fat

Feta Pockets

> 2 cups bean sprouts
> 1 small cucumber, chopped
> ½ cup (2 ounces) crumbled Wisconsin feta cheese
> ¼ cup plain low-fat yogurt
> 1 tablespoon sesame seeds, toasted
> ¼ teaspoon pepper
> 2 pita bread rounds, cut in half
> 1 medium tomato, cut into 4 slices

In medium bowl, stir together sprouts, cucumber, cheese, yogurt, sesame seeds and pepper. Spoon mixture evenly among pita bread halves. Place tomato slice on filling in each bread half.

Makes 4 servings

Favorite recipe from **Wisconsin Milk Marketing Board**

Nutrients per Serving (1 Pocket):
Calories: 145, Calories from Fat: 30%, Total Fat: 5g, Saturated Fat: 3g, Cholesterol: 14mg, Sodium: 289mg, Carbohydrate: 19g, Dietary Fiber: 3g, Protein: 7g

Dietary Exchanges: 1 Starch, 1 Vegetable, 1 Fat

Chicago Fire Italian Sausage Sandwiches

1 package BUTTERBALL® Lean Fresh Turkey Hot Italian Sausage
5 large hot dog buns
5 teaspoons yellow mustard
5 tablespoons chopped onion
5 tablespoons pickle relish
10 tomato wedges
10 hot sport peppers

Grill sausage according to package directions. Place in buns. Add mustard, onion, relish, tomato wedges and peppers to each sandwich.

Makes 5 sandwiches

Preparation Time: 15 minutes

Nutrients per Serving (1 sandwich):
Calories: 287, Calories from Fat: 33%, Total Fat: 11g, Saturated Fat: 3g, Cholesterol: 45mg, Sodium: 1,257mg, Carbohydrate: 31g, Dietary Fiber: 2g, Protein: 18g

Dietary Exchanges: 2 Starch, 2 Lean Meat, 1 Fat

recipe tip

While only part of the population is sodium-sensitive, the American Heart Association recommends healthy Americans consume less than 2400 milligrams of salt per day. Since these sandwiches are fairly high in sodium, consider eating less salty foods at other meals throughout the day.

Chicago Fire Italian Sausage Sandwich

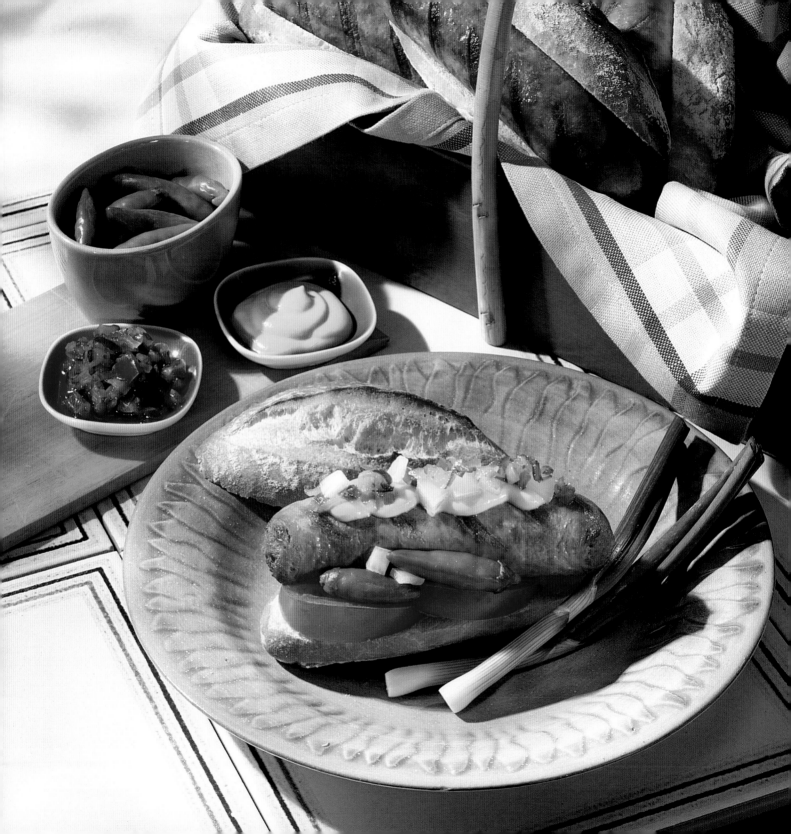

Speedy Garden Roll-Ups

Chick-Pea Spread (page 102)
4 (6-inch) flour tortillas
½ cup shredded carrot
½ cup shredded red cabbage
½ cup (2 ounces) shredded reduced-fat Cheddar cheese
4 red leaf lettuce leaves

1. Prepare Chick-Pea Spread.

2. Spread each tortilla with ¼ cup Chick-Pea Spread to about ½ inch from edge. Sprinkle evenly with 2 tablespoons each carrot, cabbage and cheese. Top with 1 lettuce leaf.

3. Roll up tortillas jelly-roll fashion. Seal with additional Chick-Pea Spread.

4. Serve immediately, or wrap tightly with plastic wrap and refrigerate up to 4 hours.

Makes 4 servings

continued on page 102

recipe tip

Great for a lunchbox meal, a Speedy Garden Roll-Up is also a fantastic low-fat and healthy midday snack.

Speedy Garden Roll-Ups

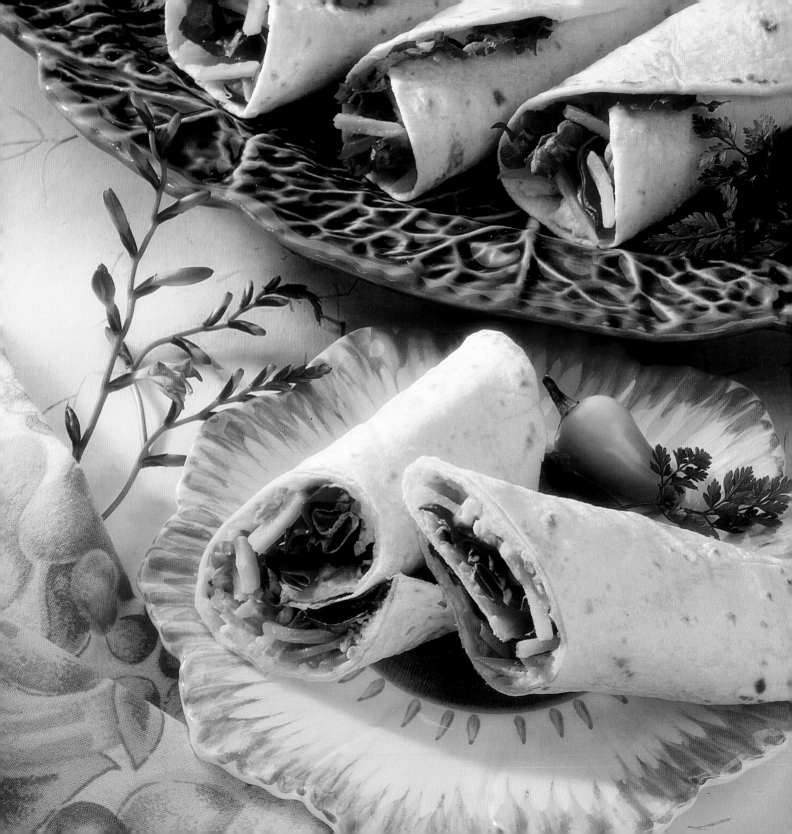

Sandwich Splendor

Chick-Pea Spread

1 can (about 15 ounces) chick-peas (garbanzo beans), rinsed and drained
¼ cup nonfat cream cheese
1 tablespoon finely chopped onion
1 tablespoon chopped fresh cilantro
2 teaspoons lemon juice
2 cloves garlic
½ teaspoon sesame oil
⅛ teaspoon black pepper

Place chick-peas, cream cheese, onion, cilantro, lemon juice, garlic, sesame oil and pepper in blender or food processor container; process until smooth.   *Makes about 1 cup*

Nutrients per Serving (1 roll-up with 1 tablespoon Chick-Pea Spread):
Calories: 280, Calories from Fat: 21%, Total Fat: 7g, Saturated Fat: 2g, Cholesterol: 10mg,
Sodium: 633mg, Carbohydrate: 40g, Dietary Fiber: 7g, Protein: 15g

Dietary Exchanges: 2 Starch, 1 Lean Meat, 1 Fat

recipe tip

Also known as garbanzo beans, chick-peas are larger than green peas. They are round, irregularly shaped tan beans with a firm texture and a mild, nutlike flavor. You can find them canned, dried and, in some parts of the country, fresh.

Salmon Pattie **Burgers**

1 can (about 14 ounces) red salmon, drained
1 egg white
2 tablespoons toasted wheat germ
1 tablespoon dried onion flakes
1 tablespoon capers, drained
½ teaspoon dried thyme leaves
¼ teaspoon black pepper
    Nonstick cooking spray
4 whole wheat buns, split
    Dijon mustard
4 tomato slices
4 thin slices red onion *or* 8 slices dill pickles
4 lettuce leaves

1. Place salmon in medium bowl; mash bones and skin with fork, and flake salmon. (If you prefer, discard bones and skin.) Add egg white, wheat germ, onion flakes, capers, thyme and pepper; mix well.

2. Divide into 4 portions and shape into firm patties. Place on plate; cover with plastic wrap and refrigerate 1 hour or until firm.

3. Spray large skillet with cooking spray. Cook patties on medium heat 5 minutes per side.

4. Spread cut sides of buns lightly with mustard. Place patties on bottoms of buns; top with tomato and onion slices, lettuce leaves and tops of buns.   *Makes 4 servings*

Nutrients per Serving (1 sandwich):
Calories: 329, Calories from Fat: 27%, Total Fat: 10g, Saturated Fat: 2g, Cholesterol: 36mg, Sodium: 719mg, Carbohydrate: 36g, Dietary Fiber: 6g, Protein: 26g

Dietary Exchanges: 2 Starch, 1 Vegetable, 3 Lean Meat

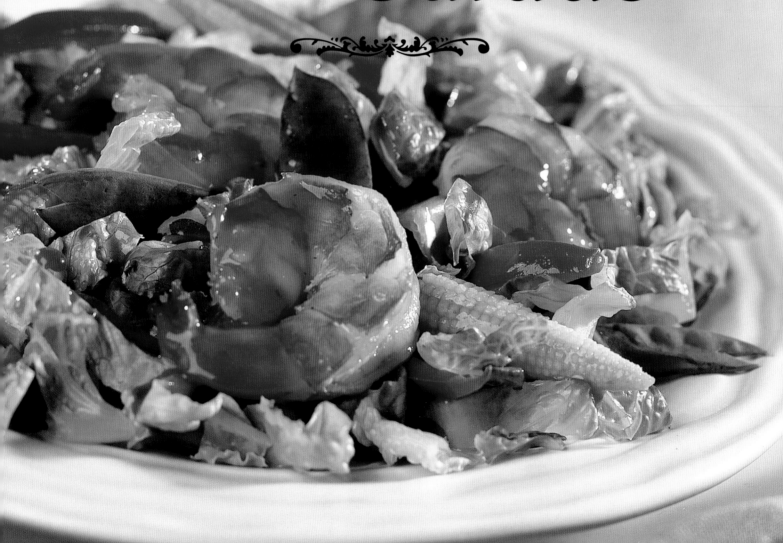

Satisfying
Salads

Spicy Asian Shrimp Salad

6 cups shredded romaine lettuce or napa cabbage

2 cups pea pods (about 6 ounces)

1 can (15 ounces) baby corn, drained

½ pound medium shrimp, cleaned, cooked

1 red pepper, cut into thin strips

½ cup KRAFT LIGHT DONE RIGHT CATALINA® Reduced Fat Dressing

1 tablespoon soy sauce

½ to 1 teaspoon hot pepper sauce

TOSS all ingredients in large bowl.   *Makes 4 servings*

Variation: Prepare as directed, substituting 2 cooked boneless skinless chicken breast halves, sliced, for shrimp.

Variation: Prepare as directed, substituting 1 cup frozen corn, thawed, for baby corn.

Prep: 15 minutes

Nutrients per Serving (¼ of total recipe):
Calories: 200, Calories from Fat: 27%, Total Fat: 6g, Saturated Fat: 1g, Cholesterol: 110mg,
Sodium: 1020mg, Carbohydrate: 21g, Dietary Fiber: 5g, Protein: 16g

Dietary Exchanges: 1 Starch, 2 Vegetable, 2 Lean Meat

Spicy Asian Shrimp Salad

Warm Chicken & Couscous Salad

1 tablespoon olive oil

1 package (about 12 ounces) chicken tenders or boneless skinless chicken
   breasts, cut into strips

2 teaspoons Cajun or blackened seasoning

1 teaspoon minced garlic

1 can (about 14 ounces) chicken broth

2 cups frozen broccoli, carrot and red bell pepper blend

1 cup uncooked couscous

3 cups packed torn spinach leaves

¼ cup poppy seed dressing

1. Heat oil in large nonstick skillet over medium-high heat. Toss chicken with Cajun seasoning. Add chicken and garlic to skillet; cook and stir 3 minutes or until chicken is no longer pink.

2. Add broth and vegetables to skillet; bring to a boil. Stir in couscous. Remove from heat; cover and let stand 5 minutes. Stir in spinach; transfer to plates. Drizzle with dressing. *Makes 4 servings*

Prep and Cook Time: 20 minutes

Nutrients per Serving (¼ of total recipe):
Calories: 406, Calories from Fat: 29%, Total Fat: 13g, Saturated Fat: 2g, Cholesterol: 52mg,
Sodium: 869mg, Carbohydrate: 42g, Dietary Fiber: 7g, Protein: 30g

Dietary Exchanges: 2 Starch, 2 Vegetable, 2 Lean Meat, 2 Fat

Warm Chicken & Couscous Salad

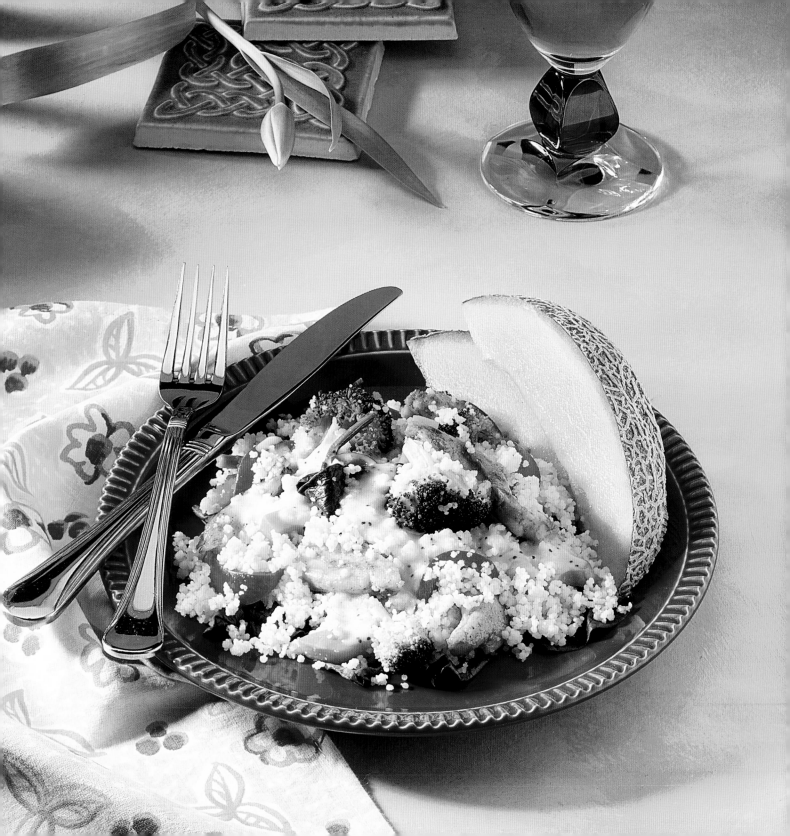

Oriental Brown Rice Salad

1 bag SUCCESS® Brown Rice
   Dijon Dressing (recipe follows)
1 pound boneless, skinless chicken pieces, cooked
1 package (10 ounces) frozen peas, thawed and drained
2 cups fresh bean sprouts
½ cup sliced celery
¼ cup sliced green onions
¼ cup green bell pepper strips

Prepare rice according to package directions. Cool. Prepare Dijon Dressing; set aside.

Place rice in large bowl. Add dressing and remaining ingredients; mix lightly to coat. Refrigerate at least 30 minutes.   *Makes 4 servings*

Dijon Dressing

¼ cup sherry
¼ cup vinegar
2 tablespoons corn oil
2 tablespoons reduced-sodium soy sauce
1½ tablespoons Dijon mustard
½ teaspoon sesame oil
⅛ teaspoon ground ginger

Place all ingredients in covered container; shake well.

Nutrients per Serving (¼ of total recipe):
Calories: 470, Calories from Fat: 19%, Total Fat: 10g, Saturated Fat: 1g, Cholesterol: 66mg, Sodium: 475mg, Carbohydrate: 55g, Dietary Fiber: 8g, Protein: 37g

Dietary Exchanges: 3 Starch, 2 Vegetable, 4 Lean Meat

Skinny Waldorf Salad

2 cups chopped cored Red Delicious apples
1 cup chopped celery
1 cup cubed cooked boneless skinless chicken breast
¼ cup chopped green onions
3 tablespoons lemon nonfat yogurt
2 teaspoons fat-free mayonnaise
1 teaspoon toasted poppy seeds
¼ teaspoon salt
  Dash pepper

Combine apples, celery, chicken and green onions in large bowl; set aside. For dressing, combine yogurt, mayonnaise, poppy seeds, salt and pepper in small bowl. Pour over apple mixture; toss to coat. Refrigerate, covered, at least 1 hour to allow flavors to blend. *Makes 4 servings*

Nutrients per Serving (¼ of total recipe):
Calories: 95, Calories from Fat: 10%, Total Fat: 1g, Saturated Fat: <1g, Cholesterol: 22mg, Sodium: 205mg, Carbohydrate: 12g, Dietary Fiber: 2g, Protein: 9g

Dietary Exchanges: ½ Fruit, ½ Vegetable, 1 Lean Meat

recipe tip

One whole chicken breast (about 10 ounces) will yield about 1 cup of chopped cooked chicken.

Pasta and Tuna **Filled Peppers**

¾ cup uncooked ditalini pasta

4 large green bell peppers

1 cup chopped seeded tomato

1 can (6 ounces) white tuna packed in water, drained and flaked

½ cup chopped celery

½ cup (2 ounces) shredded reduced-fat Cheddar cheese

¼ cup fat-free mayonnaise or salad dressing

1 teaspoon salt-free garlic and herb seasoning

2 tablespoons shredded reduced-fat Cheddar cheese (optional)

1. Cook pasta according to package directions, omitting salt. Rinse and drain. Set aside.

2. Cut thin slice from top of each pepper. Remove veins and seeds from insides of peppers. Rinse; place peppers, cut side down, on paper towels to drain.*

3. Combine pasta, tomato, tuna, celery, ½ cup cheese, mayonnaise and seasoning in large bowl until well blended; spoon evenly into pepper shells.

4. Place peppers on large microwave-safe plate; cover with waxed paper. Microwave at HIGH 7 to 8 minutes, turning halfway through cooking time. Top evenly with remaining 2 tablespoons cheese before serving, if desired. Garnish as desired.   *Makes 4 servings*

For more tender peppers, cook in boiling water 2 minutes. Rinse with cold water; drain upside down on paper towels before filling.

Nutrients per Serving (1 filled pepper):
Calories: 216, Calories from Fat: 16%, Total Fat: 4g, Saturated Fat: 1g, Cholesterol: 26mg, Sodium: 574mg, Carbohydrate: 27g, Dietary Fiber: 2g, Protein: 19g

Dietary Exchanges: 1½ Starch, 1 Vegetable, 2 Lean Meat

Pasta and Tuna Filled Pepper

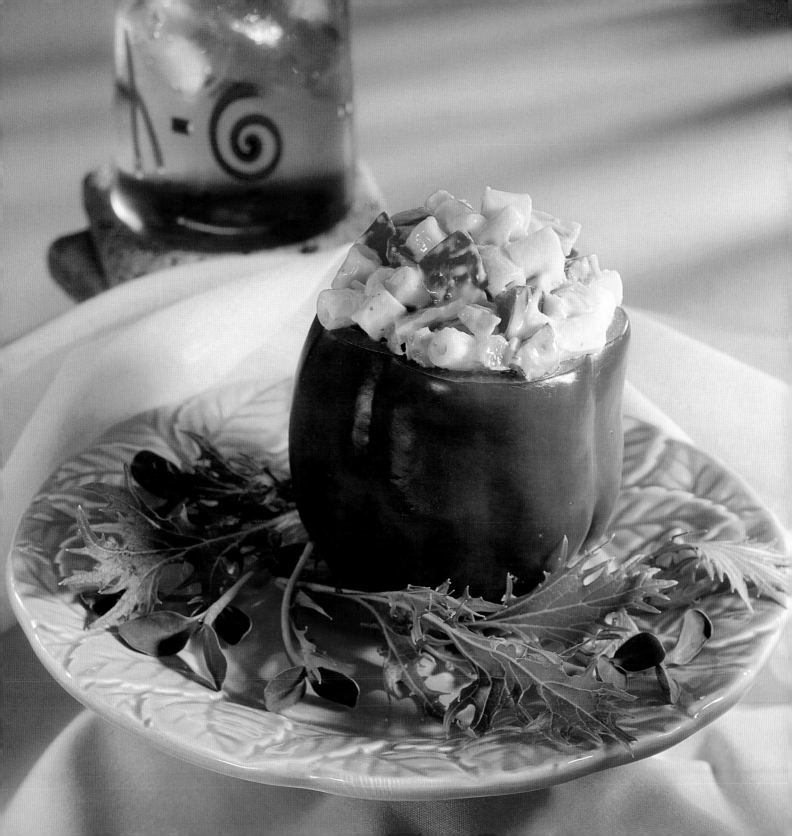

Grilled Chicken Spinach Salad

2 boneless skinless chicken breasts, grilled, cut into strips

5 cups torn spinach

1 cup sliced mushrooms

½ cup thinly sliced red onion wedges

4 slices OSCAR MAYER® Bacon, crisply cooked, crumbled

1 cup KRAFT FREE CATALINA® Fat Free Dressing

TOSS all ingredients except dressing in large bowl. Serve with dressing.

Makes 6 servings

Prep Time: 15 minutes

Nutrients per Serving (⅙ of total recipe):
Calories: 180, Calories from Fat: 23%, Total Fat: 5g, Saturated Fat: 2g, Cholesterol: 55mg, Sodium: 590mg, Carbohydrate: 13g, Dietary Fiber: 2g, Protein: 21g

Dietary Exchanges: 1 Starch, 2 Lean Meat

recipe tip

For a new flavor combination, substitute grilled shrimp for the grilled chicken in this recipe.

Grilled Chicken Spinach Salad

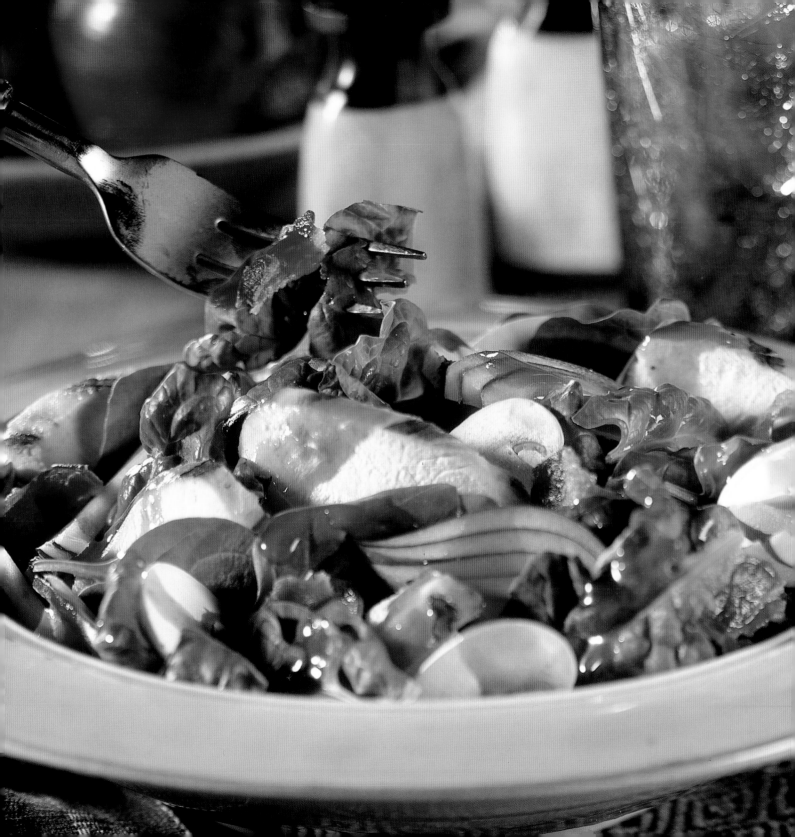

White Bean Salad with Cilantro Vinaigrette

1 medium red bell pepper

6 green onions with tops

2 cans (15 ounces each) Great Northern beans, rinsed and drained

½ cup prepared fat-free Italian salad dressing

2 tablespoons white wine vinegar

1 tablespoon dried cilantro leaves

2 teaspoons sugar

2 teaspoons olive oil

Cut bell pepper into ¼-inch strips. Cut green onions into ¼-inch slices. Combine bell pepper, green onions, beans, Italian dressing, vinegar, cilantro, sugar and oil in medium bowl. Cover; refrigerate 2 hours or overnight. Garnish with purple kale and fresh cilantro, if desired.   *Makes 8 servings*

Nutrients per Serving (⅛ of total recipe):
Calories: 155, Calories from Fat: 12%, Total Fat: 2g, Saturated Fat: <1g, Cholesterol: 0mg, Sodium: 431mg, Carbohydrate: 28g, Dietary Fiber: 1g, Protein: 8g

Dietary Exchanges: 2 Starch, ½ Vegetable

recipe tip

To cut a bell pepper into strips, stand the pepper on its end on a cutting board. Cut off 3 to 4 lengthwise slices from the sides with a utility knife, cutting close to, but not through, the stem. Discard the stem and seeds. Scrape out any remaining seeds, and rinse the inside of the pepper under cold running water. Slice each piece lengthwise into long strips.

White Bean Salad with Cilantro Vinaigrette

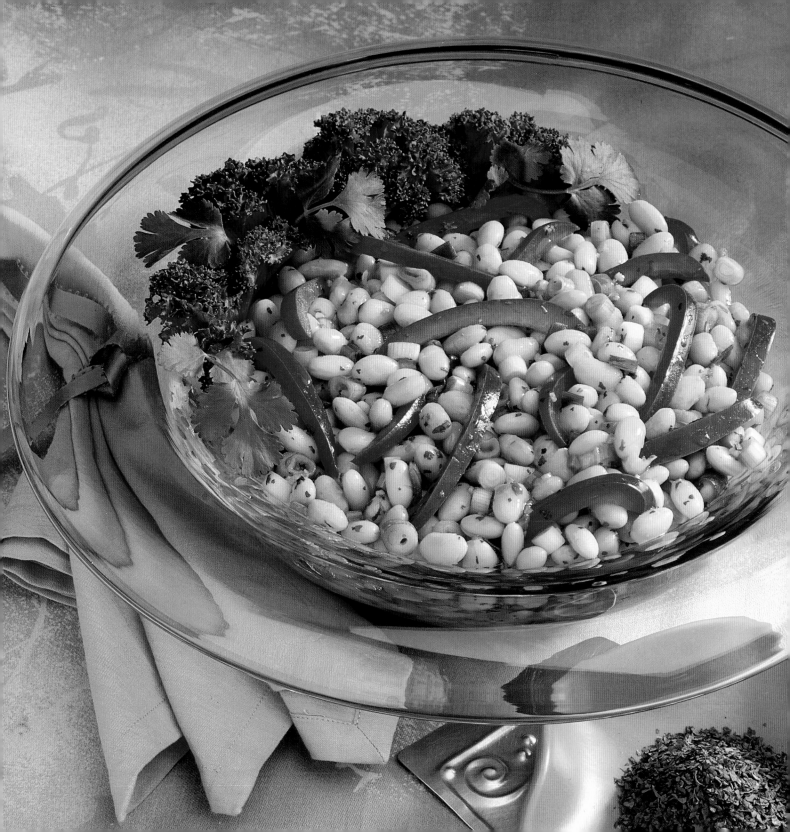

Lite Oriental Turkey & Pasta Salad

Satisfying Salads

        8 ounces uncooked capellini (angel hair pasta)
        3 tablespoons fresh lemon juice
        2 tablespoons *plus* 1½ teaspoons vegetable oil
        3 tablespoons KIKKOMAN® Lite Soy Sauce, divided
        2 tablespoons minced fresh cilantro
    1¼ teaspoons Oriental sesame oil
        1 teaspoon sugar
        1 clove garlic, pressed
        1 turkey cutlet (about ½ pound)
    ¼ pound snow peas, trimmed
        1 carrot
        1 tablespoon vegetable oil
        1 tablespoon water

Cook capellini according to package directions, omitting salt. Rinse under cold water; drain thoroughly. Cool. Blend lemon juice, 2 tablespoons *plus* 1½ teaspoons vegetable oil, 2 tablespoons lite soy sauce, cilantro, sesame oil, sugar and garlic. Pour over capellini in large bowl; toss to combine. Cover; refrigerate 30 minutes.

Meanwhile, cut turkey into thin strips; cut snow peas and carrot into julienne strips.

Heat remaining 1 tablespoon oil in wok or large skillet over high heat. Add turkey; stir-fry 2 minutes. Add snow peas, carrot and water; stir-fry 1 minute. Stir in remaining 1 tablespoon lite soy sauce until turkey and vegetables are coated with sauce. Pour over capellini; toss to combine. Garnish, if desired. Serve immediately.   *Makes 4 servings*

Nutrients per Serving (¼ of total recipe):
Calories: 428, Calories from Fat: 32%, Total Fat: 15g, Saturated Fat: 2g, Cholesterol: 34mg, Sodium: 476mg, Carbohydrate: 49g, Dietary Fiber: 3g, Protein: 22g

Dietary Exchanges: 2 Starch, 1 Vegetable, 2 Lean Meat, 2 Fat

Strawberry **Lime Mold**

2 cups boiling water
1 package (4-serving size) JELL-O® Brand Lime Flavor Sugar Free Low Calorie
   Gelatin Dessert
½ cup cold water
1 package (4-serving size) JELL-O® Brand Strawberry Flavor Sugar Free Low
   Calorie Gelatin Dessert
1 package (10 ounces) frozen strawberries in lite syrup, partially thawed
1 container (8 ounces) BREYERS® Vanilla Lowfat Yogurt

Satisfying Salads

STIR 1 cup of the boiling water into lime gelatin in medium bowl at least 2 minutes until completely dissolved. Stir in cold water. Refrigerate about 45 minutes or until slightly thickened (consistency of unbeaten egg whites).

MEANWHILE, stir remaining 1 cup boiling water into strawberry gelatin in separate medium bowl at least 2 minutes until completely dissolved. Add strawberries; stir until thawed. Pour into 5-cup mold. Refrigerate 15 minutes or until set but not firm (should stick to finger when touched and should mound).

STIR yogurt into lime gelatin with wire whisk until smooth. Spoon over gelatin in mold.

REFRIGERATE 4 hours or until firm. Unmold. Store leftover gelatin mold in refrigerator.

Makes 10 servings

Tip: To unmold, dip mold in warm water for about 15 seconds. Gently pull gelatin from around edges with moist fingers. Place moistened serving plate on top of mold. Invert mold and plate; holding mold and plate together, shake slightly to loosen. Gently remove mold and center gelatin on plate.

Nutrients per Serving (¹⁄₁₀ of total recipe):
Calories: 60, Calories from Fat: 1%, Total Fat: <1g, Saturated Fat: <1g, Cholesterol: 1mg, Sodium: 65mg, Carbohydrate: 11g, Dietary Fiber: <1g, Protein: 2g

Dietary Exchanges: 1 Starch

Sunburst Chicken Salad

1 tablespoon fat-free mayonnaise

1 tablespoon nonfat sour cream

2 teaspoons frozen orange juice concentrate, thawed

¼ teaspoon grated orange peel

1 boneless skinless chicken breast, cooked and chopped

1 large kiwi, thinly sliced

⅓ cup mandarin oranges

¼ cup finely chopped celery

4 lettuce leaves, washed

2 tablespoons coarsely chopped cashews

Combine mayonnaise, sour cream, concentrate and peel in small bowl. Add chicken, kiwi, oranges and celery; toss to coat. Cover; refrigerate 2 hours. Serve on lettuce leaves. Top with cashews.

Makes 2 servings

Nutrients per Serving (½ of total recipe):
Calories: 195, Calories from Fat: 29%, Total Fat: 6g, Saturated Fat: 1g, Cholesterol: 39mg, Sodium: 431mg, Carbohydrate: 18g, Dietary Fiber: 2g, Protein: 18g

Dietary Exchanges: 1 Fruit, 2 Lean Meat, ½ Fat

recipe tip

Ripe kiwifruit yields to gentle pressure; most need additional ripening after being purchased. To ripen, store the kiwifruit at room temperature out of direct sunlight, or place them in a paper bag. Turn them occasionally. Once ripened, the kiwis can be stored unpeeled in the refrigerator for up to one week.

Sunburst Chicken Salad

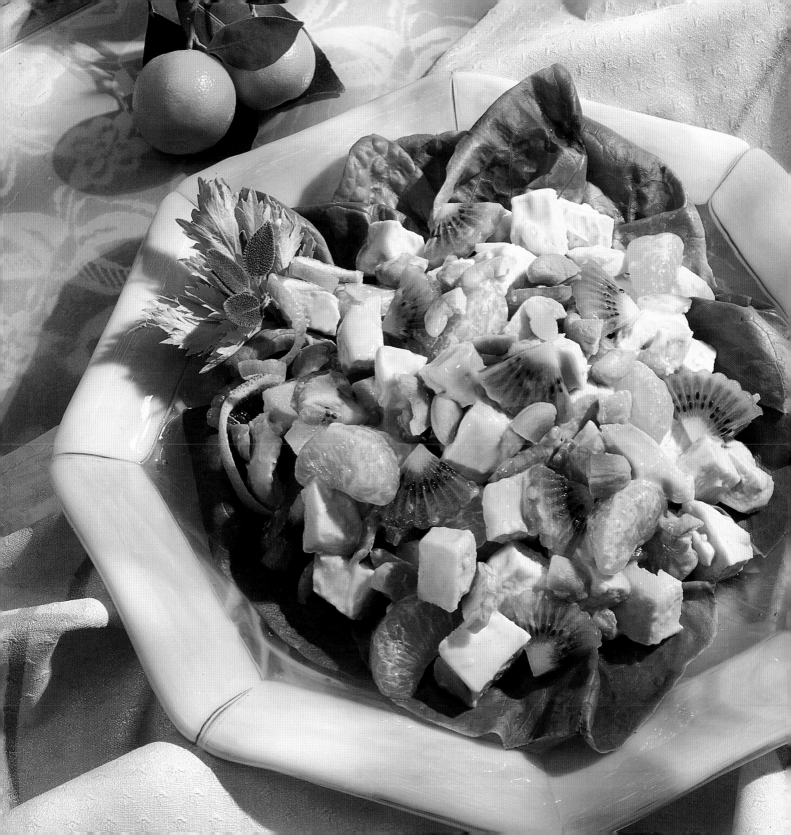

Seafood Salad

4 tablespoons olive oil, divided

½ cup diced onion

2 cloves garlic, minced

8 ounces medium shrimp, peeled, deveined

8 ounces medium scallops

¼ teaspoon salt

¼ teaspoon ground black pepper

1 cup Italian bread cubes

1 can (14.5 ounces) CONTADINA® Recipe Ready Diced Tomatoes, drained

2 cups torn salad greens

1 cup yellow bell pepper, cut into strips

2 tablespoons chopped fresh Italian parsley

1 tablespoon white wine vinegar

1. Heat 1 tablespoon oil in medium skillet. Add onion and garlic; sauté for 1 minute.

2. Add shrimp, scallops, salt and black pepper; sauté for 3 minutes. Remove from heat.

3. Heat 1 tablespoon oil in small skillet. Add bread cubes; sauté until golden brown.

4. Toss seafood mixture, tomatoes, greens, bell pepper, parsley, remaining oil and vinegar in large bowl. Top with bread cubes. *Makes 6 servings*

Prep Time: 10 minutes
Cook Time: 10 minutes

Nutrients per Serving (⅙ of total recipe):
Calories: 207, Calories from Fat: 49%, Total Fat: 11g, Saturated Fat: 1g, Cholesterol: 70mg, Sodium: 573mg, Carbohydrate: 11g, Dietary Fiber: 2g, Protein: 16g

Dietary Exchanges: 2 Vegetable, 2 Lean Meat, 1 Fat

Tex-Mex Flank Steak Salad

6 ounces beef flank steak
½ teaspoon Mexican seasoning blend or chili powder
⅛ teaspoon salt
   Nonstick olive oil cooking spray
4 cups packaged mixed salad greens
1 can (11 ounces) mandarin orange sections, drained
2 tablespoons green taco sauce

1. Slice steak very thinly across the grain. Combine beef slices, Mexican seasoning and salt in medium bowl.

2. Lightly spray large nonstick skillet with cooking spray. Heat over medium-high heat. Add steak strips. Cook and stir 1 to 2 minutes or to desired doneness.

3. Toss together greens and orange sections. Arrange on serving plates. Top with warm steak. Drizzle with taco sauce.

Makes 2 servings

Nutrients per Serving (½ of total recipe):
Calories: 240, Calories from Fat: 25%, Total Fat: 7g, Saturated Fat: 3g, Cholesterol: 37mg, Sodium: 388mg, Carbohydrate: 21g, Dietary Fiber: 2g, Protein: 25g

Dietary Exchanges: 1 Fruit, 2 Vegetable, 2 Lean Meat

recipe tip

Quick and healthy, this salad serves as the perfect dinner for a busy weeknight. Just add a whole-grain roll, and the meal's complete!

Smoked Turkey and **Fresh Vegetable Salad**

½ pound smoked turkey breast, cut into ½-inch cubes

1 cup cubed red-skinned potato, steamed

1 cup fresh broccoli florets

½ cup thinly sliced yellow squash

½ cup coarsely grated carrot

¼ cup thinly sliced red bell pepper

¼ cup green onion slices

⅓ cup reduced-calorie mayonnaise

1 teaspoon Dijon mustard

1 teaspoon lemon juice

½ teaspoon dill weed

¼ teaspoon dried parsley flakes

⅛ teaspoon garlic powder

1. Combine turkey, potato, broccoli, squash, carrot, pepper and onions in medium bowl.

2. Combine mayonnaise, mustard, lemon juice, dill, parsley and garlic powder in small bowl.

3. Add mayonnaise mixture to turkey mixture; gently toss until turkey and vegetables are coated. Cover and chill at least 1 hour.

Makes 2 servings

Favorite recipe from **National Turkey Federation**

Nutrients per Serving (½ of total recipe):
Calories: 341, Calories from Fat: 42%, Total Fat: 15g, Saturated Fat: 2g, Cholesterol: 50mg, Sodium: 1,930mg, Carbohydrate: 22g, Dietary Fiber: 4g, Protein: 25g

Dietary Exchanges: 4 Vegetable, 3 Lean Meat, 1½ Fat

Smoked Turkey and Fresh Vegetable Salad

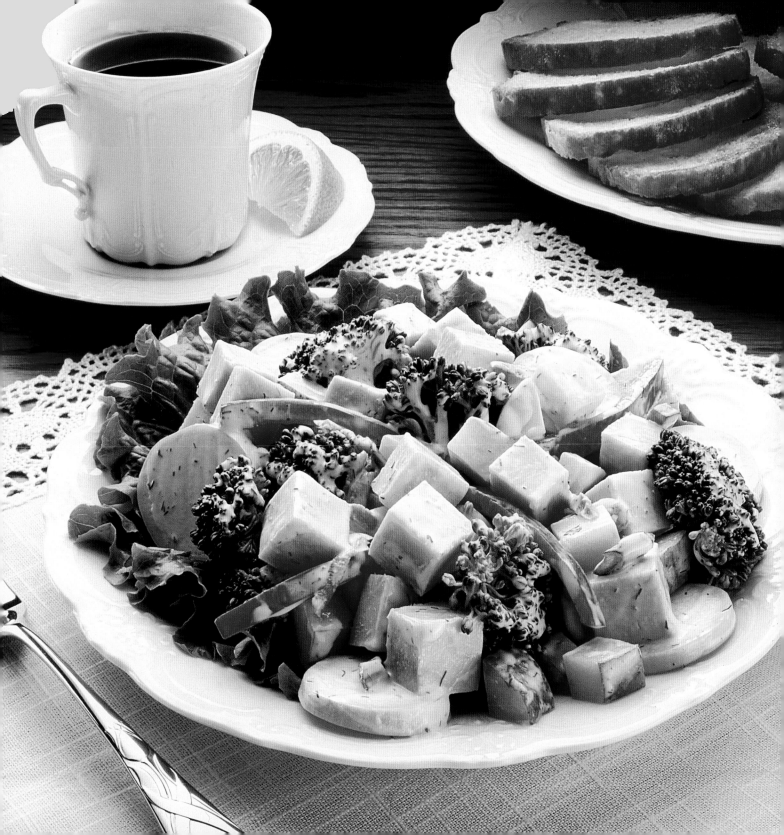

Fresh Seafood and Linguine Salad

1½ pounds small squid
4 pounds mussels, cleaned*
1½ to 3 dozen clams*
8 ounces linguine
½ cup plus 3 tablespoons olive oil, divided
¼ cup freshly squeezed lemon juice
2 cloves garlic, minced
¼ teaspoon salt
¼ teaspoon black pepper
1 red onion, thinly sliced and separated into rings for garnish (optional)
⅓ cup finely chopped Italian parsley for garnish (optional)

*Discard any opened clams or mussels.

1. Clean squid. Cut bodies crosswise into ¼-inch rings; finely chop tentacles and fins. To steam clams and mussels, bring 1 cup water to a boil in large stockpot over high heat. Add clams and mussels; cover. Reduce heat to low; steam 5 to 7 minutes or until shells open. Discard any that remain closed.

2. Meanwhile, cook pasta according to package directions; drain. Toss with 2 tablespoons olive oil.

3. Add 1 tablespoon olive oil to large saucepan. Heat over medium heat. Add squid; cook and stir 2 minutes or until opaque. Place in large bowl. Add pasta, mussels and clams.

4. Combine ½ cup olive oil, lemon juice, garlic, salt and pepper in small bowl; blend well. Pour over salad; toss gently to coat. Cover; refrigerate at least 3 hours. Season with additional lemon juice, salt and pepper, if desired. Garnish with onion rings and parsley, if desired. *Makes 6 servings*

Nutrients per Serving (⅙ of total recipe):
Calories: 385, Calories from Fat: 15%, Total Fat: 6g, Saturated Fat: 1g, Cholesterol: 321mg, Sodium: 580mg, Carbohydrate: 33g, Dietary Fiber: 2g, Protein: 46g

Dietary Exchanges: 2 Starch, 5 Lean Meat

Fresh Seafood and Linguine Salad

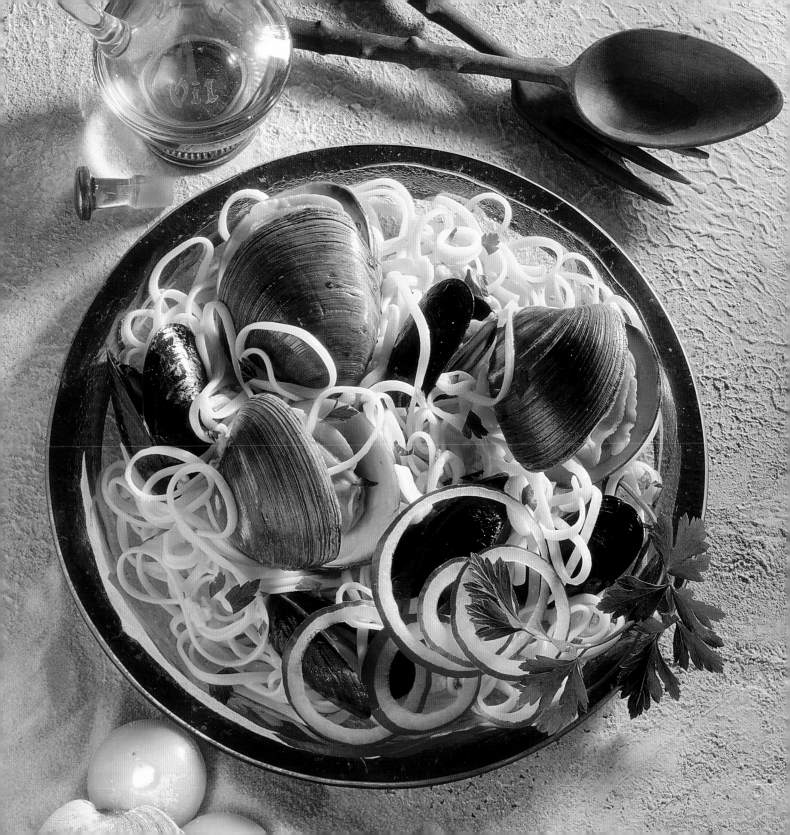

Garlic Lovers' Chicken Caesar Salad

Dressing

1 can (10¾ ounces) reduced-fat condensed cream of chicken soup, undiluted

½ cup fat-free reduced-sodium chicken broth

¼ cup balsamic vinegar

¼ cup fat-free shredded Parmesan cheese, divided

3 cloves garlic, minced

1 tablespoon low-sodium Worcestershire sauce

¼ teaspoon black pepper

Salad

2 heads romaine lettuce, torn into 2-inch pieces

4 grilled boneless skinless chicken breast halves, cut into 2-inch strips

½ cup fat-free herb-seasoned croutons

For dressing, combine soup, chicken broth, vinegar, 2 tablespoons Parmesan cheese, garlic, Worcestershire and pepper in food processor or blender; process until smooth. For salad, combine lettuce and 1 cup dressing in large salad bowl; toss well to coat. Top with chicken and croutons; sprinkle with remaining 2 tablespoons cheese. *Makes 8 servings*

Nutrients per Serving (⅛ of total recipe):
Calories: 132, Calories from Fat: 15%, Total Fat: 2g, Saturated Fat: 1g, Cholesterol: 40mg, Sodium: 185mg, Carbohydrate: 10g, Dietary Fiber: 1g, Protein: 17g

Dietary Exchanges: ½ Starch, 2 Lean Meat

Garlic Lovers' Chicken Caesar Salad

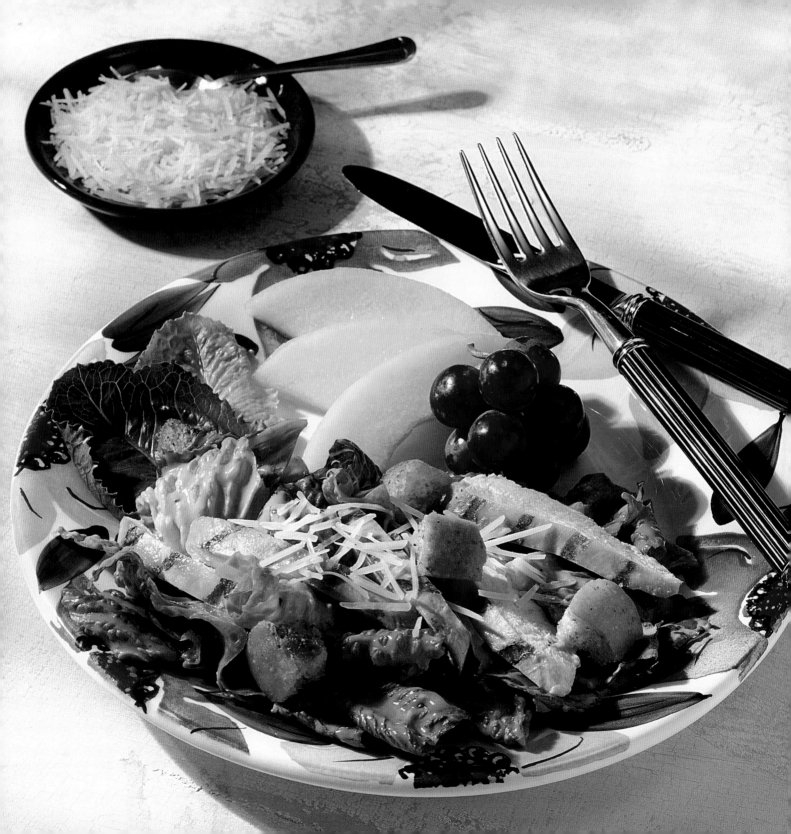

Crunchy Tuna Salad in Pepper Boats

2 large green or yellow bell peppers, halved lengthwise, seeded
½ cup **MIRACLE WHIP® FREE® Fat Free Dressing**
2 cans (6½ ounces each) tuna in water, drained, flaked
¼ **cup chopped carrot**
¼ **cup chopped celery**
¼ **cup chopped red onion**
¼ **cup chopped pecans (optional)**

• **PLACE** pepper halves on microwavable plate. Microwave on HIGH (100%) 1 minute; refrigerate.

• **MIX** remaining ingredients; refrigerate. Serve in pepper halves.   *Makes 4 servings*

Prep Time: 20 minutes plus refrigerating
Microwave Time: 1 minute

Nutrients per Serving (1 Pepper Boat):
Calories: 160, Calories from Fat: 6%, Total Fat: 1g, Saturated Fat: <1g, Cholesterol: 28mg,
Sodium: 572mg, Carbohydrate: 9g, Dietary Fiber: 2g, Protein: 24g

Dietary Exchanges: 2 Vegetable, 3 Lean Meat

recipe tip

Here are some ways to minimize tears when chopping onions:
1. Wear glasses or goggles.
2. Place the onion in your freezer 20 minutes before chopping.
3. Chew on a piece of bread.
4. Work under an exhaust fan.

Oven-Broiled Italian Style Salad

¼ cup **FILIPPO BERIO®** Olive Oil

1 clove garlic, crushed

2 medium red onions, thinly sliced into rounds

3 large beefsteak tomatoes, thinly sliced into rounds

1 (8-ounce) package thinly sliced part-skim mozzarella cheese

1 tablespoon balsamic vinegar

3 tablespoons shredded fresh basil *or* 1 tablespoon dried basil leaves

Salt and freshly ground black pepper

In small bowl, combine olive oil and garlic. Brush 2 tablespoons olive oil mixture over onion slices. In large nonstick skillet, cook onions over medium heat 5 minutes or until beginning to brown, turning halfway through cooking time. In large, shallow, heatproof serving dish, arrange slightly overlapping slices of onion, tomato and mozzarella. Whisk vinegar into remaining 2 tablespoons olive oil mixture; drizzle over onion mixture. Broil, 4 to 5 inches from heat, 4 to 5 minutes or until cheese just begins to melt. Sprinkle with basil. Season to taste with salt and pepper.   *Makes 4 servings*

Nutrients per Serving (¼ of total recipe):
Calories: 309, Calories from Fat: 65%, Total Fat: 23g, Saturated Fat: 8g, Cholesterol: 32mg, Sodium: 272mg, Carbohydrate: 12g, Dietary Fiber: 2g, Protein: 15g

Dietary Exchanges: 2 Vegetable, 2 Lean Meat, 3 Fat

Spicy Chicken Salad in Peanut Sauce

8 ounces uncooked linguine

⅔ cup chicken broth

2 tablespoons soy sauce

2 cloves garlic, crushed

½ to 1 teaspoon hot pepper sauce

⅓ cup creamy peanut butter

2 teaspoons dark sesame oil

2 cups loosely packed fresh spinach, rinsed and patted dry

2 cups shredded cooked chicken

1 cup shredded carrots

¼ cup sliced green onions

1. Cook linguine according to package directions, omitting salt. Drain.

2. Combine chicken broth, soy sauce, garlic and hot pepper sauce in medium saucepan; bring to a boil over medium heat. Remove from heat. Whisk in peanut butter and sesame oil until smooth.

3. Arrange spinach on 4 plates. Toss linguine with 3 tablespoons peanut sauce; spoon over spinach.

4. Add chicken, carrots and green onions to remaining peanut sauce. Spoon over linguine. Garnish as desired. *Makes 4 servings*

Nutrients per Serving (¼ of total recipe):
Calories: 456, Calories from Fat: 39%, Total Fat: 20g, Saturated Fat: 5g, Cholesterol: 109mg, Sodium: 869mg, Carbohydrate: 42g, Dietary Fiber: 4g, Protein: 30g

Dietary Exchanges: 2 Starch, 1 Vegetable, 3 Lean Meat, 2½ Fat

Spicy Chicken Salad in Peanut Sauce

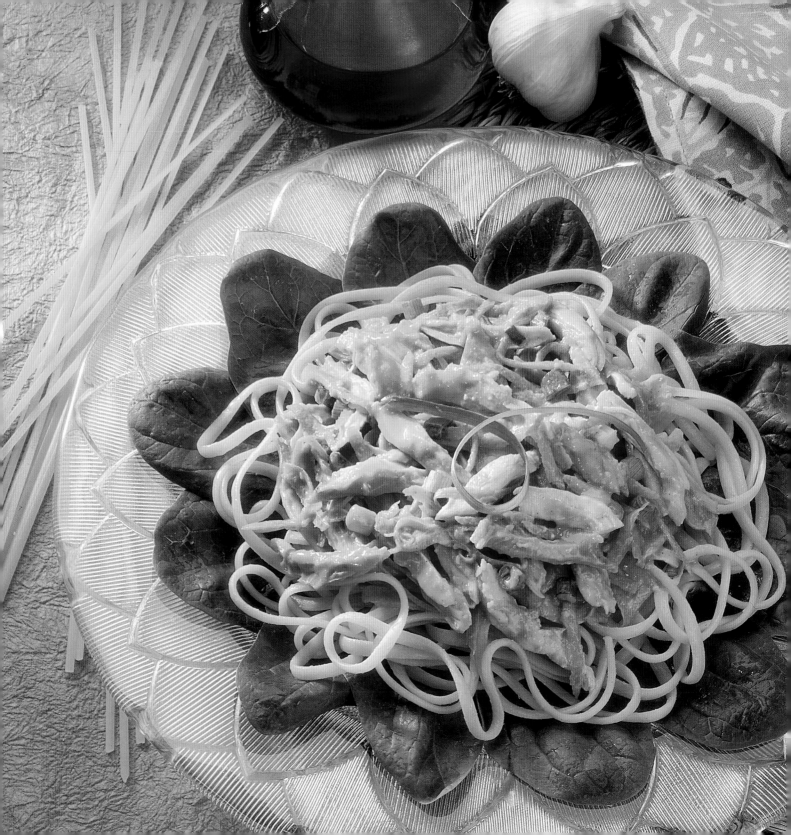

Chicken and Fruit Salad

½ cup plain nonfat yogurt

½ to 1 teaspoon lemon-pepper seasoning

½ teaspoon dry mustard

¼ teaspoon garlic salt

¼ teaspoon poppy seed

1¼ teaspoons EQUAL® FOR RECIPES *or* 4 packets EQUAL® sweetener *or*
    3 tablespoons EQUAL® SPOONFUL™

1 to 2 tablespoons orange juice

4 cups torn spinach leaves

8 ounces thinly sliced cooked chicken breast

2 cups sliced strawberries

1½ cups thinly sliced yellow summer squash

2 medium oranges, peeled and sectioned

1 cup halved seedless green grapes

½ cup toasted pecan pieces (optional)

• Combine yogurt, lemon-pepper seasoning, mustard, garlic salt, poppy seed and Equal® in small bowl. Add enough orange juice to reach drizzling consistency; set aside.

• Line platter with spinach. Arrange chicken, strawberries, squash, orange sections and grapes over spinach. Drizzle salad with dressing. Sprinkle with pecans, if desired.   *Makes 4 servings*

Nutrients per Serving (¼ of total recipe):
Calories: 197, Calories from Fat: 11%, Total Fat: 2g, Saturated Fat: <1g, Cholesterol: 44mg, Sodium: 212mg, Carbohydrate: 23g, Dietary Fiber: 6g, Protein: 23g

Dietary Exchanges: 1½ Fruit, 2 Lean Meat

Chicken and Fruit Salad

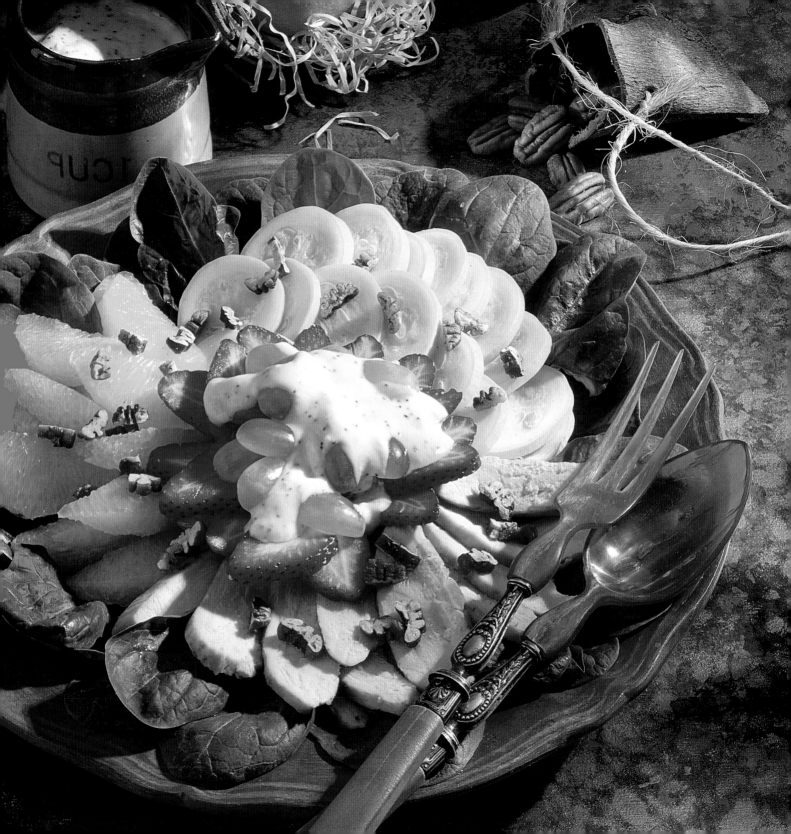

Hearty Healthy Chicken Salad

1 broiler-fryer chicken, cooked, skinned, boned and cut into chunks

1 cup small macaroni, cooked and drained

3 tomatoes, cubed

1 cup sliced celery

½ cup chopped red bell pepper

3 tablespoons chopped green onions

1 teaspoon salt

½ teaspoon black pepper

¼ teaspoon dried oregano leaves, crushed

1 cup low-sodium chicken broth

1 clove garlic, minced

¼ cup white wine vinegar

Combine chicken, macaroni, tomatoes, celery, bell pepper and onions in large bowl. Sprinkle with salt, black pepper and oregano. Place chicken broth and garlic in small saucepan. Bring to a boil over high heat for 10 minutes or until broth is reduced to ½ cup. Add wine vinegar. Pour over salad; mix well. Refrigerate until cold. *Makes 6 servings*

Favorite recipe from **National Chicken Council**

Nutrients per Serving (⅙ of total recipe):
Calories: 266, Calories from Fat: 30%, Total Fat: 9g, Saturated Fat: 2g, Cholesterol: 101mg, Sodium: 482mg, Carbohydrate: 11g, Dietary Fiber: 2g, Protein: 35g

Dietary Exchanges: ½ Starch, 1 Vegetable, 3½ Lean Meat

Spring Steak & Spinach Salad

    3 tablespoons KIKKOMAN® Lite Soy Sauce, divided

    3 tablespoons red wine vinegar, divided

    1 clove garlic, pressed

    ¼ teaspoon pepper

    ¾ pound boneless tender beef steak, ¾ inch thick

    ¼ cup vegetable oil

    ¼ teaspoon dried oregano leaves, crumbled

    1 pound fresh spinach, washed, stems removed and leaves torn into bite-size pieces

    6 ounces fresh mushrooms, sliced

    3 medium oranges, peeled and sectioned

Blend 2 tablespoons lite soy sauce, 1 tablespoon vinegar, garlic and pepper; pour over steak in large plastic food storage bag. Press air out of bag; close top securely. Turn bag over several times to coat both sides of steak. Marinate 30 minutes, turning bag over occasionally.

Meanwhile, combine remaining 1 tablespoon lite soy sauce, 2 tablespoons vinegar, oil and oregano; set aside.

Remove steak from marinade; place on grill 4 to 5 inches from hot coals. Cook 4 minutes on each side (for medium-rare), or to desired doneness. (Or, place steak on rack of broiler pan. Broil 4 minutes on each side [for medium-rare], or to desired doneness.) Cut steak across grain into thin slices; combine with spinach, mushrooms and oranges in large bowl. Blend soy sauce mixture; pour over spinach mixture. Toss to coat.

Makes 4 servings

Nutrients per Serving (¼ of total recipe):
Calories: 302, Calories from Fat: 50%, Total Fat: 17g, Saturated Fat: 3g, Cholesterol: 40mg, Sodium: 621mg, Carbohydrate: 15g, Dietary Fiber: 13g, Protein: 24g

Dietary Exchanges: 1 Fruit, 3 Lean Meat, 2 Fat

Colorful Turkey Pasta Salad

2½ cups tri-colored rotini pasta, cooked (without salt) and drained

2 cups cubed cooked turkey, white meat preferred

½ cup thinly sliced green onions

¼ cup chopped celery

¼ cup chopped fresh parsley

1½ teaspoons chopped fresh tarragon *or* ½ teaspoon dried tarragon leaves

2 tablespoons reduced-calorie mayonnaise

2 tablespoons tarragon vinegar

1 tablespoon fresh lemon juice

1 tablespoon canola or olive oil

1. In large bowl, combine pasta, turkey, onions, celery, parsley and tarragon.

2. In small bowl, mix together mayonnaise, vinegar, lemon juice and oil. Add to turkey mixture.

3. Mix well, coating all surfaces. Cover and refrigerate 1 to 2 hours or until chilled throughout.

Makes 4 servings

Favorite recipe from **California Poultry Federation**

Nutrients per Serving (¼ of total recipe):
Calories: 353, Calories from Fat: 26%, Total Fat: 10g, Saturated Fat: 2g, Cholesterol: 56mg, Sodium: 116mg, Carbohydrate: 37g, Dietary Fiber: 2g, Protein: 27g

Dietary Exchanges: 2 Starch, 1 Vegetable, 3 Lean Meat

Colorful Turkey Pasta Salad

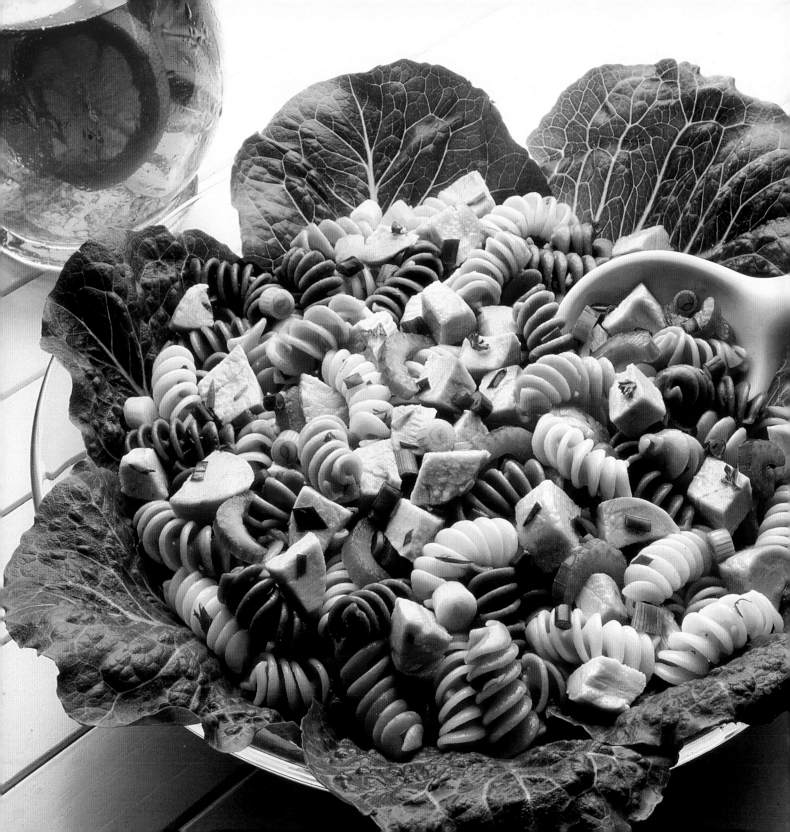

Grilled Chicken au Poivre Salad

4 boneless skinless chicken breast halves (about 1¼ pounds)

¼ cup plus 3 tablespoons olive oil, divided

¼ cup finely chopped onion

3 cloves garlic, minced

2½ tablespoons white wine vinegar, divided

2 teaspoons cracked or coarse ground black pepper

½ teaspoon salt

¼ teaspoon poultry seasoning

1 tablespoon Dijon mustard

Dash sugar

1 bag (10 ounces) prewashed salad greens

4 cherry tomatoes

1. Place chicken, ¼ cup oil, onion, garlic, 1 tablespoon vinegar, pepper, salt and poultry seasoning in resealable plastic food storage bag. Seal bag; knead to coat chicken. Refrigerate at least 2 hours or overnight.

2. Grill chicken on covered grill over medium-hot coals 10 to 15 minutes or until chicken is no longer pink in center.

3. Combine remaining 3 tablespoons oil, 1½ tablespoons vinegar, mustard and sugar in small bowl; whisk until smooth.

4. Arrange salad greens and cherry tomatoes on 4 plates. Cut chicken crosswise into strips. Arrange strips on top of greens. Drizzle with dressing. *Makes 4 servings*

Nutrients per Serving (¼ of total recipe):
Calories: 252, Calories from Fat: 55%, Total Fat: 15g, Saturated Fat: 2g, Cholesterol: 53mg, Sodium: 439mg, Carbohydrate: 5g, Dietary Fiber: 2g, Protein: 23g

Dietary Exchanges: 1 Vegetable, 3 Lean Meat, 1 Fat

Grilled Chicken au Poivre Salad

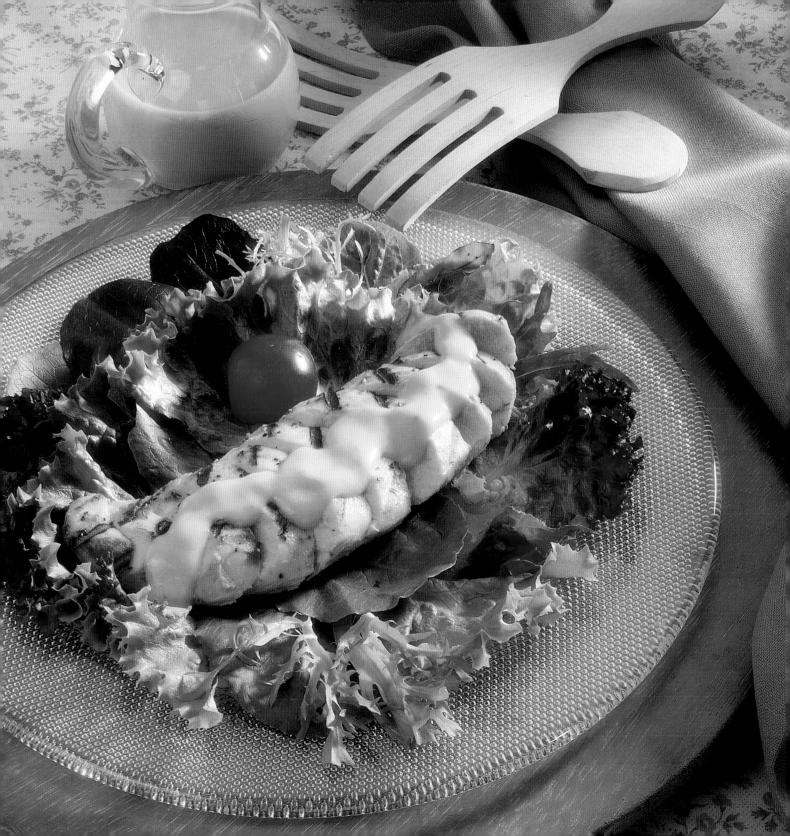

Hot Chinese Chicken Salad

8 ounces fresh or steamed Chinese egg noodles

¼ cup fat-free reduced-sodium chicken broth

2 tablespoons reduced-sodium soy sauce

2 tablespoons rice wine vinegar

1 tablespoon rice wine or dry sherry

1 teaspoon sugar

½ teaspoon red pepper flakes

1 tablespoon vegetable oil, divided

1 clove garlic, minced

1½ cups fresh pea pods, sliced diagonally

1 cup thinly sliced green or red bell pepper

1 pound boneless skinless chicken breasts, cut into ½-inch pieces

1 cup thinly sliced red or green cabbage

2 green onions, thinly sliced

1. Cook noodles in boiling water 4 to 5 minutes or until tender. Drain; set aside. Blend chicken broth, soy sauce, vinegar, rice wine, sugar and red pepper flakes in small bowl; set aside.

2. Heat 1 teaspoon oil in large nonstick skillet or wok. Add garlic, pea pods and bell pepper; cook 1 to 2 minutes or until vegetables are crisp-tender. Set aside.

3. Heat remaining 2 teaspoons oil in skillet. Add chicken; cook 3 to 4 minutes or until chicken is no longer pink. Add cabbage, cooked vegetables and noodles. Stir in sauce; toss until well blended. Cook and stir 1 to 2 minutes or until heated through. Sprinkle with green onions before serving.

Makes 6 servings

Nutrients per Serving (1⅓ cups):
Calories: 164, Calories from Fat: 30%, Total Fat: 6g, Saturated Fat: 1g, Cholesterol: 45mg, Sodium: 353mg, Carbohydrate: 12g, Dietary Fiber: 2g, Protein: 17g

Dietary Exchanges: ½ Starch, 1 Vegetable, 2 Lean Meat

Hot Chinese Chicken Salad

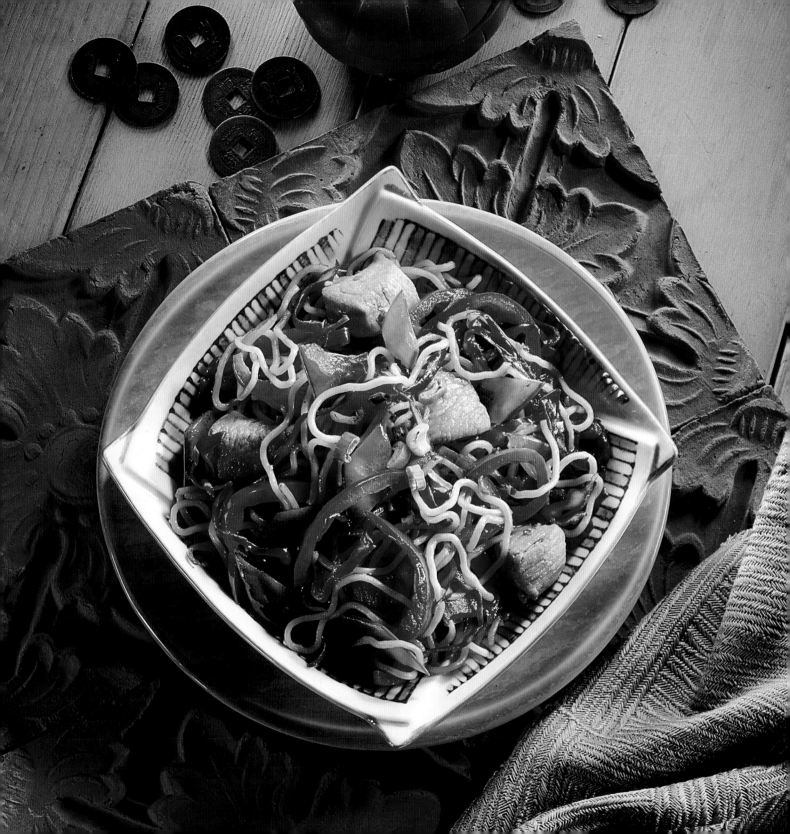

Scallop and Spinach Salad

1 package (10 ounces) spinach leaves, washed, stemmed and torn
3 thin slices red onion, halved and separated
12 ounces sea scallops
    Ground red pepper
    Paprika
    Nonstick cooking spray
½ cup prepared fat-free Italian salad dressing
¼ cup crumbled blue cheese
2 tablespoons toasted walnuts

1. Pat spinach dry; place in large bowl with red onion. Cover; set aside.

2. Rinse scallops. Cut in half horizontally (to make 2 thin rounds); pat dry. Sprinkle top side lightly with red pepper and paprika. Spray large nonstick skillet with cooking spray; heat over high heat until very hot. Add half of scallops, seasoned side down, in single layer, placing ½ inch or more apart. Sprinkle with red pepper and paprika. Cook 2 minutes or until browned on bottom. Turn scallops; cook 1 to 2 minutes or until opaque in center. Transfer to plate; cover to keep warm. Wipe skillet clean; repeat procedure with remaining scallops.

3. Place dressing in small saucepan; bring to a boil over high heat. Pour dressing over spinach and onion; toss to coat. Divide among 4 plates. Place scallops on top of spinach; sprinkle with blue cheese and walnuts.

Makes 4 servings

Nutrients per Serving: (¼ of total recipe)
Calories: 169, Calories from Fat: 29%, Total Fat: 6g, Saturated Fat: 2g, Cholesterol: 50mg, Sodium: 660mg, Carbohydrate: 6g, Dietary Fiber: 2g, Protein: 24g

Dietary Exchanges: 1 Vegetable, 3 Lean Meat

Scallop and Spinach Salad

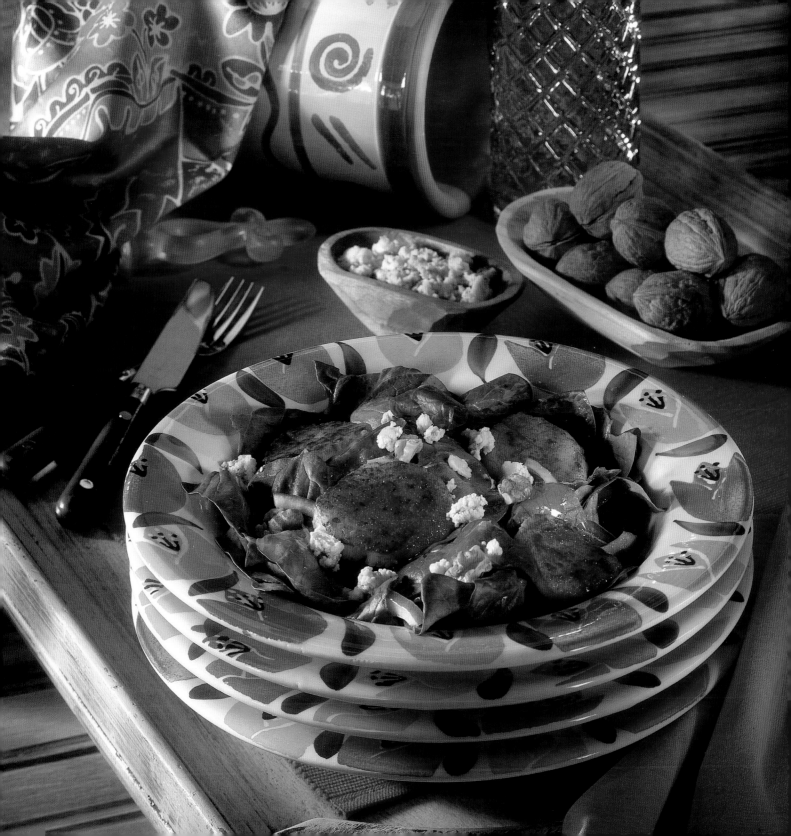

Warm Salad Valencia

1 package (1¼ pounds) PERDUE® FIT 'N EASY® Fresh Skinless and Boneless
    OVEN STUFFER® Roaster Thighs
3 tablespoons olive oil, divided
1 teaspoon dried thyme leaves
   Salt and ground black pepper to taste
2 red bell peppers, quartered and seeded
3 tablespoons orange juice
1 tablespoon *each* grainy Dijon mustard, balsamic vinegar and fresh lemon juice
1 head Boston or Bibb lettuce
1 head frisée or curly chicory
2 oranges, peeled and sectioned
2 tablespoons thinly sliced scallions

Prepare outdoor grill for cooking, or preheat broiler. Rub chicken with 1 tablespoon oil; season both sides with thyme, salt and black pepper. Grill or broil chicken 6 to 8 inches from heat source 25 to 35 minutes until cooked through, turning once. Slice chicken, reserving juices; set aside. Place bell peppers on edge of grill or on broiler pan. Cook 5 to 10 minutes until tender, turning occasionally. Remove peppers from heat; slice and set aside.

Meanwhile, in small saucepan on side of grill or over low heat, combine orange juice, mustard, vinegar and lemon juice. Whisk in remaining 2 tablespoons oil and any juices from chicken; bring to a simmer. Season mixture with salt and pepper to taste.

To serve on dinner plates, arrange greens and orange sections; top with chicken and pepper slices. Drizzle dressing over salad. Sprinkle with scallions and serve immediately. *Makes 5 servings*

Nutrients per Serving (⅕ of total recipe):
Calories: 268, Calories from Fat: 43%, Total Fat: 13g, Saturated Fat: 2g, Cholesterol: 94mg, Sodium: 167mg, Carbohydrate: 14g, Dietary Fiber: 4g, Protein: 24g

Dietary Exchanges: ½ Fruit, 1 Vegetable, 3 Lean Meat, 1 Fat

Satisfying Salads

Strawberry Banana Salad

1½ cups boiling water
1 package (8-serving size) *or* 2 packages (4-serving size each) JELL-O® Brand
    Strawberry or Strawberry Banana Flavor Sugar Free Low Calorie Gelatin
2 cups cold water
1 cup chopped strawberries
1 banana, sliced

STIR boiling water into gelatin in large bowl at least 2 minutes until completely dissolved. Stir in cold water. Refrigerate about 1½ hours or until thickened (spoon drawn through leaves definite impression).

STIR in strawberries and banana. Pour into 5-cup mold that has been sprayed with no stick cooking spray.

REFRIGERATE 4 hours or until firm. Unmold. Store leftover gelatin mold in refrigerator.

Makes 10 servings

Prep Time: 15 minutes
Refrigerate Time: 5½ hours

Nutrients per Serving (½ cup):
Calories: 22, Calories from Fat: 4%, Total Fat: <1g, Saturated Fat: <1g, Cholesterol: 0mg, Sodium: 44mg, Carbohydrate: 4g, Dietary Fiber: 1g, Protein: 1g

Dietary Exchanges: ½ Fruit

Fajita Salad

1 beef sirloin steak (6 ounces)
¼ cup fresh lime juice
2 tablespoons chopped fresh cilantro
1 clove garlic, minced
1 teaspoon chili powder
2 medium red bell peppers
1 medium onion
1 teaspoon olive oil
1 cup garbanzo beans, rinsed and drained
4 cups mixed salad greens
1 medium tomato, cut into wedges
1 cup salsa
   Sour cream (optional)
   Cilantro sprigs (optional)

1. Cut beef into thin strips. Place in resealable plastic food storage bag. Combine lime juice, cilantro, garlic and chili powder in small bowl; pour over beef. Seal bag. Let stand 10 minutes, turning once.

2. Cut peppers into strips. Slice onion. Heat oil in large nonstick skillet over medium-high heat. Add peppers and onion. Cook and stir 6 minutes or until vegetables are crisp-tender. Remove from skillet. Add beef and marinade to skillet. Cook and stir 3 minutes or until meat is cooked through. Remove from heat. Add peppers, onion and beans to skillet; toss to coat with pan juices. Cool slightly.

3. Divide salad greens evenly among serving plates. Top with beef mixture and tomato wedges. Serve with salsa. Garnish with sour cream and sprigs of cilantro, if desired.   *Makes 4 servings*

Nutrients per Serving (¼ of total recipe):
Calories: 181, Calories from Fat: 18%, Total Fat: 4g, Saturated Fat: 1g, Cholesterol: 22mg, Sodium: 698mg, Carbohydrate: 25g, Dietary Fiber: 6g, Protein: 16g

Dietary Exchanges: 1½ Starch, 1½ Lean Meat

Fajita Salad

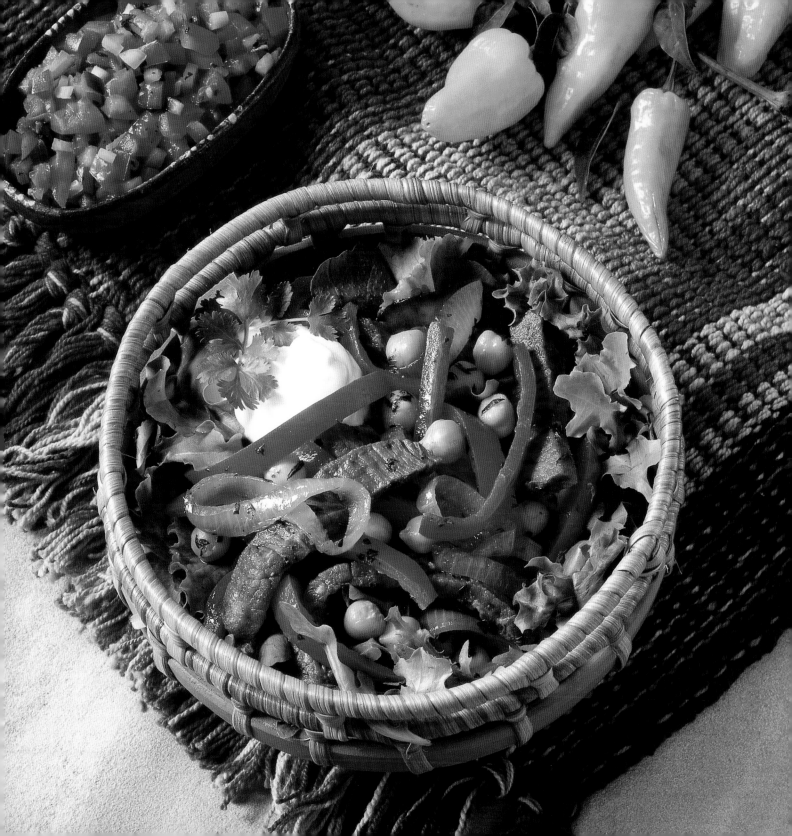

Mandarin Turkey Salad with Buttermilk-Herb Dressing

Buttermilk-Herb Dressing (page 150)
1 can (about 14 ounces) fat-free reduced-sodium chicken broth
1¼ pounds turkey tenderloins, cut in half lengthwise
½ teaspoon dried basil leaves
½ pound (about 8 cups) mesclun salad greens, washed and dried
2 pounds (about 10 cups) raw cut-up salad bar vegetables such as broccoli florets,
red or yellow bell peppers, carrots and red onion
1 can (11 ounces) mandarin orange segments, drained

1. Prepare Buttermilk-Herb Dressing. Set aside.

2. Place broth in medium saucepan; bring to a boil over high heat. Add turkey and basil. Return to a boil; reduce heat. Simmer, covered, 12 to 14 minutes or until turkey is no longer pink.

3. Remove turkey from broth. When cool enough to handle, shred turkey into strips.

4. Arrange salad greens on individual plates. Divide turkey evenly over salad greens. Arrange vegetables and orange segments around turkey; drizzle each serving with 2 tablespoons Buttermilk-Herb Dressing.

Makes 6 servings

continued on page 150

Mandarin Turkey Salad with Buttermilk-Herb Dressing

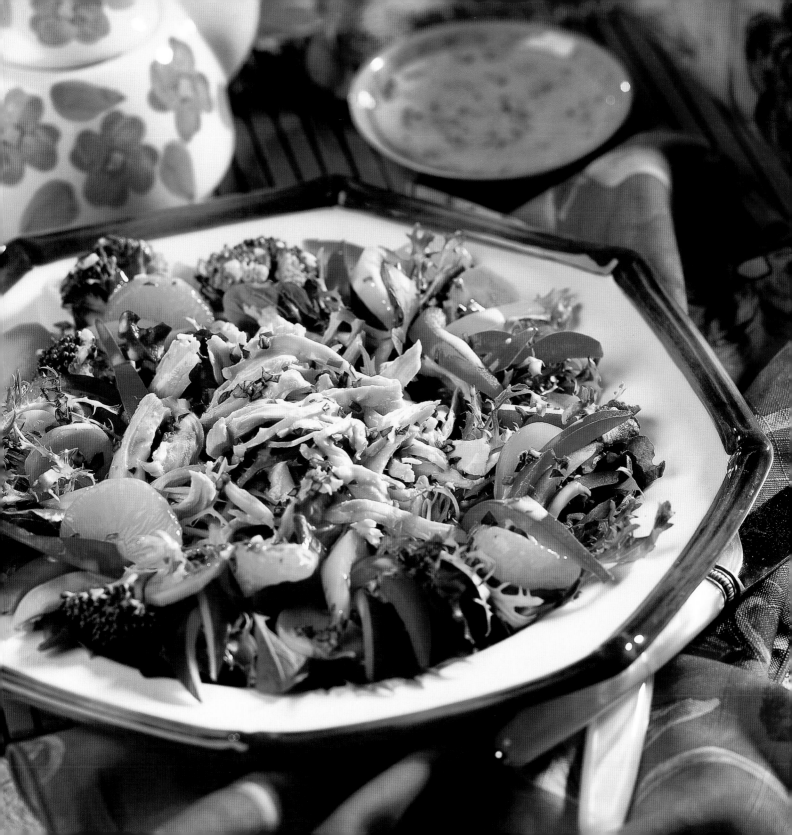

Buttermilk-Herb Dressing

½ cup plus 1 tablespoon low-fat buttermilk
3 tablespoons raspberry-flavored vinegar
1 tablespoon chopped fresh basil leaves
1½ teaspoons snipped fresh chives
¼ teaspoon minced garlic

Place all ingredients in small bowl; stir to combine.   *Makes about ¾ cup*

Nutrients per Serving: (⅙ of salad with 2 tablespoons dressing):
Calories: 182, Calories from Fat: 10%, Total Fat: 2g, Saturated Fat: 1g, Cholesterol: 38mg,
Sodium: 140mg, Carbohydrate: 19g, Dietary Fiber: 4g, Protein: 22g

Dietary Exchanges: ½ Fruit, 2 Vegetable, 2 Lean Meat

recipe tip

The Buttermilk-Herb Dressing in this recipe makes a great addition to many different salads. Try it on another one of your favorites. It can be stored, covered, in the refrigerator for up to one day.

Tuna Salad Stuffed Eggs

8 eggs
1 can (9 ounces) tuna packed in water, drained
½ cup diced celery
¼ cup mayonnaise
3 tablespoons drained sweet pickle relish
2 tablespoons minced onion
¼ teaspoon lemon-pepper seasoning
⅛ teaspoon salt
3 cups shredded iceberg lettuce
2 cups red seedless grapes

1. Place eggs in single layer in large saucepan; cover with cold water. Bring to a boil over medium-high heat. Cover; remove from heat and let stand 20 minutes. Drain and cool.

2. Peel shells from eggs; discard shells. Cut eggs in half lengthwise; carefully separate yolks from whites, leaving whites intact. Crumble 4 yolks, saving remaining yolks for another use, if desired.

3. Combine tuna, yolks, celery, mayonnaise, relish, onion, lemon-pepper and salt in medium bowl; stir until blended.

4. Carefully spoon heaping tablespoon tuna mixture into each egg white portion. Place filled egg halves together, forming complete egg. Press gently to adhere. Repeat with remaining egg halves.

5. Cover and refrigerate at least 2 hours or up to 24 hours. Serve eggs over lettuce with grapes.

Makes 4 servings

Nutrients per Serving (2 stuffed eggs plus ½ cup grapes):
Calories: 348, Calories from Fat: 26%, Total Fat: 10g, Saturated Fat: 5g, Cholesterol: 218mg, Sodium: 526mg, Carbohydrate: 35g, Dietary Fiber: 2g, Protein: 30g

Dietary Exchanges: 2 Fruit, 1 Vegetable, 3½ Lean Meat

Healthy Grilled Chicken Salad

½ cup A.1.® Steak Sauce
½ cup prepared Italian salad dressing
1 teaspoon dried basil leaves
1 pound boneless chicken breast halves
6 cups mixed salad greens
¼ pound snow peas, blanched and halved
1 cup sliced mushrooms
1 medium red bell pepper, thinly sliced
   Parmesan cheese, optional

Blend steak sauce, dressing and basil. Place chicken in glass dish; coat with ¼ cup marinade. Cover; refrigerate 1 hour, turning occasionally.

Arrange salad greens, snow peas, mushrooms and pepper slices on 6 individual salad plates; set aside.

Heat remaining marinade mixture in small saucepan over medium heat; keep warm.

Remove chicken from marinade; discard marinade. Grill over medium heat for 8 to 10 minutes or until done, turning occasionally. Thinly slice chicken; arrange over salad greens. Drizzle warm dressing over prepared salad. Serve immediately, sprinkled with Parmesan cheese if desired.   *Makes 6 servings*

Nutrients per Serving (⅙ of total recipe):
Calories: 211, Calories from Fat: 46%, Total Fat: 11g, Saturated Fat: 2g, Cholesterol: 44mg, Sodium: 488mg, Carbohydrate: 10g, Dietary Fiber: 2g, Protein: 19g

Dietary Exchanges: 2 Vegetable, 2 Lean Meat, 1 Fat

Healthy Grilled Chicken Salad

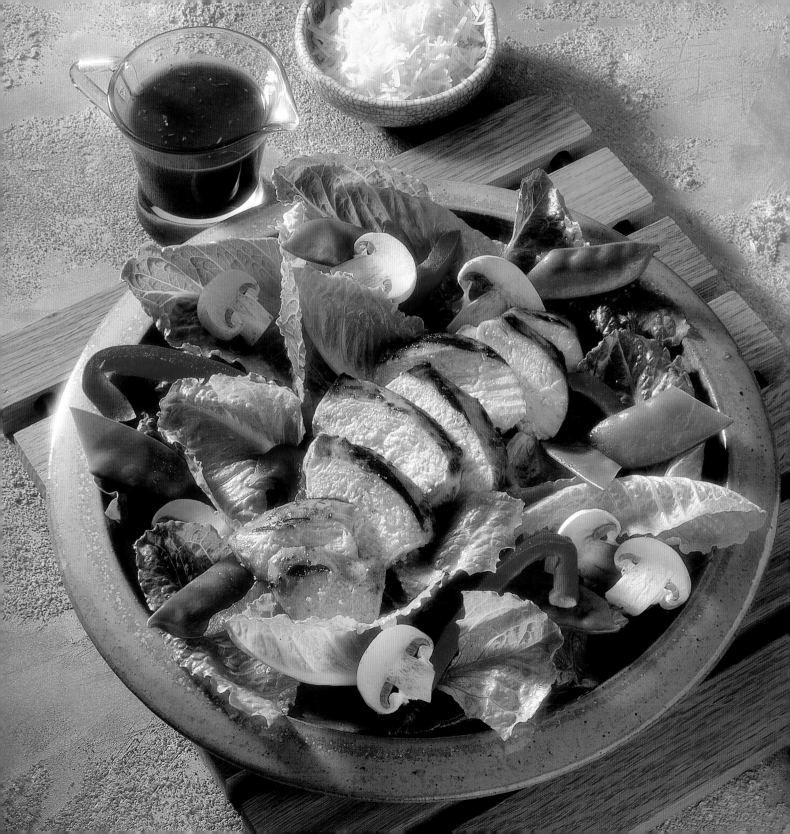

Warm Blackened Tuna Salad

Satisfying Salads

   5 cups torn washed romaine lettuce

   2 cups coarsely shredded red cabbage

   2 medium yellow or green bell peppers, cut into strips

1½ cups sliced zucchini

   1 teaspoon onion powder

   ½ teaspoon *each* garlic powder, black pepper, ground red pepper and dried thyme
      leaves, crushed

12 ounces fresh or thawed frozen tuna steaks, cut 1 inch thick

   ⅓ cup water

   ¾ cup onion slices

   2 tablespoons balsamic vinegar

1½ teaspoons Dijon-style mustard

   1 teaspoon canola or vegetable oil

   ½ teaspoon chicken bouillon granules

1. Preheat broiler. Combine all vegetables (except onion) in large bowl; set aside. Combine onion powder, garlic powder, black pepper, ground red pepper and thyme in small bowl. Rub spice mixture onto tuna. Place on broiler pan. Broil 4 inches below heat 6 minutes. Turn tuna; broil 5 to 8 minutes more or until tuna begins to flake when tested with a fork. Cut into bite-size pieces; set aside.

2. For dressing, bring water to a boil in small saucepan over high heat. Add onion slices; reduce heat to medium-low. Simmer, covered, 4 to 5 minutes or until onion is tender. Add vinegar, mustard, oil and bouillon granules; cook and stir until heated through.

3. Place romaine mixture on four salad plates; arrange tuna on top. Drizzle with dressing. Serve warm.

Makes 4 servings

Nutrients per Serving (¼ of total recipe):
Calories: 196, Calories from Fat: 27%, Total Fat: 6g, Saturated Fat: 1g, Cholesterol: 32mg,
Sodium: 185mg, Carbohydrate: 13g, Dietary Fiber: 4g, Protein: 23g

Dietary Exchanges: 2 Vegetable, 2½ Lean Meat

Thai Chicken Broccoli Salad

4 ounces uncooked linguine
  Nonstick cooking spray
½ pound boneless skinless chicken breasts, cut into 2×½-inch pieces
2 cups broccoli florets
⅔ cup chopped red bell pepper
6 green onions, sliced diagonally into 1-inch pieces
¼ cup reduced-fat creamy peanut butter
2 tablespoons hot water
2 tablespoons reduced-sodium soy sauce
2 teaspoons dark sesame oil
½ teaspoon red pepper flakes
⅛ teaspoon garlic powder
¼ cup unsalted peanuts, chopped

1. Cook pasta according to package directions, omitting salt. Drain; set aside.

2. Spray large nonstick skillet with cooking spray; heat over medium-high heat until hot. Add chicken; stir-fry 5 minutes or until chicken is no longer pink. Remove chicken from skillet.

3. Add broccoli and 2 tablespoons cold water to skillet. Cook, covered, 2 minutes. Uncover; cook and stir 2 minutes or until broccoli is crisp-tender. Remove broccoli from skillet. Combine pasta, chicken, broccoli, bell pepper and onions in large bowl.

4. Combine peanut butter, hot water, soy sauce, oil, red pepper and garlic powder in small bowl until well blended. Drizzle over pasta mixture; toss to coat. Top with peanuts before serving.

Makes 4 servings

Nutrients per Serving (¼ of total recipe):
Calories: 275, Calories from Fat: 29%, Total Fat: 9g, Saturated Fat: 2g, Cholesterol: 29mg, Sodium: 314mg, Carbohydrate: 29g, Dietary Fiber: 4g, Protein: 20g

Dietary Exchanges: 1½ Starch, 1 Vegetable, 2 Lean Meat, ½ Fat

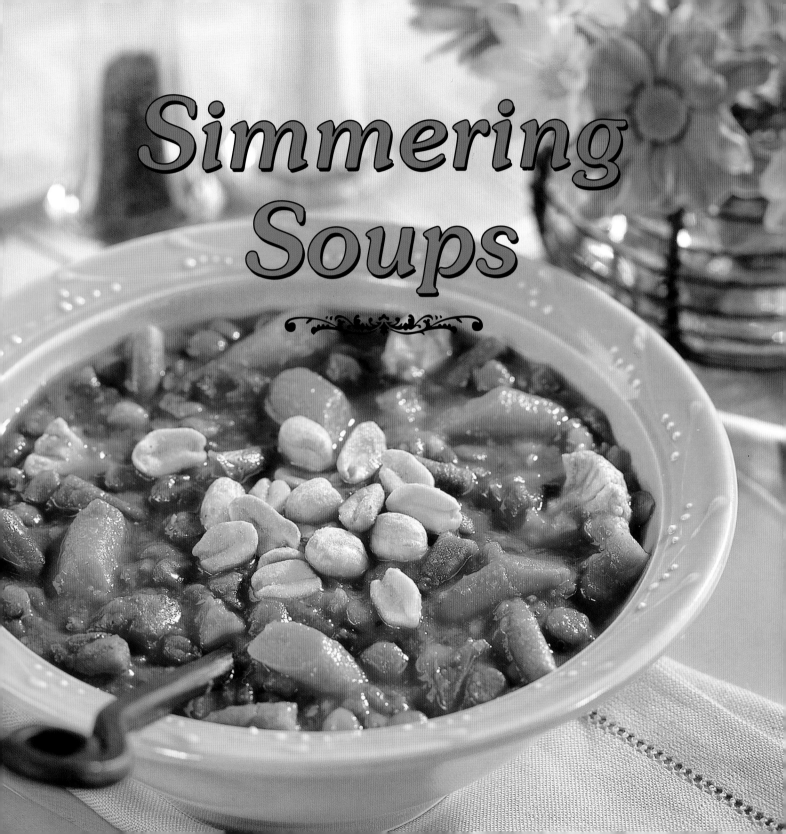

Simmering Soups

Hearty Lentil Stew

1 cup dried lentils, rinsed and drained

1 package (16 ounces) frozen green beans

2 cups cauliflower florets

1 cup chopped onion

1 cup baby carrots, cut in half crosswise

3 cups fat-free reduced-sodium chicken broth

2 teaspoons ground cumin

¾ teaspoon ground ginger

1 can (15 ounces) chunky tomato sauce with garlic and herbs

½ cup dry-roasted peanuts

Slow Cooker Directions

1. Place lentils in slow cooker. Top with green beans, cauliflower, onion and carrots. Combine broth, cumin and ginger in large bowl; mix well. Pour mixture over vegetables. Cover and cook on LOW 9 to 11 hours.

2. Stir in tomato sauce. Cover and cook on LOW 10 minutes. Ladle stew into bowls. Sprinkle peanuts evenly over each serving.

Makes 6 servings

Nutrients per Serving (⅙ of stew):
Calories: 264, Calories from Fat: 22%, Total Fat: 7g, Saturated Fat: <1g, Cholesterol: 0mg, Sodium: 667mg, Carbohydrate: 35g, Dietary Fiber: 16g, Protein: 19g

Dietary Exchanges: 2 Starch, 1 Vegetable, 1 Lean Meat, 1 Fat

Hearty Lentil Stew

New England Vegetable-Clam Chowder

2 slices uncooked turkey bacon

2 teaspoons vegetable oil

3 medium carrots, chopped

2 ribs celery, chopped

1 medium red bell pepper, seeded and diced

1 large onion, chopped

2 cans (6½ ounces each) chopped clams, drained and juice reserved

1 bottle (8 ounces) clam juice

½ cup low-fat (1%) milk

¼ cup vermouth or fat-free reduced-sodium chicken broth

1 teaspoon dried thyme leaves

¼ teaspoon salt

⅛ teaspoon white pepper

1½ cups mashed potatoes, made without salt or butter, *or* rehydrated instant
   potatoes to equal 1½ cups

1. Heat medium saucepan or Dutch oven over medium-high heat. Add bacon; brown. Remove from saucepan; cut into ½-inch pieces. Set aside.

2. Heat oil in same saucepan. Add carrots, celery, bell pepper and onion. Cook and stir 5 minutes. Add bacon, reserved juice from clams, bottled clam juice, milk, vermouth, thyme, salt and white pepper. Bring to a boil. Reduce heat; cover. Simmer 10 to 15 minutes or until vegetables are tender.

3. Gently stir mashed potatoes into chowder until well blended. Simmer 5 to 10 minutes or until chowder is slightly thickened. Stir in clams; heat thoroughly. Garnish as desired.   *Makes 4 servings*

Nutrients per Serving (¼ of chowder):
Calories: 299, Calories from Fat: 21%, Total Fat: 7g, Saturated Fat: 1g, Cholesterol: 62mg, Sodium: 462mg, Carbohydrate: 28g, Dietary Fiber: 3g, Protein: 28g

Dietary Exchanges: 1 Starch, 2 Vegetable, 2½ Lean Meat, 1 Fat

*New England
Vegetable-Clam Chowder*

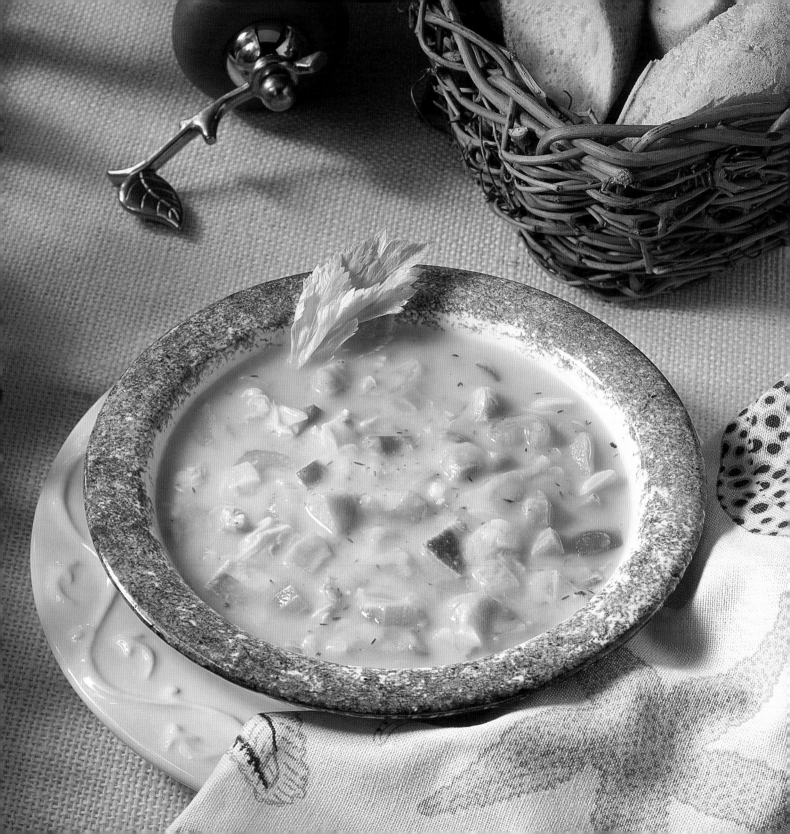

Southwestern Chicken Soup

½ teaspoon salt

¼ teaspoon garlic powder

¼ teaspoon black pepper

1 pound boneless skinless chicken breast halves

1 tablespoon olive oil

1 medium onion, halved and sliced

1 small hot chili pepper,* seeded and chopped (optional)

4 cans (about 14 ounces each) fat-free reduced-sodium chicken broth

2 cups peeled and diced potatoes

2 small zucchini, sliced

1½ cups frozen corn

1 cup diced tomato

2 tablespoons lime or lemon juice

1 tablespoon chopped fresh cilantro

Hot chili peppers can sting and irritate the skin; wear rubber gloves when handling peppers and do not touch eyes. Wash hands after handling.

1. Combine salt, garlic powder and black pepper in small bowl; sprinkle evenly over chicken.

2. Heat oil in Dutch oven over medium-high heat. Add chicken; cook, without stirring, 2 minutes or until golden. Turn chicken and cook 2 minutes more. Add onion and chili pepper, if desired; cook 2 minutes longer, adding a little chicken broth if needed to prevent burning.

3. Add chicken broth; bring to a boil. Stir in potatoes. Reduce heat to a simmer; cook 5 minutes. Add zucchini, corn and tomato; cook 10 minutes longer or until vegetables are tender. Just before serving, stir in lime juice and cilantro.   *Makes 6 servings*

Nutrients per Serving (⅙ of soup):
Calories: 210, Calories from Fat: 29%, Total Fat: 7g, Saturated Fat: 2g, Cholesterol: 46mg, Sodium: 270mg, Carbohydrate: 19g, Dietary Fiber: 2g, Protein: 22g

Dietary Exchanges: 1 Starch, 1 Vegetable, 2 Lean Meat

Southwestern Chicken Soup

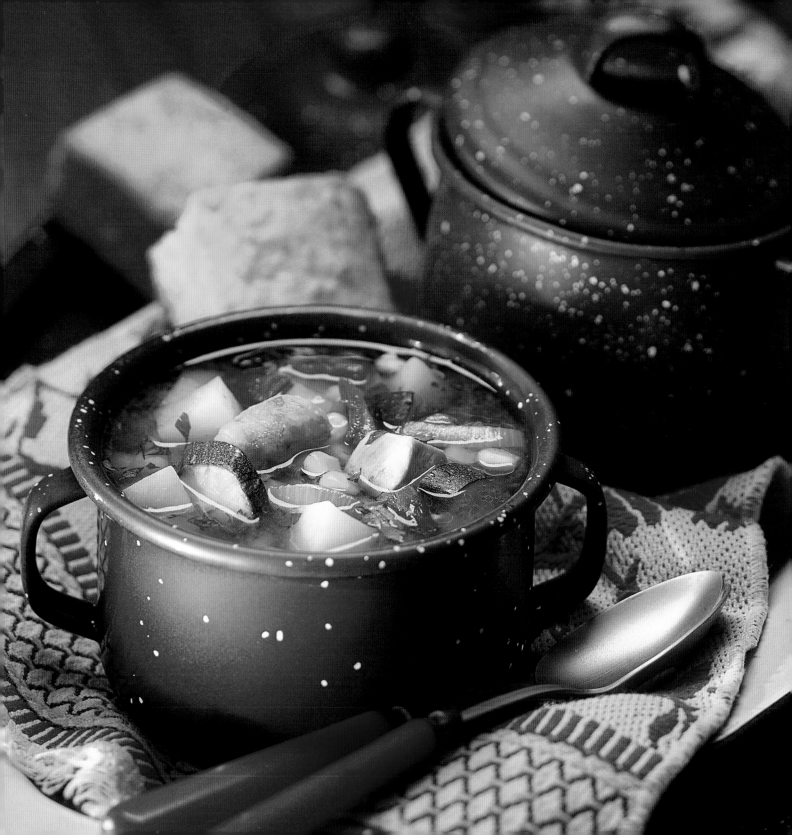

Asian Ramen Noodle Soup

2 cans (about 14 ounces each) fat-free reduced-sodium chicken broth
4 ounces boneless pork loin, sliced into thin strips
¾ cup thinly sliced mushrooms
½ cup firm tofu, cut into ¼-inch cubes (optional)
3 tablespoons white vinegar
3 tablespoons sherry
1 tablespoon reduced-sodium soy sauce
½ teaspoon ground red pepper
2 ounces uncooked low-fat ramen noodles
1 egg, beaten
¼ cup finely chopped green onions, green tops only

1. Bring chicken broth to a boil in large saucepan over high heat; add pork, mushrooms and tofu, if desired. Reduce heat to medium-low; simmer, covered, 5 minutes. Stir in vinegar, sherry, soy sauce and pepper.

2. Return broth mixture to a boil over high heat; stir in ramen noodles. Cook, stirring occasionally, 5 to 7 minutes or until noodles are tender. Slowly stir in beaten egg and green onions; remove from heat. Ladle soup into individual bowls. *Makes 4 servings*

Nutrients per Serving (¾ cup):
Calories: 148, Calories from Fat: 24%, Total Fat: 4g, Saturated Fat: 1g, Cholesterol: 66mg, Sodium: 269mg, Carbohydrate: 15g, Dietary Fiber: 1g, Protein: 10g

Dietary Exchanges: ½ Starch, 1 Vegetable, 1½ Lean Meat

Simmering Soups

Chicken, Barley and Vegetable Soup

½ pound boneless skinless chicken breasts, cut into ½-inch pieces
½ pound boneless skinless chicken thighs, cut into ½-inch pieces
¾ teaspoon salt
¼ teaspoon black pepper
1 tablespoon olive oil
½ cup uncooked pearl barley
4 cans (about 14 ounces each) fat-free reduced-sodium chicken broth
2 cups water
1 bay leaf
2 cups peeled whole baby carrots
2 cups diced peeled potatoes
2 cups sliced mushrooms
2 cups frozen peas
3 tablespoons reduced-fat sour cream
1 tablespoon chopped fresh dill *or* 1 teaspoon dried dill weed

1. Sprinkle chicken with salt and pepper. Heat oil in Dutch oven over medium-high heat. Add chicken; cook, without stirring, 2 minutes or until golden. Turn chicken; cook 2 minutes more. Remove chicken.

2. Add barley to Dutch oven; cook and stir 1 to 2 minutes or until barley starts to brown, adding a little chicken broth if needed to prevent burning. Add chicken broth, water and bay leaf; bring to a boil. Reduce heat to low; simmer, covered, 30 minutes.

3. Add chicken, carrots, potatoes and mushrooms; cook 10 minutes or until vegetables are tender. Add peas and cook 2 minutes longer. Remove bay leaf; discard.

4. Stir in sour cream and dill; serve immediately. Garnish with fresh dill, if desired.

Makes 6 servings

Nutrients per Serving (⅙ of soup):
Calories: 317, Calories from Fat: 26%, Total Fat: 9g, Saturated Fat: 2g, Cholesterol: 46mg, Sodium: 435mg, Carbohydrate: 37g, Dietary Fiber: 6g, Protein: 22g

Dietary Exchanges: 2 Starch, 1 Vegetable, 2 Lean Meat, 1 Fat

Beef Stew in Red Wine

1½ pounds boneless beef round, cut into 1-inch cubes

1½ cups dry red wine

2 teaspoons olive oil

Peel of half an orange

2 large cloves garlic, thinly sliced

1 bay leaf

½ teaspoon dried thyme leaves

⅛ teaspoon black pepper

8 ounces fresh mushrooms, quartered

8 sun-dried tomatoes, quartered

1 can (about 14 ounces) fat-free reduced-sodium beef broth

6 small potatoes, unpeeled, cut into wedges

1 cup baby carrots

1 cup fresh pearl onions, outer skins removed

1 tablespoon cornstarch mixed with 2 tablespoons water

1. Combine beef, wine, oil, orange peel, garlic, bay leaf, thyme and pepper in large glass bowl. Refrigerate, covered, at least 2 hours or overnight.

2. Place beef mixture, mushrooms and tomatoes in large nonstick skillet. Add enough beef broth to just cover ingredients. Bring to a boil over high heat. Cover; reduce heat to low. Simmer 1 hour. Add potatoes, carrots and onions; cover and cook 20 to 25 minutes or until vegetables are tender and meat is no longer pink. Remove meat and vegetables from skillet with slotted spoon; cover and set aside. Remove orange peel and bay leaf; discard. Stir cornstarch mixture into skillet with sauce. Increase heat to medium; cook and stir until sauce is slightly thickened. Return meat and vegetables to sauce; heat thoroughly.

Makes 6 servings

Nutrients per Serving (⅙ of stew):
Calories: 313, Calories from Fat: 16%, Total Fat: 6g, Saturated Fat: 1g, Cholesterol: 55mg, Sodium: 304mg, Carbohydrate: 31g, Dietary Fiber: 3g, Protein: 26g

Dietary Exchanges: 1½ Starch, 1½ Vegetable, 3 Lean Meat

Beef Stew in Red Wine

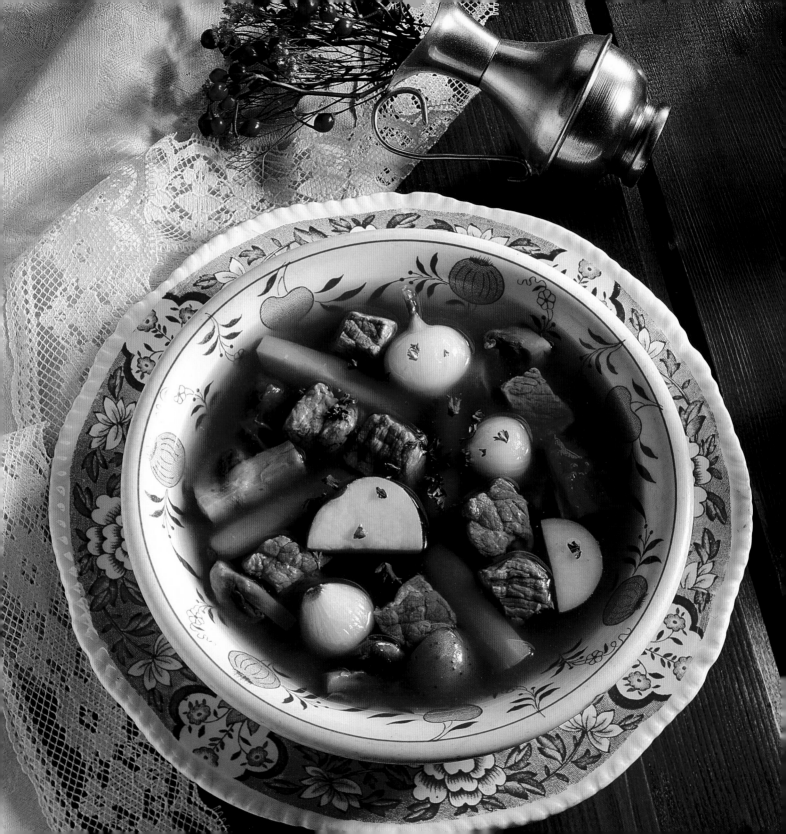

Spicy Pumpkin Soup with Green Chili Swirl

1 can (4 ounces) diced green chilies
¼ cup reduced-fat sour cream
¼ cup fresh cilantro leaves
1 can (15 ounces) solid-pack pumpkin
1 can (about 14 ounces) fat-free reduced-sodium chicken broth
½ cup water
1 teaspoon ground cumin
½ teaspoon chili powder
¼ teaspoon garlic powder
⅛ teaspoon ground red pepper (optional)
Additional sour cream (optional)

1. Combine green chilies, ¼ cup sour cream and cilantro in food processor or blender; process until smooth.*

2. Combine pumpkin, chicken broth, water, cumin, chili powder, garlic powder and red pepper, if desired, in medium saucepan; stir in ¼ cup green chili mixture. Bring to a boil; reduce heat to medium. Simmer uncovered 5 minutes, stirring occasionally.

3. Pour into serving bowls. Top each serving with small dollops of remaining green chili mixture and additional sour cream, if desired. Run tip of spoon through dollops to swirl. *Makes 4 servings*

Omit food processor step by adding green chilies directly to soup. Finely chop cilantro and combine with sour cream. Dollop with sour cream-cilantro mixture as directed.

Nutrients per Serving (¼ of soup):
Calories: 72, Calories from Fat: 17%, Total Fat: 1g, Saturated Fat: <1g, Cholesterol: 5mg, Sodium: 276mg, Carbohydrate: 12g, Dietary Fiber: 4g, Protein: 4g

Dietary Exchanges: 1 Starch

Spicy Pumpkin Soup with Green Chili Swirl

Simmering Soups

166

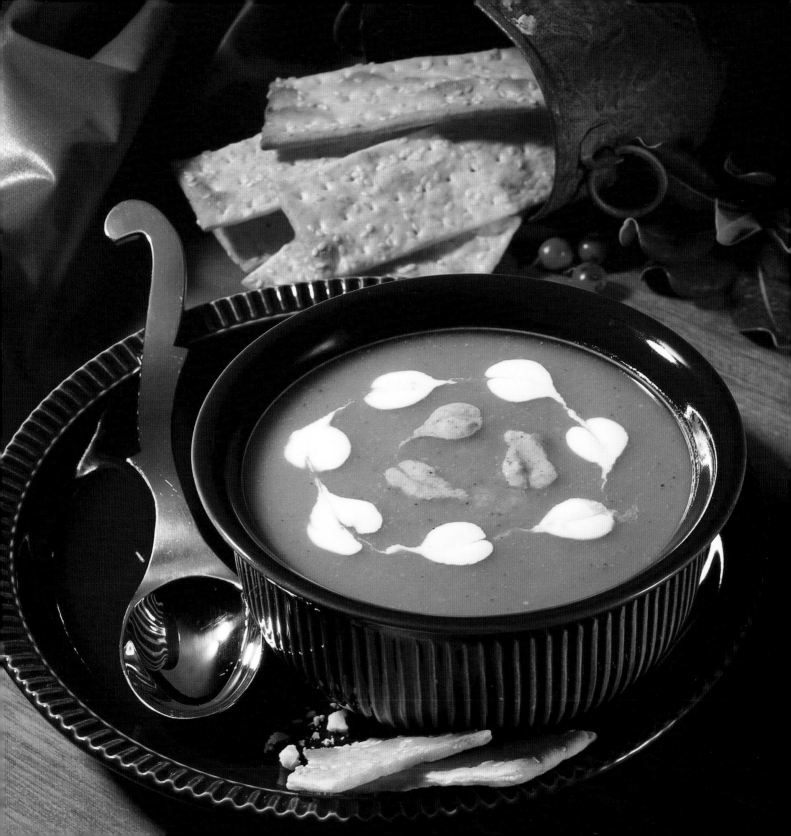

Cajun-Style Chicken Gumbo

1 pound boneless skinless chicken breasts

1 teaspoon Cajun or Creole seasoning

1 teaspoon dried thyme leaves

2 tablespoons vegetable oil

1 medium onion, coarsely chopped

1 medium green bell pepper, coarsely chopped

1 cup thinly sliced or julienned carrots

½ cup thinly sliced celery

4 cloves garlic, minced

2 tablespoons all-purpose flour

1 can (about 14 ounces) fat-free reduced-sodium chicken broth

1 can (14½ ounces) no-salt-added stewed tomatoes, undrained

½ teaspoon hot pepper sauce

2 cups hot cooked rice

¼ cup chopped fresh parsley (optional)

Additional hot pepper sauce (optional)

1. Cut chicken into 1-inch pieces; place in medium bowl. Sprinkle with seasoning and thyme; toss well. Set aside.

2. Heat oil in large saucepan over medium-high heat. Add onion, bell pepper, carrots, celery and garlic to saucepan; cover and cook 10 minutes or until vegetables are crisp-tender, stirring once. Add chicken; cook 3 minutes, stirring occasionally. Sprinkle mixture with flour; cook 1 minute, stirring frequently. Add chicken broth, tomatoes and pepper sauce; bring to a boil over high heat. Reduce heat to medium; simmer, uncovered, 10 minutes or until chicken is no longer pink in center, vegetables are tender and sauce is slightly thickened.

3. Ladle gumbo into 4 shallow bowls; top each with a scoop of rice. Sprinkle with parsley and serve with additional pepper sauce, if desired. *Makes 4 servings*

Nutrients per Serving (¼ of gumbo):
Calories: 388, Calories from Fat: 22%, Total Fat: 10g, Saturated Fat: 1g, Cholesterol: 76mg, Sodium: 219mg, Carbohydrate: 41g, Dietary Fiber: 4g, Protein: 34g

Dietary Exchanges: 2 Starch, 2 Vegetable, 3 Meat, ½ Fat

Italian Wonton Soup

2 tablespoons pine nuts

8 ounces boneless skinless chicken breast, ground

2 tablespoons sun-dried tomatoes (not oil-packed), minced

1 teaspoon fennel seed, crushed

1 teaspoon grated lemon peel

1 teaspoon water plus ½ teaspoon cornstarch

16 wonton wrappers

3 cups fat-free reduced-sodium chicken broth

1 cup dry white wine

2 tablespoons pesto

½ medium red bell pepper, diced

1. Heat Dutch oven over low heat 2 to 3 minutes. Add pine nuts; cook 2 to 3 minutes, stirring every 30 seconds, until golden. Remove; set aside.

2. Combine chicken, tomatoes, fennel and lemon peel in medium bowl. Separate wrappers and lay on work surface in single layer. Spoon 1 tablespoon filling in center of each wrapper. Blend water into cornstarch in small bowl. Brush edges of 1 wrapper. Lift 1 corner and fold over filling to meet opposite corner. Align edges and press to seal, forming triangle. Repeat with remaining wontons.

3. Pour chicken broth and wine into Dutch oven. Heat over high heat; bring to a boil. Carefully place wontons in chicken broth. Simmer 2 to 3 minutes or until chicken in center of wontons is no longer pink. Remove Dutch oven from heat. Place wontons in bowls. Stir pesto into chicken broth; ladle over wontons. Sprinkle with red bell pepper and pine nuts. *Makes 4 servings*

Nutrients per Serving (¼ of soup):
Calories: 298, Calories from Fat: 27%, Total Fat: 9g, Saturated Fat: 2g, Cholesterol: 40mg, Sodium: 356mg, Carbohydrate: 25g, Dietary Fiber: 1g, Protein: 20g

Dietary Exchanges: 1½ Starch, 1 Vegetable, 2 Lean Meat, 1 Fat

Turkey Chili

Nonstick cooking spray
1 pound extra-lean ground turkey breast
1 cup chopped onion
1 cup chopped green bell pepper
3 cloves garlic, minced
3 cans (14½ ounces each) chopped tomatoes, undrained
½ cup water
1 tablespoon chili powder
1 teaspoon ground cinnamon
1 teaspoon ground cumin
½ teaspoon paprika
½ teaspoon dried oregano leaves, crushed
½ teaspoon black pepper
¼ teaspoon salt
1 can (16 ounces) pinto beans, rinsed and drained

1. Spray large skillet with cooking spray. Cook turkey, onion, bell pepper and garlic over medium-high heat about 5 minutes or until turkey begins to brown, stirring frequently and breaking up turkey with back of spoon.

2. Stir in tomatoes; cook 5 minutes. Add water, chili powder, cinnamon, cumin, paprika, oregano, black pepper and salt; mix well. Stir in beans.

3. Bring to a boil; reduce heat to medium-low. Simmer about 30 minutes or until chili thickens. Garnish, if desired.

Makes 4 servings

Nutrients per Serving (¼ of chili):
Calories: 361, Calories from Fat: 29%, Total Fat: 12g, Saturated Fat: 4g, Cholesterol: 96mg, Sodium: 1048mg, Carbohydrate: 39g, Dietary Fiber: 11g, Protein: 28g

Dietary Exchanges: 2½ Starch, 3 Lean Meat, ½ Fat

Turkey Chili

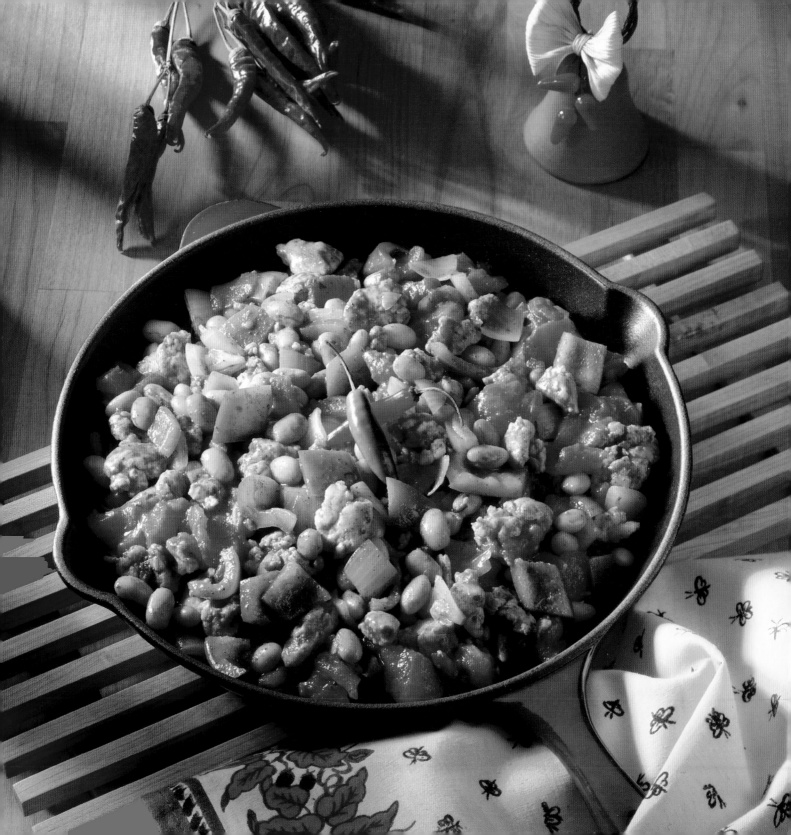

Cheddared Farmhouse Chowder

Simmering Soups

1 can (10½ ounces) condensed reduced-fat cream of mushroom soup, undiluted
1½ cups fat-free (skim) milk or fat-free evaporated milk
1 bag (16 ounces) frozen corn, carrots and broccoli, thawed
2 medium baking potatoes, cut into ½-inch cubes
½ teaspoon dried thyme leaves
⅛ teaspoon ground red pepper (optional)
¼ teaspoon black pepper
½ cup frozen peas, thawed
¼ teaspoon salt
¾ cup (3 ounces) shredded reduced-fat sharp Cheddar cheese

Whisk together soup and milk in large saucepan until well blended. Bring to a boil over medium-high heat, stirring frequently. Add corn mixture, potatoes, thyme, ground red pepper, if desired, and black pepper. Return to a boil. Reduce heat; cover. Simmer 15 minutes or until carrots are just tender, stirring frequently with a spatula. Remove from heat; stir in peas and salt. Let stand 5 minutes to absorb flavors. Ladle equal amounts into soup bowls and top each with equal amount shredded cheese.

Makes 5 servings

Nutrients per Serving (1 cup with shredded cheese):
Calories: 266, Calories from Fat: 19%, Total Fat: 6g, Saturated Fat: 3g, Cholesterol: 18mg, Sodium: 577mg, Carbohydrate: 43g, Dietary Fiber: 5g, Protein: 12g

Dietary Exchanges: 3 Starch, 1 Fat

Cheddared Farmhouse Chowder

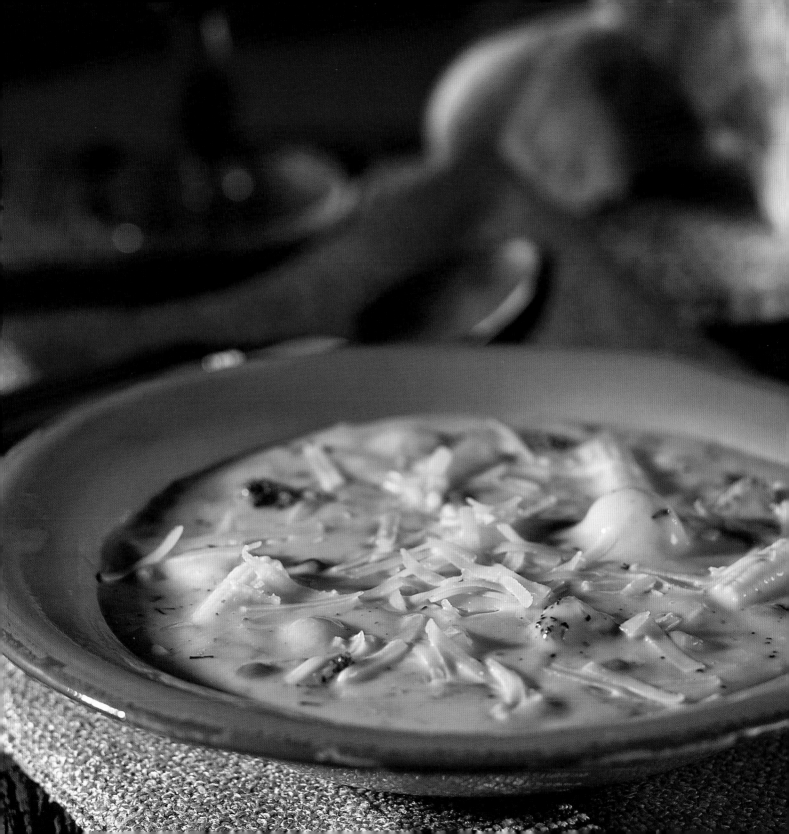

Skillet Chicken Soup

¾ pound boneless skinless chicken breasts or thighs, cut into ¾-inch pieces

1 teaspoon paprika

½ teaspoon salt

¼ teaspoon black pepper

2 teaspoons vegetable oil

1 large onion, chopped

1 medium red bell pepper, cut into ½-inch pieces

3 cloves garlic, minced

1 cup canned fat-free reduced-sodium chicken broth

1 can (19 ounces) cannellini beans or small white beans, rinsed and drained

3 cups sliced savoy or napa cabbage

½ cup fat-free herb-flavored croutons, slightly crushed

1. Toss chicken with paprika, salt and black pepper in medium bowl until coated.

2. Heat oil in large, deep nonstick skillet over medium-high heat until hot. Add chicken, onion, bell pepper and garlic. Cook until chicken is no longer pink, stirring frequently.

3. Add broth and beans; bring to a simmer. Cover and simmer 5 minutes or until chicken is cooked through. Stir in cabbage; cover and simmer 3 additional minutes or until cabbage is wilted. Ladle into shallow bowls; distribute crushed croutons evenly over top of bowls. *Makes 4 servings*

Nutrients per Serving (¼ of soup):
Calories: 284, Calories from Fat: 16%, Total Fat: 5g, Saturated Fat: 1g, Cholesterol: 52mg, Sodium: 721mg, Carbohydrate: 30g, Dietary Fiber: 8g, Protein: 28g

Dietary Exchanges: 1 Starch, 2 Vegetable, 3 Lean Meat

Skillet Chicken Soup

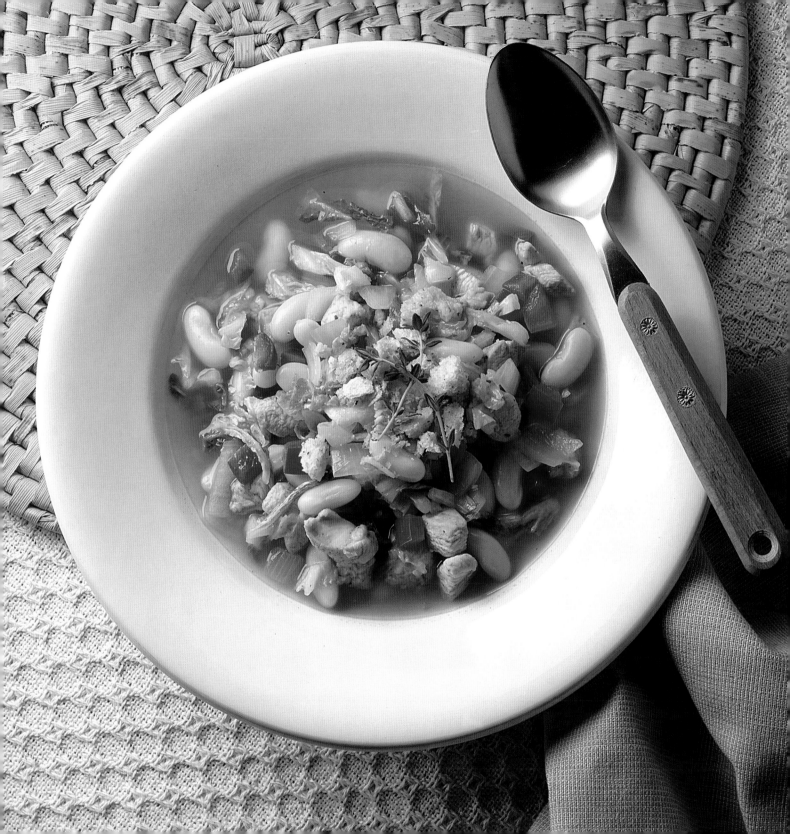

Spicy Crab Soup

1 pound crabmeat, cooked, flaked and cartilage removed*

1 can (28 ounces) crushed tomatoes in tomato purée, undrained

2 cups water

1 can (10¾ ounces) fat-free reduced-sodium chicken broth

¾ cup chopped celery

¾ cup diced onion

1 teaspoon seafood seasoning

¼ teaspoon lemon-pepper

1 package (10 ounces) frozen corn, thawed

1 package (10 ounces) frozen peas, thawed

*Purchase flake-style or mixture of flake and chunk crabmeat if purchasing blue crab or surimi blended seafood.

Combine tomatoes with purée, water, broth, celery, onion, seafood seasoning and lemon-pepper in 6-quart saucepan. Bring to a boil over high heat. Reduce heat to low. Cover and simmer 20 to 30 minutes. Add corn and peas; simmer 10 minutes more. Add crabmeat; simmer until heated through.

Makes 6 servings

*Favorite recipe from **National Fisheries Institute***

Nutrients per Serving (⅙ of soup):
Calories: 214, Calories from Fat: 9%, Total Fat: 2g, Saturated Fat: <1g, Cholesterol: 81mg, Sodium: 509mg, Carbohydrate: 28g, Dietary Fiber: 7g, Protein: 23g

Dietary Exchanges: 1 Starch, 1 Vegetable, 2 Lean Meat

Triathlete's Turkey Chili

2 tablespoons vegetable oil

2 medium onions, finely chopped

2 small red or green bell peppers, finely chopped

2 pounds lean ground turkey

2 cans (14 ounces each) diced tomatoes, undrained

1 can (14 ounces) beef broth

1 cup water

4 tablespoons tomato paste

2 teaspoons chili powder

Salt and black pepper

1 can (15 ounces) kidney beans, rinsed and drained

1 can (15 ounces) pinto beans, rinsed and drained

Cooked rice or cornbread (optional)

Sour cream (optional)

1. Heat oil in Dutch oven. Add onions and bell peppers; cook and stir 3 minutes over medium heat. Add turkey; cook for another 3 minutes, stirring to break up meat. Stir in tomatoes with juice, broth, water, tomato paste, chili powder, salt and black pepper to taste. Bring to a boil. Reduce heat and simmer 30 minutes, stirring often. If chili is too thick, add water, ½ cup at a time, until desired consistency is achieved.

2. Add beans; cook 10 minutes or until beans are hot. Serve with rice or cornbread; garnish with sour cream, if desired. *Makes 8 servings*

Prep Time: 30 minutes
Cook Time: 40 minutes

Nutrients per Serving (⅛ of chili):
Calories: 337, Calories from Fat: 37%, Total Fat: 14g, Saturated Fat: 3g, Cholesterol: 90mg, Sodium: 979mg, Carbohydrate: 25g, Dietary Fiber: 8g, Protein: 27g

Dietary Exchanges: 1 Starch, 2 Vegetable, 3 Lean Meat, 1 Fat

Bounty Soup

½ pound yellow crookneck squash

2 cups frozen mixed vegetables

1 teaspoon dried parsley flakes

⅛ teaspoon dried rosemary

⅛ teaspoon dried thyme leaves

⅛ teaspoon salt

⅛ teaspoon black pepper

2 teaspoons vegetable oil

3 boneless skinless chicken breast halves (about ¾ pound), chopped

1 can (about 14 ounces) fat-free reduced-sodium chicken broth

1 can (14½ ounces) stewed tomatoes, undrained

1. Cut wide part of squash in half lengthwise; lay halves flat and cut crosswise into ¼-inch slices. Place squash, mixed vegetables, parsley, rosemary, thyme, salt and pepper in medium bowl.

2. Heat oil in large saucepan over medium-high heat. Add chicken; stir-fry 2 minutes. Stir in vegetables and seasonings. Add broth and tomatoes with juice, breaking large tomatoes apart. Cover; bring to a boil. Reduce heat to low. Cover; cook 5 minutes or until vegetables are tender.

Makes 4 servings

Prep and Cook Time: 30 minutes

Nutrients per Serving (¼ of soup):
Calories: 225, Calories from Fat: 17%, Total Fat: 4g, Saturated Fat: 1g, Cholesterol: 60mg, Sodium: 490mg, Carbohydrate: 20g, Dietary Fiber: 6g, Protein: 27g

Dietary Exchanges: 4 Vegetable, 2 Lean Meat, ½ Fat

Bounty Soup

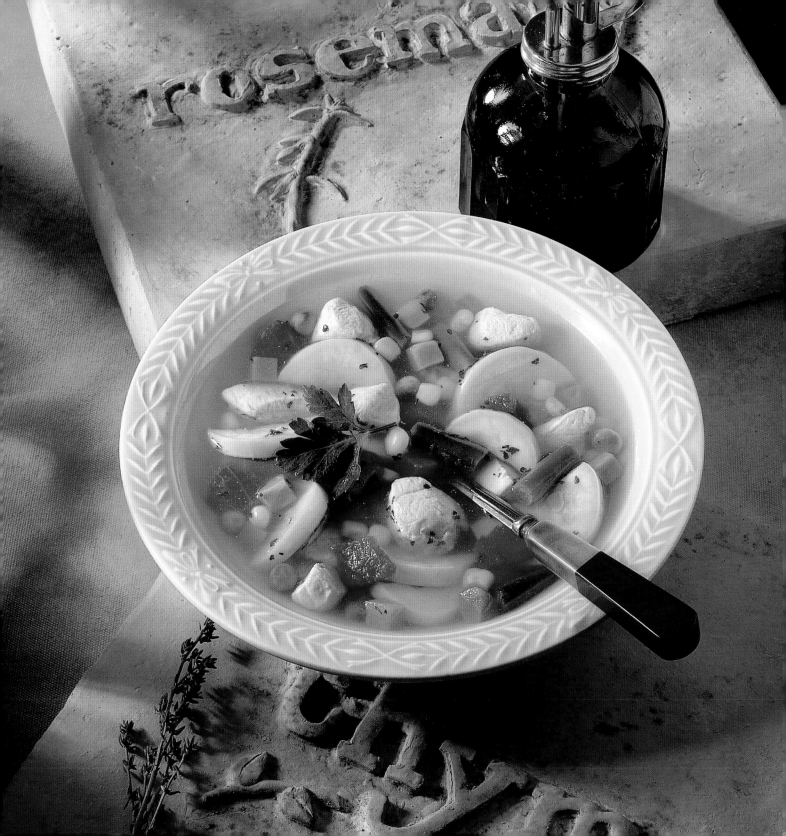

Confetti Chicken Chili

1 pound 90% fat-free ground chicken or 93% fat-free ground turkey

1 large onion, chopped

2 cans (about 14 ounces each) fat-free reduced-sodium chicken broth

1 can (15 ounces) Great Northern beans, rinsed and drained

2 medium carrots, chopped

1 medium green bell pepper, chopped

2 plum tomatoes, chopped

1 jalapeño pepper,* finely chopped (optional)

2 teaspoons chili powder

½ teaspoon ground red pepper

Jalapeño peppers can sting and irritate the skin; wear rubber gloves when handling peppers and do not touch eyes. Wash hands after handling.

1. Heat large nonstick saucepan over medium heat until hot. Add chicken and onion; cook and stir 5 minutes or until chicken is browned. Drain fat from saucepan.

2. Add remaining ingredients to saucepan. Bring to a boil. Reduce heat to low and simmer 15 minutes. *Makes 5 servings*

Prep & Cook Time: 30 minutes

Nutrients per Serving (⅕ of chili):
Calories: 282, Calories from Fat: 28%, Total Fat: 9g, Saturated Fat: 3g, Cholesterol: 67mg, Sodium: 136mg, Carbohydrate: 28g, Dietary Fiber: 3g, Protein: 25g

Dietary Exchanges: 1 Starch, 2 Vegetable, 2½ Lean Meat, ½ Fat

Confetti Chicken Chili

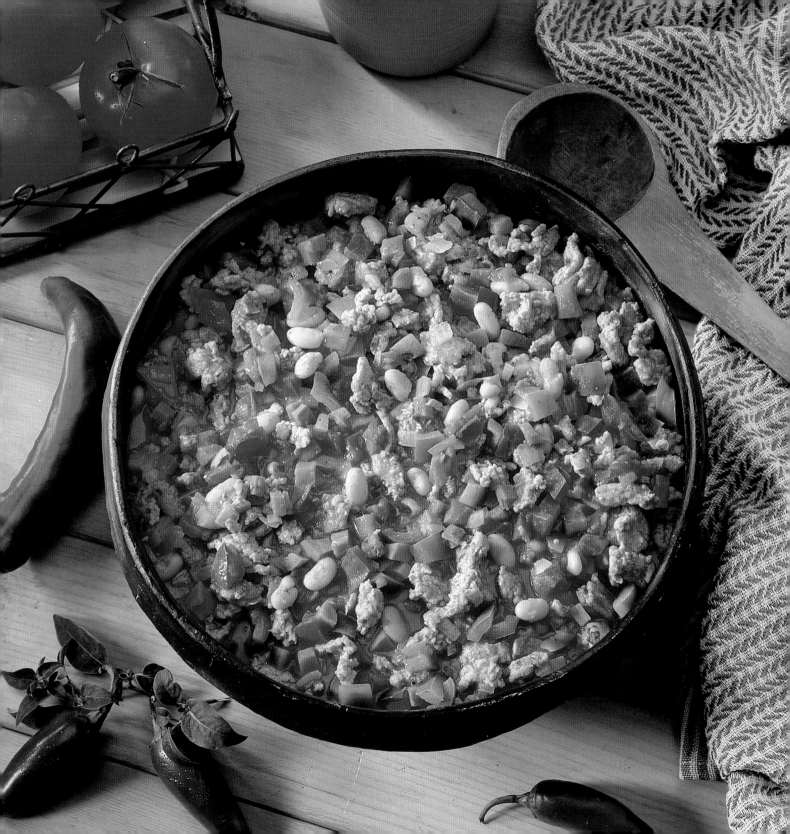

Pasta Meatball Soup

10 ounces lean ground sirloin

5 tablespoons acini di pepe pasta, uncooked, divided

¼ cup fresh, finely crushed bread crumbs

1 egg

2 tablespoons finely chopped fresh parsley, divided

1 teaspoon dried basil leaves, divided

¼ teaspoon salt

⅛ teaspoon black pepper

1 clove garlic, minced

2 cans (about 14 ounces each) fat-free reduced-sodium beef broth

1 (8-ounce) can tomato sauce

⅓ cup chopped onion

1. Combine beef, 2 tablespoons pasta, bread crumbs, egg, 1 tablespoon parsley, ½ teaspoon basil, salt, pepper and garlic in medium bowl. Form into approximately 28 to 30 (1-inch) meatballs.

2. Bring beef broth, tomato sauce, onion and remaining ½ teaspoon basil to a boil in large saucepan over medium-high heat. Carefully add meatballs to broth. Reduce heat to medium-low; simmer, covered, 20 minutes. Add remaining 3 tablespoons pasta; cook 10 minutes or until tender. Garnish with remaining 1 tablespoon parsley.

Makes 4 servings

Nutrients per Serving (1½ cups):
Calories: 216, Calories from Fat: 30%, Total Fat: 7g, Saturated Fat: 2g, Cholesterol: 89mg, Sodium: 599mg, Carbohydrate: 15g, Dietary Fiber: 1g, Protein: 22g

Dietary Exchanges: 1 Starch, 2½ Lean Meat

Pasta Meatball Soup

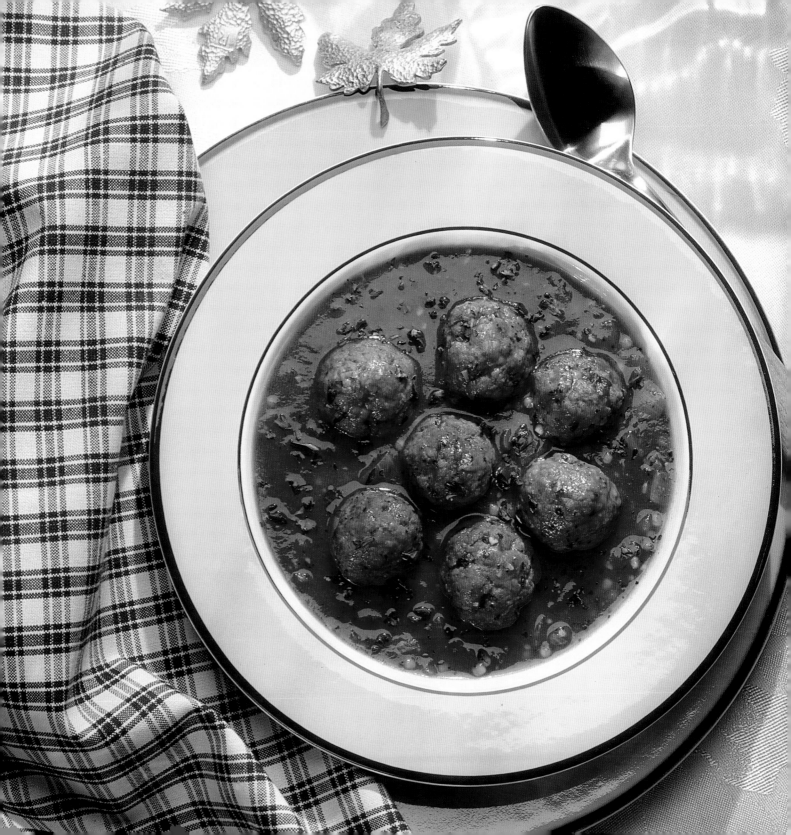

Chunky Chicken Stew

1 teaspoon olive oil

1 small onion, chopped

1 cup thinly sliced carrots

1 cup fat-free reduced-sodium chicken broth

1 can (14½ ounces) no-salt-added diced tomatoes, undrained

1 cup diced cooked chicken breast

3 cups sliced kale or baby spinach leaves

1. Heat oil in large saucepan over medium-high heat. Add onion; cook and stir about 5 minutes or until golden brown, stirring occasionally. Stir in carrots, then broth; bring to a boil.

2. Reduce heat and simmer, uncovered, 5 minutes. Add tomatoes; simmer 5 minutes or until carrots are tender. Add chicken; heat through. Add kale, stirring until kale is wilted. Simmer 1 minute. Ladle into soup bowls.

Makes 2 servings

Nutrients per Serving (½ of stew):
Calories: 274, Calories from Fat: 21%, Total Fat: 6g, Saturated Fat: 1g, Cholesterol: 0mg, Sodium: 209mg, Carbohydrate: 25g, Dietary Fiber: 7g, Protein: 30g

Dietary Exchanges: 4 Vegetable, 3 Lean Meat

recipe tip
One cup of diced cooked chicken is equal to about 1 whole 10-ounce chicken breast.

Country Bean Soup

1¼ cups dried navy beans or lima beans, rinsed and drained
4 ounces salt pork or fully cooked ham, chopped
¼ cup chopped onion
½ teaspoon dried oregano leaves
¼ teaspoon salt
¼ teaspoon ground ginger
¼ teaspoon dried sage
¼ teaspoon black pepper
2 cups fat-free (skim) milk
2 tablespoons butter
Additional salt and pepper (optional)

1. Place navy beans in large saucepan; add enough water to cover beans. Bring to a boil; reduce heat and simmer 2 minutes. Remove from heat; cover and let stand 1 hour. (Or, cover beans with water and soak overnight.)

2. Drain beans and return to saucepan. Stir in 2½ cups water, salt pork, onion, oregano, ¼ teaspoon salt, ginger, sage and ¼ teaspoon pepper. Bring to a boil; reduce heat. Cover and simmer 2 to 2½ hours or until beans are tender. (If necessary, add more water during cooking.) Add milk and butter, stirring until mixture is heated through and butter is melted. Season with additional salt and pepper, if desired.

Makes 6 servings

Nutrients per Serving (⅙ of soup):
Calories: 230, Calories from Fat: 27%, Total Fat: 7g, Saturated Fat: 4g, Cholesterol: 27mg, Sodium: 420mg, Carbohydrate: 27g, Dietary Fiber: <1g, Protein: 15g

Dietary Exchanges: 1½ Starch, ½ Milk, 1 Lean Meat, 1 Fat

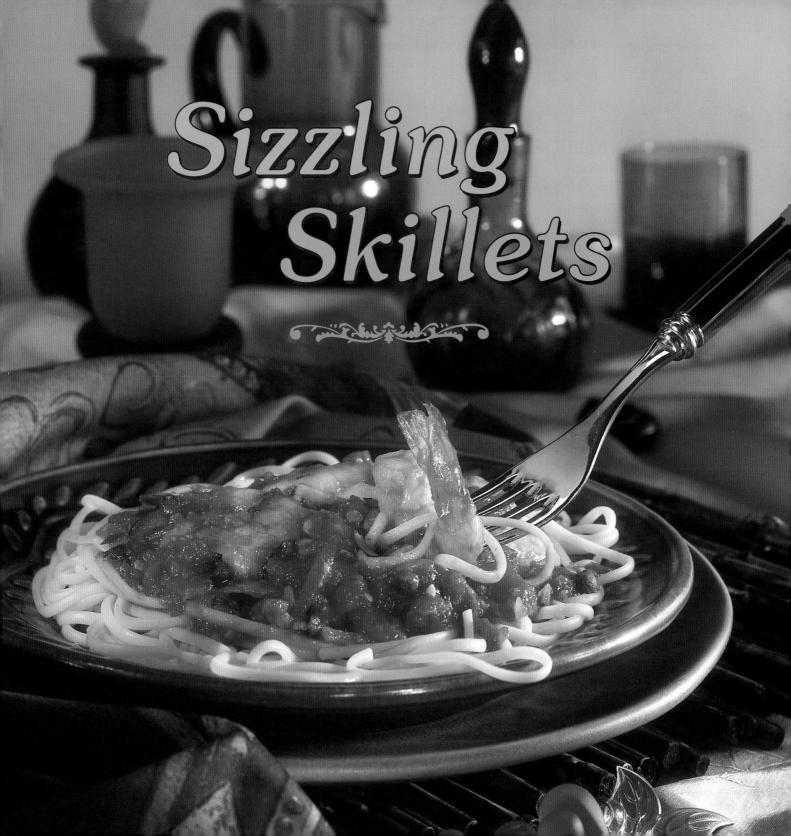

Sizzling Skillets

Spicy Shrimp Puttanesca

8 ounces uncooked linguine, capellini or spaghetti

1 tablespoon olive oil

12 ounces medium shrimp, peeled and deveined

4 cloves garlic, minced

¾ teaspoon red pepper flakes

1 cup finely chopped onion

1 can (14½ ounces) no-salt-added stewed tomatoes, undrained

2 tablespoons tomato paste

2 tablespoons chopped pitted calamata or black olives

1 tablespoon drained capers

¼ cup chopped fresh basil or parsley

1. Cook linguine according to package directions, omitting salt. Drain; set aside.

2. Meanwhile, heat oil in large nonstick skillet over medium-high heat. Add shrimp, garlic and red pepper flakes; cook and stir 3 to 4 minutes or until shrimp are opaque. Transfer shrimp mixture to large bowl; set aside.

3. Add onion to same skillet; cook over medium heat 5 minutes, stirring occasionally. Add tomatoes with juice, tomato paste, olives and capers; simmer, uncovered, 5 minutes.

4. Return shrimp mixture to skillet; simmer 1 minute. Stir in basil; simmer 1 minute. Place linguine in large serving bowl; top with shrimp mixture. *Makes 4 servings*

Nutrients per Serving (¼ of Puttanesca):
Calories: 343, Calories from Fat: 18%, Total Fat: 7g, Saturated Fat: 1g, Cholesterol: 129mg, Sodium: 482mg, Carbohydrate: 43g, Dietary Fiber: 5g, Protein: 26g

Dietary Exchanges: 2 Starch, 2 Vegetable, 2 Meat

Spicy Shrimp Puttanesca

Beef 'n' Broccoli

½ cup A.1.® Steak Sauce

¼ cup soy sauce

2 cloves garlic, crushed

1 pound top round steak, thinly sliced

1 (16-ounce) bag frozen broccoli, red bell peppers, bamboo shoots and
 mushrooms, thawed*

Hot cooked rice (optional)

*1 (16-ounce) bag frozen broccoli cuts, thawed, may be substituted.

In small bowl, combine steak sauce, soy sauce and garlic. Pour marinade over steak in nonmetal dish. Cover; refrigerate 1 hour, stirring occasionally.

Remove steak from marinade; reserve marinade. In large lightly oiled skillet, over medium-high heat, stir-fry steak 3 to 4 minutes or until steak is no longer pink. Remove steak with slotted spoon; keep warm.

In same skillet, heat vegetables and reserved marinade to a boil; reduce heat to low. Cover; simmer for 2 to 3 minutes. Stir in steak. Serve over rice, if desired.   *Makes 4 servings*

Nutrients per Serving (¼ of total recipe without rice):
Calories: 231, Calories from Fat: 20%, Total Fat: 5g, Saturated Fat: 2g, Cholesterol: 56mg, Sodium: 1654mg, Carbohydrate: 14g, Dietary Fiber: 3g, Protein: 28g

Dietary Exchanges: 2 Vegetable, 3 Lean Meat

Beef 'n' Broccoli

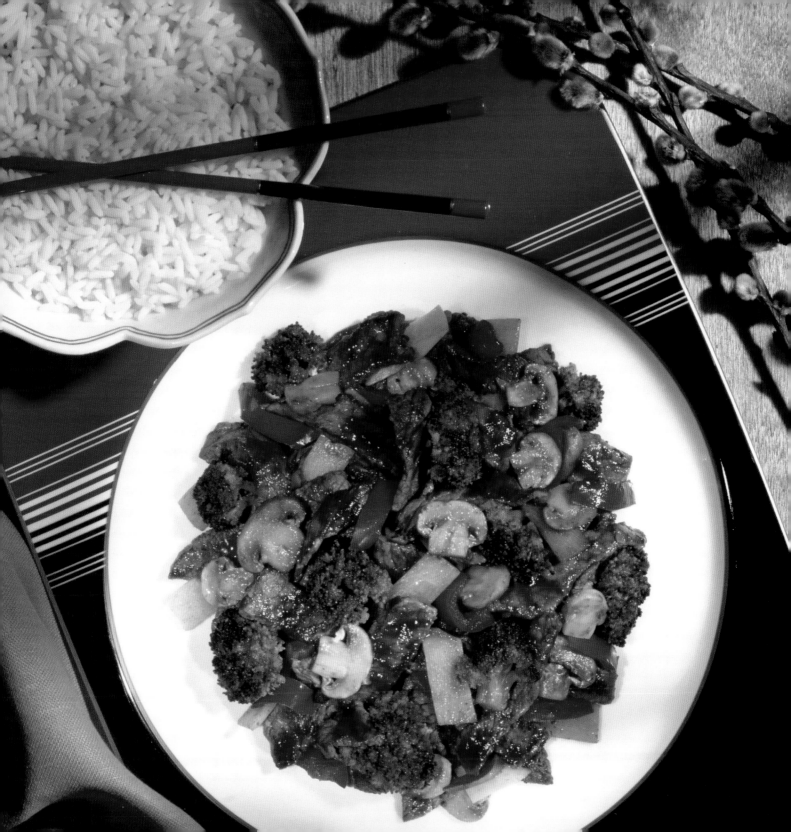

Lemony Vegetable Salmon Pasta

½ pound salmon fillet

Juice of 1 SUNKIST® lemon, divided

2 cups broccoli florets

2 medium carrots, thinly sliced diagonally

1 cup reduced-sodium chicken broth

1 teaspoon sesame oil

1 tablespoon cornstarch

1½ cups (4 ounces) uncooked spiral-shaped pasta, cooked and drained

In large non-stick skillet, cover salmon with water. Add juice of ½ lemon. Bring to a boil; reduce heat and simmer 10 to 12 minutes or until fish flakes easily with fork. Remove salmon; cool enough to remove skin and flake fish. Discard liquid and, in clean skillet, combine broccoli, carrots, chicken broth and sesame oil. Bring to a boil. Reduce heat; cover and briskly simmer 5 minutes or until vegetables are just tender. Combine cornstarch with remaining juice of ½ lemon; stir into vegetable mixture. Cook, stirring until mixture thickens. Add cooked pasta and reserved salmon; heat. Serve with lemon wedges, if desired.

Makes 4 servings

Nutrients per Serving (¼ of total recipe):
Calories: 281, Calories from Fat: 19%, Total Fat: 6g, Saturated Fat: 1g, Cholesterol: 31mg, Sodium: 105mg, Carbohydrate: 40g, Dietary Fiber: 3g, Protein: 17g

Dietary Exchanges: 2 Starch, 2 Vegetable, 2 Lean Meat

recipe tip

Salmon is filled with healthy Omega-3 fatty acids. Research has shown these fatty acid powerhouses can help lower your chances of getting heart disease and can help reduce symptoms of arthritis and psoriasis. Serve up some of this delicious fish, and start enjoying its health-protective benefits!

Sizzling Skillets

Turkey Jambalaya

1 teaspoon vegetable oil
1 cup chopped onion
1 medium green bell pepper, chopped
½ cup chopped celery
3 cloves garlic, finely chopped
1¾ cups fat-free reduced-sodium chicken broth
1 cup chopped seeded tomato
¼ pound cooked ground turkey breast
¼ pound cooked turkey sausage
3 tablespoons tomato paste
1 bay leaf
1 teaspoon dried basil leaves
¼ teaspoon ground red pepper
1 cup uncooked white rice
¼ cup chopped fresh parsley

1. Heat oil in large nonstick skillet over medium-high heat until hot. Add onion, bell pepper, celery and garlic. Cook and stir 5 minutes or until vegetables are tender.

2. Add chicken broth, tomato, turkey, turkey sausage, tomato paste, bay leaf, basil and red pepper. Stir in rice. Bring to a boil over high heat, stirring occasionally. Reduce heat to medium-low. Simmer, covered, 20 minutes or until rice is tender.

3. Remove skillet from heat. Remove and discard bay leaf. Top servings with parsley. Serve immediately.

Makes 4 servings

Nutrients per Serving (¼ of Jambalaya):
Calories: 416, Calories from Fat: 18%, Total Fat: 9g, Saturated Fat: 2g, Cholesterol: 74mg, Sodium: 384mg, Carbohydrate: 51g, Dietary Fiber: 3g, Protein: 28g

Dietary Exchanges: 2½ Starch, 2½ Vegetable, 2 Lean Meat, ½ Fat

20 Minute Chicken & Brown Rice Pilaf

1 tablespoon vegetable oil
4 boneless skinless chicken breast halves
1 can (10½ ounces) condensed chicken broth
½ cup water
1 cup sliced fresh mushrooms
1 small onion, chopped
1 cup frozen peas
2 cups MINUTE® Brown Rice, uncooked

HEAT oil in skillet. Add chicken; cook until browned. Remove chicken.

ADD chicken broth and water to skillet; stir. Bring to boil.

STIR in mushrooms, onion, peas and rice. Top with chicken; cover. Cook on low heat 5 minutes or until chicken is cooked through. Let stand 5 minutes. *Makes 4 servings*

Take a Shortcut: Omit oil. Substitute 1 package (6 ounces) LOUIS RICH® Grilled Chicken Breast Strips for the cooked chicken breasts. Bring chicken broth and water to a boil in large skillet. Stir in chicken breast strips with the mushrooms, onion, peas and rice. Cook over low heat until mixture is thoroughly heated, stirring occasionally.

Prep/Cook Time: 20 minutes

Nutrients per Serving (¼ of total recipe):
Calories: 500, Calories from Fat: 18%, Total Fat: 10g, Saturated Fat: 2g, Cholesterol: 90mg, Sodium: 780mg, Carbohydrate: 55g, Dietary Fiber: 5g, Protein: 45g

Dietary Exchanges: 3 Starch, 2 Vegetable, 5 Lean Meat, 1 Fat

*20 Minute Chicken
& Brown Rice Pilaf*

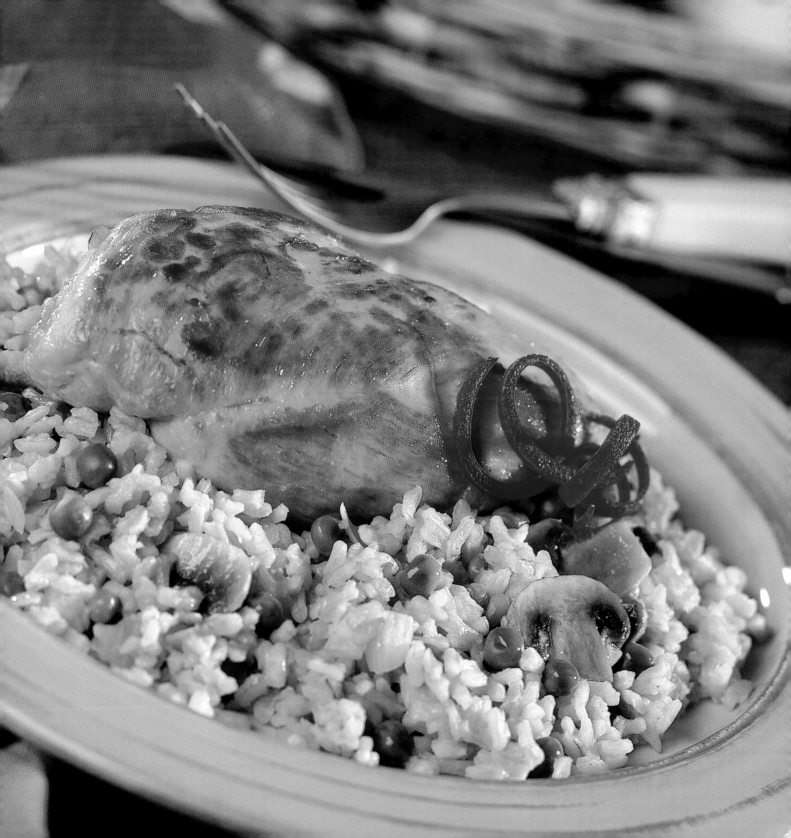

Pasta Pizza

4 ounces Italian turkey sausage
   Nonstick cooking spray
1 medium green bell pepper, chopped
1 cup sliced cremini or white mushrooms
½ cup chopped onion
2 cloves garlic, minced
2 teaspoons dried Italian seasoning
1 teaspoon dried oregano leaves
2 tablespoons reduced-sodium tomato sauce
8 ounces thin spaghetti, cooked and kept warm
2 egg whites, beaten
1 tomato, sliced
½ (3-ounce) can pitted ripe olives, rinsed, drained and halved (optional)
¾ cup (3 ounces) shredded reduced-fat mozzarella cheese
2 tablespoons finely chopped fresh basil or parsley

1. Cook sausage in small skillet until browned. Drain well; crumble. Set aside. Spray large nonstick skillet with cooking spray. Heat over medium heat until hot. Add bell pepper, mushrooms, onion, garlic, Italian seasoning and oregano; cook and stir 5 to 8 minutes or until vegetables are tender. Stir in tomato sauce. Combine vegetable mixture, sausage and spaghetti in large bowl; mix in egg whites.

2. Spray same large nonstick skillet with cooking spray. Heat over medium heat. Add spaghetti mixture; pat evenly. Cook, covered, about 5 minutes or until bottom is browned. Loosen pasta; invert onto plate. Slide back into skillet. Arrange tomato slices and olives over top; sprinkle with cheese. Cook, covered, about 5 minutes or until cheese is melted. Sprinkle with basil. *Makes 4 servings*

Nutrients per Serving (¼ of total recipe):
Calories: 417, Calories from Fat: 22%, Total Fat: 10g, Saturated Fat: 3g, Cholesterol: 34mg, Sodium: 383mg, Carbohydrate: 58g, Dietary Fiber: 1g, Protein: 23g

Dietary Exchanges: 3 Starch, 3 Vegetable, 2 Lean Meat, ½ Fat

Pasta Pizza

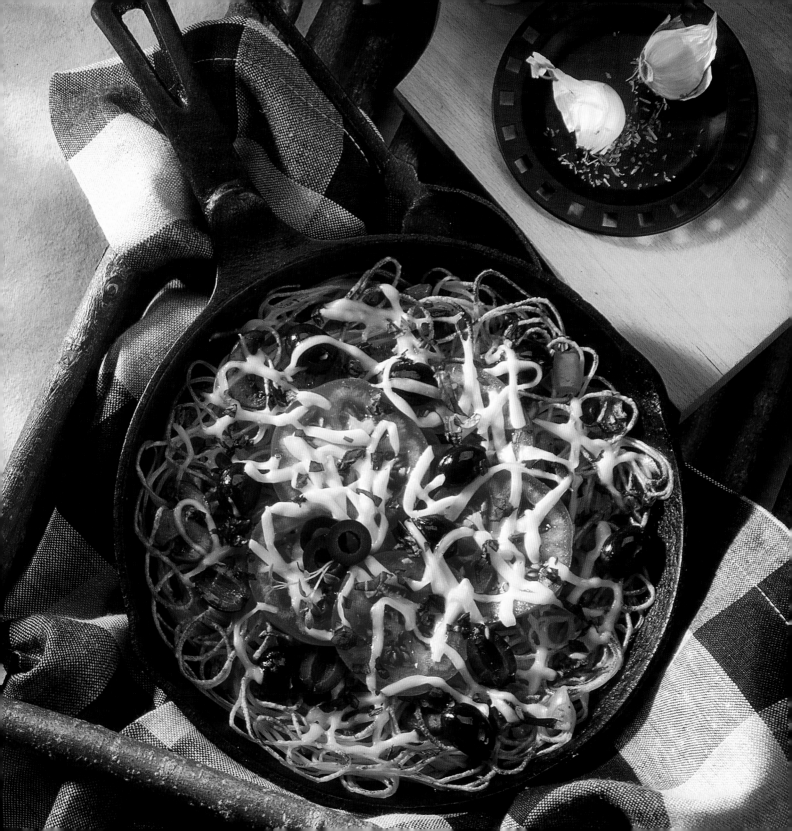

Shrimp Creole Pronto

2 tablespoons oil

1 cup chopped onions

1 cup chopped celery

1 green bell pepper, chopped

2 garlic cloves, minced

2 cups chopped, peeled tomatoes

1 can (8 ounces) tomato sauce

½ cup HOLLAND HOUSE® Marsala Cooking Wine

¼ teaspoon freshly ground black pepper

1 pound fresh or frozen, thawed, uncooked shrimp, peeled, deveined

¼ to ½ teaspoon hot pepper sauce

4 cups hot cooked rice *or* 1 (10-ounce) package of egg noodles, cooked without salt, drained

Heat oil in large saucepan over medium-high heat. Add onions, celery, bell pepper and garlic; cook 2 to 3 minutes. Add tomatoes; cook 2 to 3 minutes, stirring occasionally. Add remaining ingredients except rice; cook 2 to 3 minutes or until shrimp turn pink. Serve over hot cooked rice.   *Makes 4 servings*

Nutrients per Serving (¼ of total recipe):
Calories: 473, Calories from Fat: 19%, Total Fat: 10g, Saturated Fat: 1g, Cholesterol: 172mg, Sodium: 552mg, Carbohydrate: 61g, Dietary Fiber: 4g, Protein: 30g

Dietary Exchanges: 3 Starch, 3 Vegetable, 3 Lean Meat

Shrimp Creole Pronto

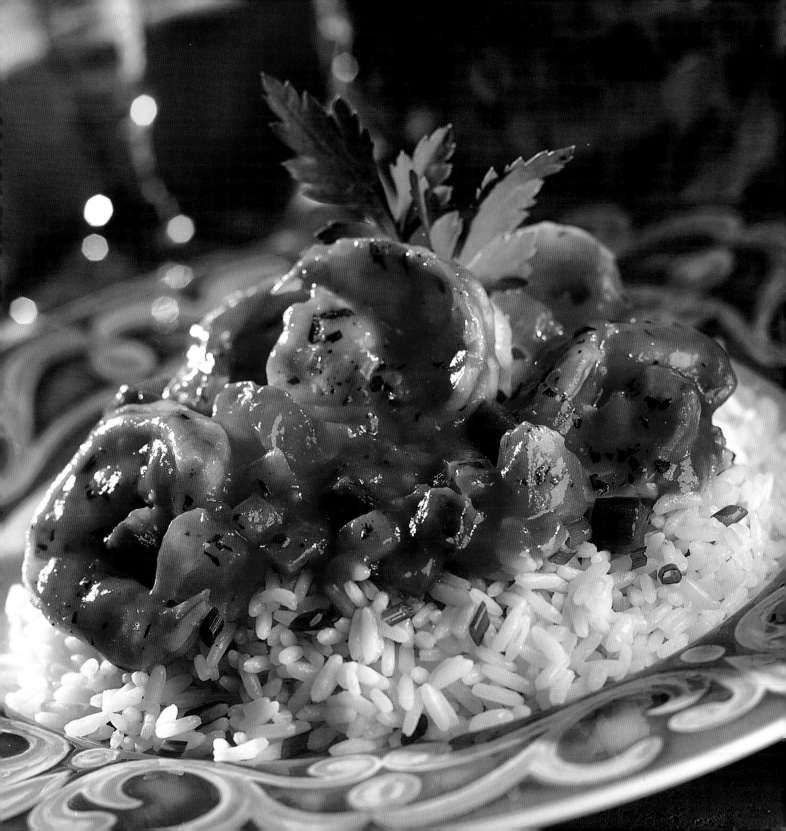

Mediterranean Chicken and Rice

4 **TYSON® Fresh or Individually Fresh Frozen® Boneless, Skinless Chicken Breasts**
2 cups **UNCLE BEN'S® Instant Brown Rice**
1 tablespoon olive oil
1 teaspoon minced garlic
1 can (15 ounces) diced tomatoes, undrained
1½ cups water
½ teaspoon dried oregano leaves
16 pitted kalamata olives
2 ounces feta cheese, crumbled

PREP: CLEAN: Wash hands. Remove protective ice glaze from frozen chicken by holding under cool running water 1 to 2 minutes. CLEAN: Wash hands.

COOK: In large nonstick skillet, heat olive oil and garlic; add chicken. Cook over medium heat 4 to 6 minutes (5 to 7 minutes if using frozen chicken) or until chicken is browned. Stir in tomatoes, water and oregano; cover. Reduce heat to low; simmer 10 minutes. Stir in rice; cover. Cook 10 minutes or until rice is cooked and internal juices of chicken run clear. (Or insert instant-read meat thermometer in thickest part of chicken. Temperature should read 170° F.) Stir in olives and sprinkle with cheese.

SERVE: For a complete Mediterranean-style meal, serve with a green salad tossed with Italian vinaigrette.

CHILL: Refrigerate leftovers immediately.

Makes 4 servings

Prep Time: 5 minutes
Cook Time: 30 minutes

Nutrients per Serving (¼ of total recipe):
Calories: 556, Calories from Fat: 19%, Total Fat: 12g, Saturated Fat: 3g, Cholesterol: 78mg, Sodium: 871mg, Carbohydrate: 75g, Dietary Fiber: 3g, Protein: 37g

Dietary Exchanges: 5 Starch, 3 Lean Meat, ½ Fat

Vegetable Pork Skillet

1 tablespoon CRISCO® Oil*

4 (4 ounces each) lean, boneless, center-cut pork loin chops, ½ inch thick

2 medium onions, thinly sliced and separated into rings

1 can (14½ ounces) whole tomatoes, undrained

¾ cup water

2 teaspoons paprika

1 teaspoon salt

½ teaspoon celery seed

¼ teaspoon pepper

¼ teaspoon garlic powder

3 medium unpeeled potatoes, chopped

1 package (9 ounces) frozen cut green beans

Use your favorite Crisco Oil product.

1. Heat oil in large skillet on medium heat. Add meat. Cook until browned on both sides. Remove from skillet.

2. Add onions to skillet. Cook and stir until tender. Add tomatoes, water, paprika, salt, celery seed, pepper and garlic powder. Bring to a boil.

3. Return meat to skillet. Reduce heat to low. Cover. Simmer 15 minutes.

4. Add potatoes. Cover. Simmer 15 minutes.

5. Add beans. Cover. Simmer 5 to 7 minutes or until potatoes and beans are tender.

Makes 4 servings

Nutrients per Serving (¼ of total recipe):
Calories: 351, Calories from Fat: 28%, Total Fat: 11g, Saturated Fat: 3g, Cholesterol: 62mg, Sodium: 800mg, Carbohydrate: 34g, Dietary Fiber: 6g, Protein: 29g

Dietary Exchanges: 2 Starch, 1 Vegetable, 3 Lean Meat

Steak Diane with Couscous

1 can (about 14 ounces) beef broth, divided
1 cup frozen peas
1 cup uncooked couscous
2 tablespoons margarine or butter, divided
4 boneless beef tenderloin or top loin steaks, 1 inch thick (5 to 6 ounces each)
¼ teaspoon black pepper
8 ounces sliced button or wild mushrooms, such as portobello or shiitake
½ cup chopped onion
1 tablespoon Dijon mustard
1 tablespoon Worcestershire sauce

1. Reserve ¼ cup broth. Bring remaining broth and peas to a boil in medium saucepan over high heat. Stir in couscous; cover and remove from heat. Let stand while preparing steaks.

2. Melt 1 tablespoon margarine in medium skillet over medium-high heat. Sprinkle both sides of steaks with pepper; add to skillet. Cook 2 to 3 minutes per side for medium-rare or to desired doneness. Transfer to plate; set aside.

3. Melt remaining 1 tablespoon margarine in same skillet; add mushrooms and onion. Cook 2 minutes, stirring occasionally. Stir in reserved ¼ cup broth, mustard and Worcestershire sauce. Simmer 2 minutes or until sauce thickens. Return steaks to skillet; heat through, turning steaks and stirring mushrooms once.

4. Divide couscous mixture evenly among 4 serving plates. Top with steaks and sauce.

Makes 4 servings

Nutrients per Serving (¼ of total recipe):
Calories: 652, Calories from Fat: 48%, Total Fat: 35g, Saturated Fat: 12g, Cholesterol: 98mg, Sodium: 608mg, Carbohydrate: 47g, Dietary Fiber: 6g, Protein: 36g

Dietary Exchanges: 3 Starch, 4 Lean Meat, 4½ Fat

Steak Diane with Couscous

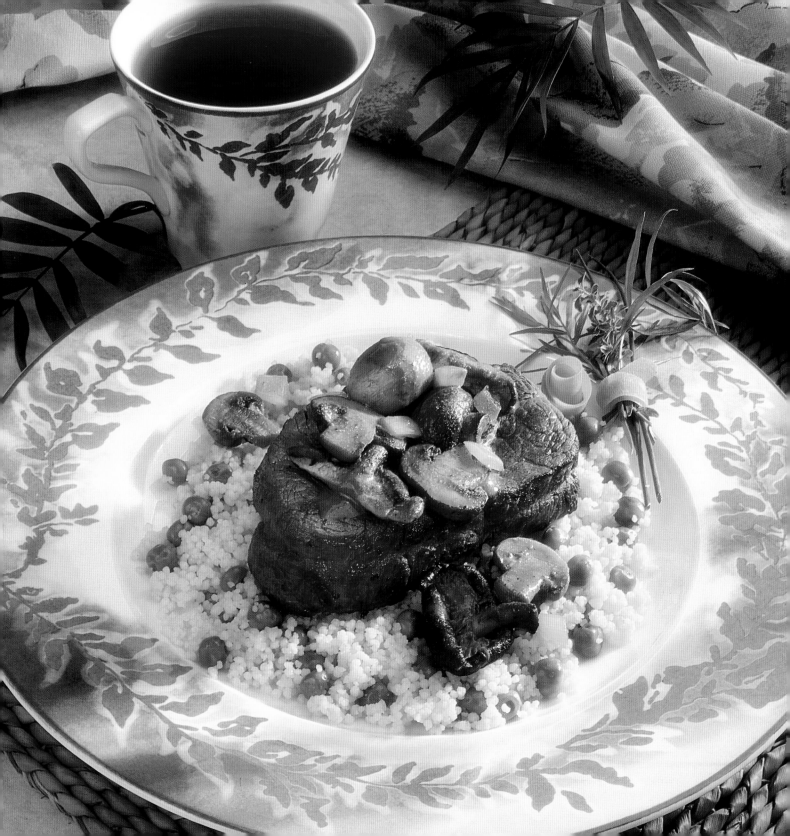

Mexican Turkey Chili Mac

1 pound ground turkey

1 package (1¼ ounces) reduced-sodium taco seasoning mix

1 can (14½ ounces) reduced-sodium stewed tomatoes

1 can (11 ounces) corn with red and green peppers, undrained

1½ cups cooked elbow macaroni (cooked without salt), drained

1 ounce low-salt corn chips, crushed

½ cup shredded reduced-fat Cheddar cheese

1. In large nonstick skillet, over medium-high heat, sauté turkey 5 to 6 minutes or until no longer pink; drain. Stir in taco seasoning, tomatoes, corn and macaroni. Reduce heat to medium and cook 4 to 5 minutes until heated throughout.

2. Sprinkle corn chips over meat mixture and top with cheese. Cover and heat 1 to 2 minutes or until cheese is melted. *Makes 6 servings*

Favorite recipe from **National Turkey Federation**

Nutrients per Serving (⅙ of total recipe):
Calories: 279, Calories from Fat: 29%, Total Fat: 9g, Saturated Fat: 3g, Cholesterol: 66mg, Sodium: 660mg, Carbohydrate: 29g, Dietary Fiber: 3g, Protein: 19g

Dietary Exchanges: 2 Starch, 2 Lean Meat, ½ Fat

recipe tip

Have you ever tried whole-wheat pasta? Substitute it for regular pasta in a recipe and you'll be doubling the amount of fiber in the dish!

Creamy Shrimp & Vegetable Casserole

1 can (10¾ ounces) reduced-fat cream of celery soup, undiluted
1 pound fresh or thawed frozen shrimp, shelled and deveined
½ cup fresh asparagus or thawed frozen asparagus, cut diagonally into 1-inch
    pieces
½ cup sliced mushrooms
¼ cup sliced green onions
¼ cup diced red bell pepper
1 clove garlic, minced
¾ teaspoon dried thyme leaves
¼ teaspoon black pepper
    Hot cooked rice or orzo (optional)

1. Preheat oven to 375°F. Coat 2-quart baking dish with nonstick cooking spray.

2. Combine soup, shrimp, asparagus, mushrooms, green onions, bell pepper, garlic, thyme and black pepper in large bowl; mix well. Place in prepared baking dish.

3. Cover and bake 30 minutes. Serve over rice, if desired.

Makes 4 servings

Nutrients per Serving (¼ of total recipe without rice):
Calories: 141, Calories from Fat: 14%, Total Fat: 2g, Saturated Fat: 1g, Cholesterol: 176mg, Sodium: 496mg, Carbohydrate: 11g, Dietary Fiber: 3g, Protein: 20g

Dietary Exchanges: 2 Vegetable, 2 Lean Meat

Sizzling Skillets

Tri-Pepper Chicken

3 tablespoons olive or vegetable oil, divided
1 small onion, chopped
1½ cups (4 ounces) sliced mushrooms
6 boneless skinless chicken breast halves (about 1½ pounds)
1 jar (12 ounces) roasted red peppers, drained and cut into strips
1 medium green bell pepper, seeded and cut into 1-inch pieces
¼ teaspoon red pepper flakes
1 jar (26 ounces) BARILLA® Lasagna & Casserole Sauce or Marinara Pasta Sauce
1 package (16 ounces) BARILLA® Linguine

1. Heat 1 tablespoon oil in large skillet. Add onion; cook over medium heat 3 minutes, stirring occasionally. Add mushrooms; cook and stir 5 minutes or until tender. Remove vegetables from skillet; set aside. Add remaining 2 tablespoons oil to skillet; add chicken and cook about 15 minutes over medium-high heat, turning until evenly brown.

2. Reduce heat to low. Return vegetables to skillet. Stir in roasted peppers, bell pepper and red pepper flakes. Pour lasagna sauce over chicken and vegetables; cover and simmer 30 minutes. Uncover and continue to cook, stirring occasionally, until chicken is tender and no longer pink when tested with tip of knife.

3. Meanwhile, cook linguine according to package directions, omitting salt; drain. Serve chicken with linguine.   *Makes 6 servings*

Nutrients per Serving (⅙ of total recipe):
Calories: 528, Calories from Fat: 25%, Total Fat: 15g, Saturated Fat: 3g, Cholesterol: 150mg, Sodium: 667mg, Carbohydrate: 63g, Dietary Fiber: 6g, Protein: 38g

Dietary Exchanges: 4 Starch, 1 Vegetable, 3 Lean Meat, 1 Fat

Tri-Pepper Chicken

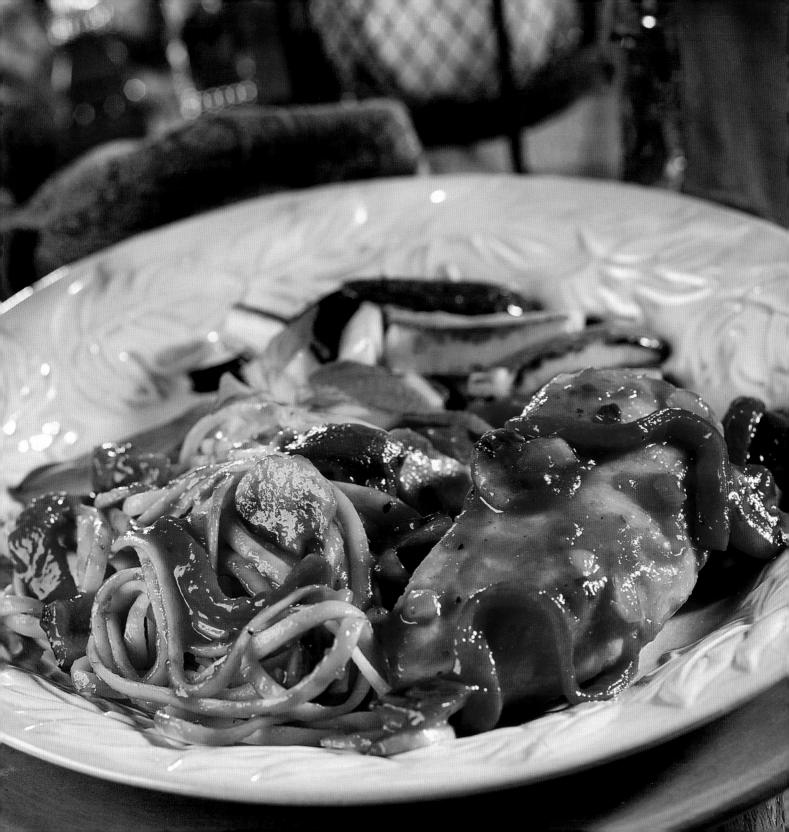

Italian Pork Cutlets

1 teaspoon CRISCO® Oil*
6 (4 ounces each) lean, boneless center-cut pork loin slices, ¾ inch thick
1 can (8 ounces) tomato sauce
1½ cups sliced fresh mushrooms
1 small green bell pepper, cut into strips
½ cup sliced green onions with tops
1 teaspoon Italian seasoning
½ teaspoon salt
⅛ teaspoon black pepper
¼ cup water
1 teaspoon cornstarch
½ cup (2 ounces) shredded low-moisture part-skim mozzarella cheese
2⅔ cups hot cooked rice (cooked without salt or fat)

*Use your favorite Crisco Oil product.

1. Heat oil in large skillet on medium heat. Add meat. Cook until browned on both sides.

2. Add tomato sauce, mushrooms, green bell pepper, onions, Italian seasoning, salt and black pepper. Reduce heat to low. Cover. Simmer 30 minutes or until meat is tender.

3. Combine water and cornstarch in small bowl. Stir until well blended. Add to juices in skillet. Cook and stir until thickened.

4. Sprinkle cheese over meat mixture. Cover. Heat until cheese melts. Serve with rice.

Makes 6 servings

Nutrients per Serving (⅙ of total recipe):
Calories: 302, Calories from Fat: 24%, Total Fat: 8g, Saturated Fat: 3g, Cholesterol: 77mg, Sodium: 544mg, Carbohydrate: 25g, Dietary Fiber: 1g, Protein: 30g

Dietary Exchanges: 1 Starch, 2 Vegetable, 3 Lean Meat

Italian Pork Cutlets

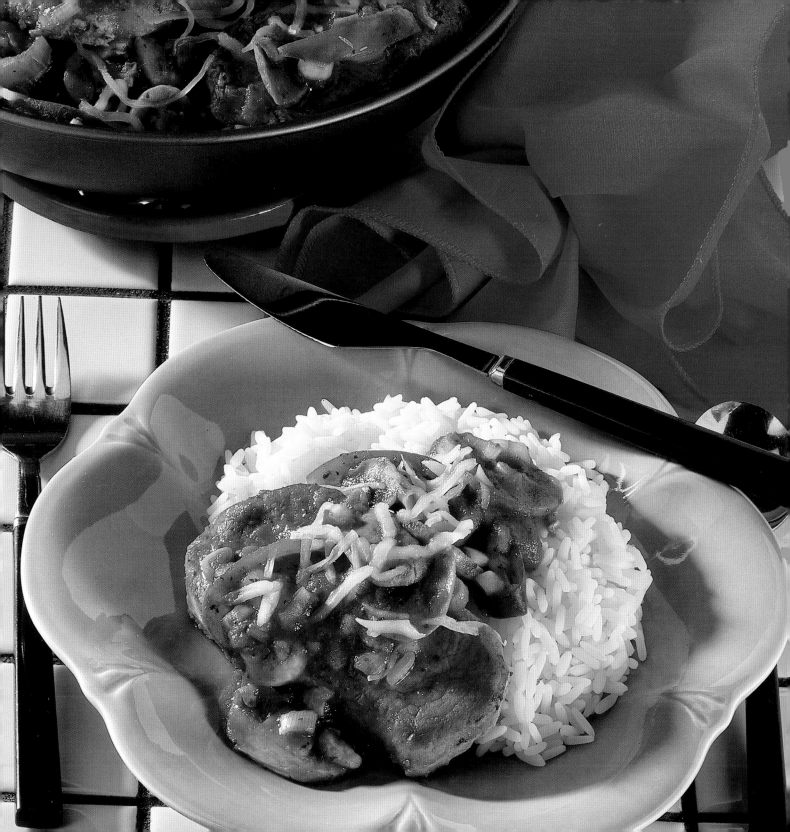

Stir-Fried Pasta with Chicken 'n' Vegetables

> 6 ounces angel hair pasta, broken in thirds (about 3 cups)
> ¼ cup *Frank's® RedHot®* Cayenne Pepper Sauce
> 3 tablespoons soy sauce
> 2 teaspoons cornstarch
> 1 tablespoon sugar
> ½ teaspoon garlic powder
> 1 pound boneless skinless chicken, cut in ¾-inch cubes
> 1 package (16 ounces) frozen stir-fry vegetables

1. Cook pasta in boiling water until just tender. Drain. Combine *Frank's RedHot* Sauce, *¼ cup water*, soy sauce, cornstarch, sugar and garlic powder in small bowl; set aside.

2. Heat *1 tablespoon oil* in large nonstick skillet over high heat. Stir-fry chicken 3 minutes. Add vegetables; stir-fry 3 minutes or until crisp-tender. Add *Frank's RedHot* Sauce mixture. Heat to boiling. Reduce heat to medium-low. Cook, stirring, 1 to 2 minutes or until sauce is thickened.

3. Stir pasta into skillet; toss to coat evenly. Serve hot.   *Makes 4 servings*

Prep Time: 5 minutes
Cook Time: 15 minutes

Nutrients per Serving (¼ of total recipe):
Calories: 345, Calories from Fat: 13%, Total Fat: 5g, Saturated Fat: 1g, Cholesterol: 123mg, Sodium: 1482mg, Carbohydrate: 39g, Dietary Fiber: 3g, Protein: 36g

Dietary Exchanges: 2 Starch, 2 Vegetable, 3 Lean Meat

Turkey Tacos

1 pound ground turkey
2 tablespoons minced dried onion
1 tablespoon chili powder
1 teaspoon paprika
½ teaspoon cumin
½ teaspoon dried oregano
½ teaspoon salt
¼ teaspoon garlic powder
⅛ teaspoon black pepper
10 taco shells
1 to 2 tomatoes, chopped
2 to 3 cups shredded lettuce
⅔ cup shredded reduced-fat Cheddar cheese

In large nonstick skillet over medium-high heat, combine turkey, onion and seasonings; cook 7 to 8 minutes or until turkey is no longer pink. Spoon mixture evenly into taco shells and top with tomatoes, lettuce and cheese.

Makes 5 servings

Favorite recipe from **National Turkey Federation**

Nutrients per Serving (2 tacos):
Calories: 331, Calories from Fat: 47%, Total Fat: 17g, Saturated Fat: 5g, Cholesterol: 82mg, Sodium: 543mg, Carbohydrate: 22g, Dietary Fiber: 4g, Protein: 22g

Dietary Exchanges: 1 Starch, 1 Vegetable, 3 Lean Meat, 1½ Fat

Curried Chicken & Vegetables with Rice

1 pound chicken tenders or boneless skinless chicken breasts, cut crosswise into ½-inch slices

2 teaspoons curry powder

¼ teaspoon *each* salt and ground red pepper

1 tablespoon vegetable oil

1 medium onion, chopped

3 cloves garlic, minced

1¼ cups canned fat-free reduced-sodium chicken broth, divided

2 tablespoons tomato paste

1 package (16 ounces) frozen mixed vegetable medley, such as broccoli, red bell peppers, cauliflower and sugar snap peas, thawed

2 teaspoons cornstarch

3 cups hot cooked white rice

½ cup plain nonfat yogurt

⅓ cup chopped fresh cilantro

1. Toss chicken with curry powder, salt and ground red pepper in medium bowl; set aside. Heat oil in large skillet over medium heat. Add onion; cook 5 minutes, stirring occasionally. Add chicken and garlic; cook 4 minutes or until chicken is no longer pink in center, stirring occasionally. Add 1 cup chicken broth, tomato paste and vegetables; bring to a boil over high heat. Reduce heat to medium; simmer, uncovered, 3 to 4 minutes or until vegetables are crisp-tender.

2. Combine remaining ¼ cup chicken broth and cornstarch, mixing until smooth. Stir into chicken mixture; simmer 2 minutes or until sauce thickens, stirring occasionally. Serve over rice; top with yogurt and cilantro.   *Makes 4 servings*

Nutrients per Serving (¼ of total recipe):
Calories: 404, Calories from Fat: 16%, Total Fat: 7g, Saturated Fat: 1g, Cholesterol: 69mg, Sodium: 299mg, Carbohydrate: 50g, Dietary Fiber: 4g, Protein: 34g

Dietary Exchanges: 2½ Starch, 2 Vegetable, 3 Lean Meat

*Curried Chicken &
Vegetables with Rice*

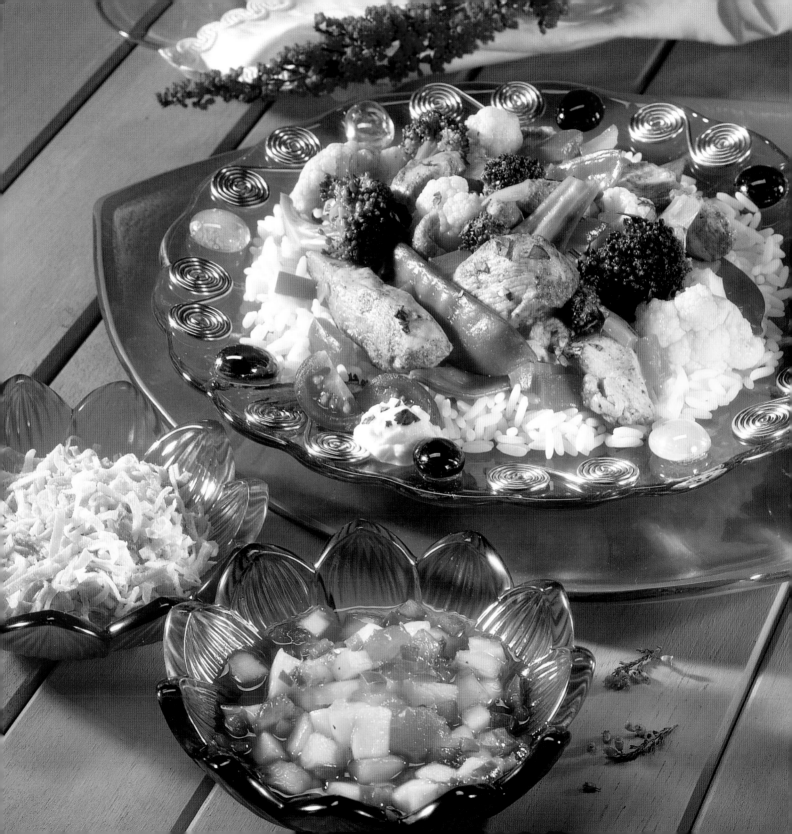

Mushroom Pasta Scampi

8 ounces uncooked linguine

2 tablespoons olive oil

1 pound fresh white mushrooms, sliced

1 tablespoon chopped garlic

1 pound frozen, peeled and deveined raw large shrimp, thawed*

10 ounces fresh spinach, trimmed and torn into pieces (about 7 cups)

¼ cup grated Parmesan cheese

¼ teaspoon crushed red pepper

To quickly thaw shrimp: Place in a colander with cold running water for about 8 minutes; drain thoroughly.

Cook linguine according to package directions, omitting salt. Drain, reserving ½ cup pasta water; set aside. Meanwhile, heat olive oil in large skillet. Add mushrooms and garlic; cook and stir about 5 minutes or until tender and mushroom liquid is almost evaporated. Add shrimp; cover and cook about 5 minutes or until shrimp is almost cooked through. Stir in spinach and reserved ½ cup pasta water. Cover and cook about 1 minute or until spinach is wilted. Place pasta in serving bowl; stir in mushroom and shrimp mixture, Parmesan cheese and red pepper. Toss to combine. Season as desired.

Makes 4 servings

Preparation and Cooking Time: about 15 minutes

*Favorite recipe from **Mushroom Council***

Nutrients per Serving (¼ of total recipe):
Calories: 415, Calories from Fat: 29%, Total Fat: 13g, Saturated Fat: 3g, Cholesterol: 240mg, Sodium: 370mg, Carbohydrate: 38g, Dietary Fiber: 9g, Protein: 37g

Dietary Exchanges: 2 Starch, 1 Vegetable, 4 Lean Meat, ½ Fat

Mushroom Pasta Scampi

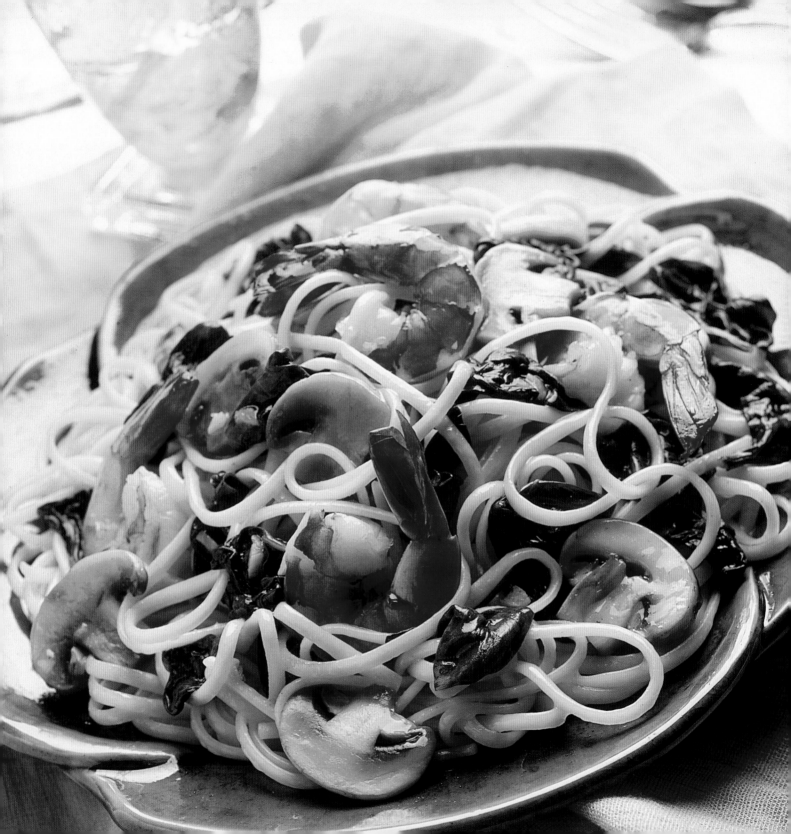

Pork & Rice Provençal

 4 well-trimmed boneless pork loin chops, ¾ inch thick (about 1 pound)
 1 teaspoon dried basil
 ½ teaspoon dried thyme
 ½ teaspoon garlic salt
 ¼ teaspoon ground black pepper
 2 tablespoons margarine or butter, divided
 1 (6.8-ounce) package RICE-A-RONI® Beef Flavor
 ½ cup chopped onion
 1 clove garlic, minced
 1 (14½-ounce) can seasoned diced tomatoes, undrained
 1 (2¼-ounce) can sliced ripe olives, drained, *or* ⅓ cup sliced pitted kalamata olives

1. Sprinkle pork chops with basil, thyme, garlic salt and pepper; set aside. In large skillet over medium-high heat, melt 1 tablespoon margarine. Add pork chops; cook 3 minutes. Reduce heat to medium; turn pork chops over and cook 3 minutes. Remove from skillet; set aside.

2. In same skillet over medium heat, sauté rice-vermicelli mix, onion and garlic with remaining 1 tablespoon margarine until vermicelli is golden brown.

3. Slowly stir in 1¾ cups water, tomatoes and Special Seasonings; bring to a boil. Cover; reduce heat to low. Simmer 10 minutes.

4. Add pork chops and olives. Cover; simmer 10 minutes or until rice is tender and pork chops are no longer pink inside.

Makes 4 servings

Prep Time: 10 minutes
Cook Time: 40 minutes

Nutrients per Serving (¼ of total recipe):
Calories: 402, Calories from Fat: 20%, Total Fat: 9g, Saturated Fat: 3g, Cholesterol: 67mg, Sodium: 1604mg, Carbohydrate: 48g, Dietary Fiber: 3g, Protein: 32g

Dietary Exchanges: 3 Starch, 1 Vegetable, 3 Lean Meat

Pork & Rice Provençal

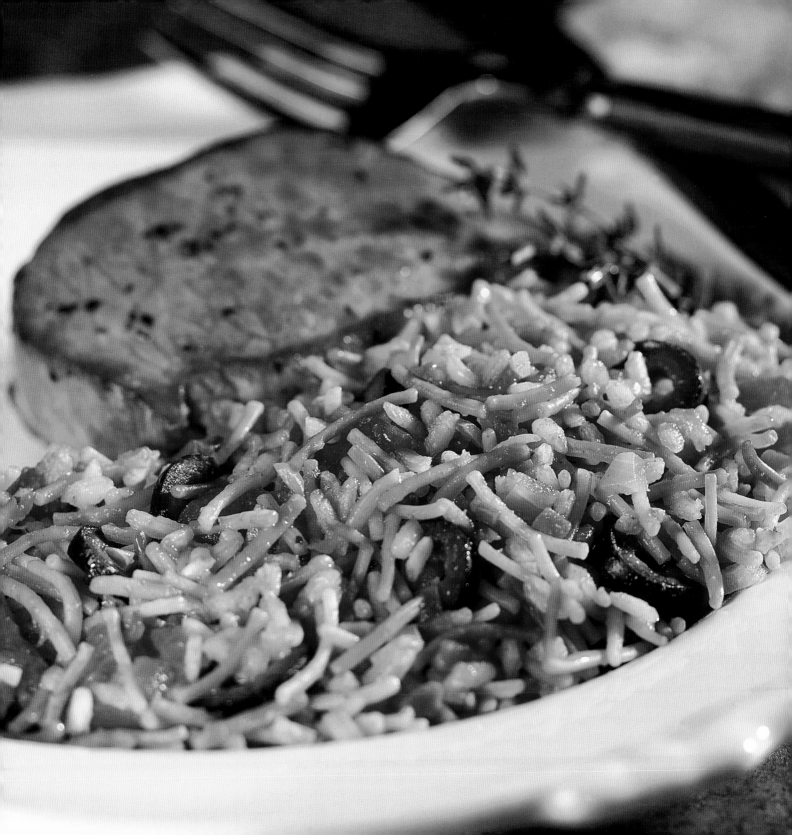

Spicy Chicken Burritos

1 medium onion, halved and sliced

1 small green bell pepper, diced

1 tablespoon FLEISCHMANN'S® Original Margarine

½ pound shredded cooked chicken (1¼ cups)

1 medium tomato, diced

1½ cups EGG BEATERS® Healthy Real Egg Product

½ teaspoon seasoned pepper

¼ teaspoon garlic powder

½ cup (2 ounces) shredded reduced-fat Cheddar cheese

6 (10-inch) flour tortillas, warmed

½ cup thick and chunky salsa

Additional thick and chunky salsa, optional

In large nonstick skillet, over medium heat, sauté onion and bell pepper in margarine until tender. Add chicken and tomato; stir until heated through. Remove from skillet; keep warm.

In same skillet, over medium heat, cook Egg Beaters®, seasoned pepper and garlic powder, stirring occasionally until mixture is set. Stir in chicken mixture; sprinkle with cheese. Evenly divide and spoon mixture onto warm tortillas; top each with salsa. Fold two opposite ends of each tortilla over filling, then fold in sides like an envelope. Serve with additional salsa if desired.   *Makes 6 servings*

Prep Time: 20 minutes
Cook Time: 20 minutes

Nutrients per Serving (1 burrito without additional salsa):
Calories: 260, Calories from Fat: 27%, Total Fat: 7g, Saturated Fat: 3g, Cholesterol: 36mg, Sodium: 535mg, Carbohydrate: 24g, Dietary Fiber: 2g, Protein: 23g

Dietary Exchanges: 1 Starch, 1 Vegetable, 3 Lean Meat

Beef Stroganoff with Rice

½ cup UNCLE BEN'S® ORIGINAL CONVERTED® Brand Rice
12 ounces sirloin steak
 1 teaspoon olive oil
 1 small onion, sliced
 2 cups sliced mushrooms
½ cup reduced-fat sour cream
¼ teaspoon dill weed
½ cup sliced green onions

1. Cook rice according to package directions.

2. Meanwhile, cut beef into thin strips. Heat oil in large skillet over medium heat. Add beef, onion and mushrooms. Cook and stir 5 minutes or until beef is cooked through. Add sour cream, dill weed and cooked rice.

3. Garnish stroganoff with green onions.

Makes 4 servings

Nutrients per Serving (¼ of total recipe):
Calories: 241, Calories from Fat: 29%, Total Fat: 8g, Saturated Fat: 4g, Cholesterol: 55mg, Sodium: 58mg, Carbohydrate: 22g, Dietary Fiber: 1g, Protein: 20g

Dietary Exchanges: 1½ Starch, 2 Lean Meat, ½ Fat

recipe tip

Beef, full of high-quality protein and also an excellent source of dietary iron and zinc, can fit into a healthy meal plan. Try to choose lean cuts, ones with "loin" or "round" in the name. Sirloin, tenderloin and top round are some of the leanest cuts.

Spinach & Turkey Skillet

6 ounces turkey breast tenderloin

⅛ teaspoon salt

2 teaspoons olive oil

¼ cup chopped onion

2 cloves garlic, minced

⅓ cup uncooked rice

¾ teaspoon dried Italian seasoning

¼ teaspoon black pepper

1 cup fat-free reduced-sodium chicken broth, divided

2 cups torn fresh spinach

⅔ cup diced plum tomatoes

3 tablespoons freshly grated Parmesan cheese

1. Cut turkey tenderloins into bite-size slices; sprinkle with salt. Heat oil in medium skillet over medium-high heat.

2. Add turkey slices; cook and stir until lightly browned. Remove from skillet. Reduce heat to low. Add onion and garlic; cook and stir until tender. Return turkey to skillet. Stir in rice, Italian seasoning and pepper.

3. Reserve 2 tablespoons chicken broth. Stir remaining broth into mixture in skillet. Bring to a boil. Reduce heat. Simmer, covered, 14 minutes. Stir in spinach and reserved broth. Cover and cook 2 to 3 minutes more or until liquid is absorbed and spinach is wilted. Stir in tomatoes. Heat through. Serve with Parmesan cheese.

Makes 2 servings

Nutrients per Serving (½ of total recipe):
Calories: 316, Calories from Fat: 26%, Total Fat: 9g, Saturated Fat: 3g, Cholesterol: 39mg, Sodium: 309mg, Carbohydrate: 33g, Dietary Fiber: 3g, Protein: 25g

Dietary Exchanges: 2 Starch, 3 Lean Meat

Spinach & Turkey Skillet

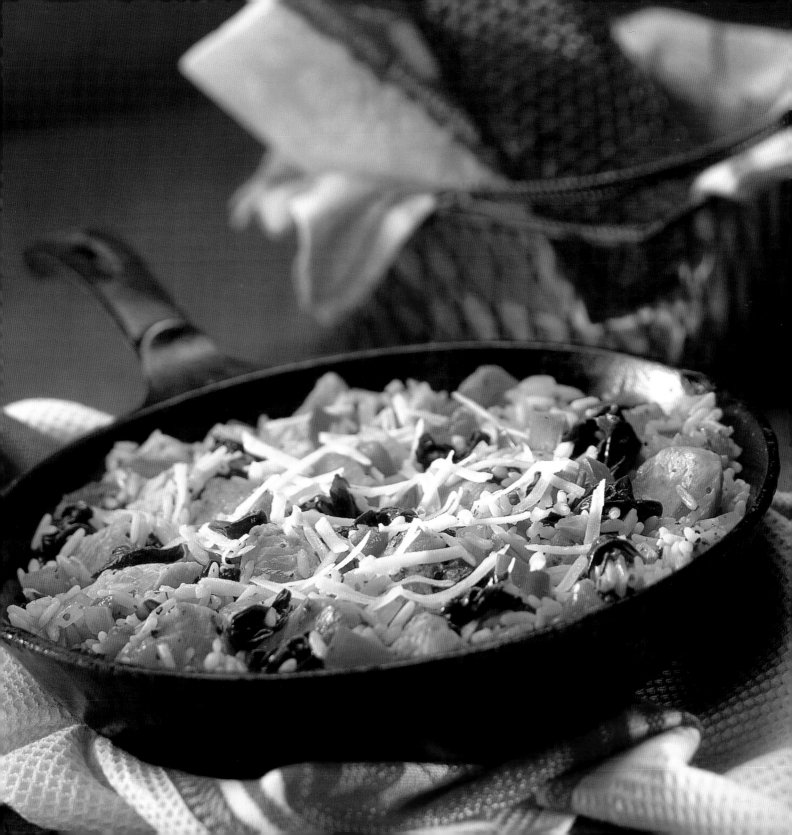

Sausage & Mushroom Pasta

1 can (10¾ ounces) reduced-fat condensed tomato soup, undiluted
¼ cup fat-free (skim) milk
   Nonstick cooking spray
½ cup chopped onion
½ cup chopped green bell pepper
2 cloves garlic, minced
1 teaspoon dried Italian seasoning
1 cup sliced mushrooms
½ teaspoon salt (optional)
1 (7-ounce) package reduced-fat smoked turkey sausage, cut into ⅛-inch slices
4 cups cooked bow-tie pasta

1. Combine soup and milk in small bowl; mix well. Set aside.

2. Spray large nonstick skillet with cooking spray; heat over medium-high heat until hot. Add onion, pepper, garlic and Italian seasoning; cook and stir until onion and pepper are tender.

3. Add mushrooms and salt, if desired; cook and stir 2 to 3 minutes.

4. Add sausage; mix well. Reduce heat; cover and simmer an additional 2 minutes. Add pasta; toss until coated with sauce.

Makes 6 servings

Nutrients per Serving (⅙ of total recipe without ½ teaspoon of salt):
Calories: 203, Calories from Fat: 11%, Total Fat: 3g, Saturated Fat: 1g, Cholesterol: 15mg, Sodium: 486mg, Carbohydrate: 36g, Dietary Fiber: 3g, Protein: 10g

Dietary Exchanges: 1 Starch, 3 Vegetable, 1 Lean Meat

Sausage & Mushroom Pasta

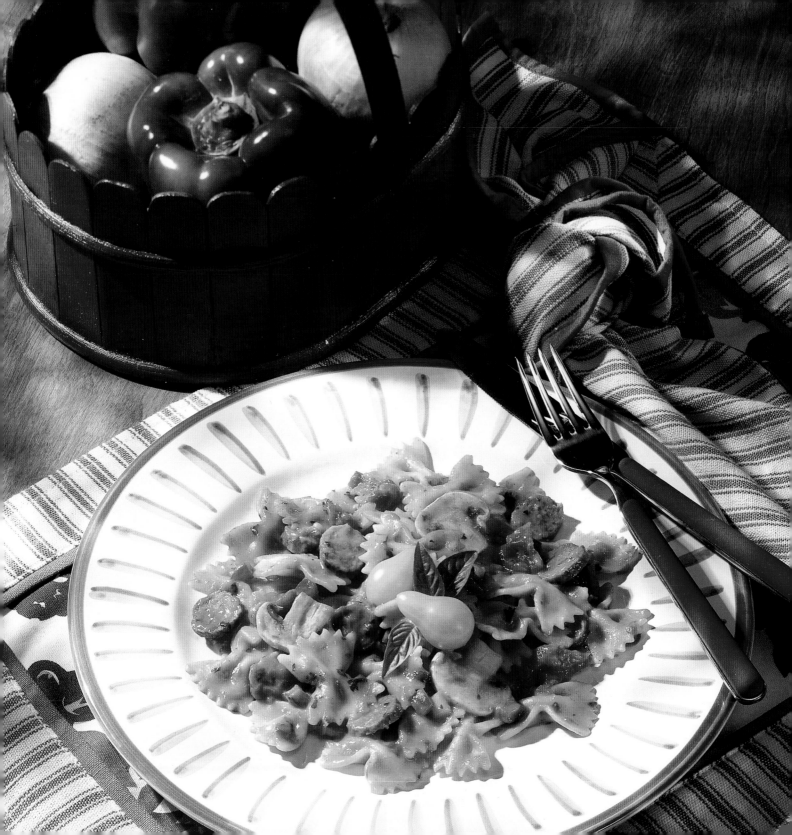

Browned Pork Chops with Gravy

4 boneless pork loin chops (12 ounces)
½ teaspoon dried sage leaves
½ teaspoon dried marjoram leaves
¼ teaspoon black pepper
⅛ teaspoon salt
  Nonstick olive oil cooking spray
¼ cup coarsely chopped onion
1 clove garlic, minced
1 cup sliced mushrooms
¾ cup beef broth
⅓ cup nonfat sour cream
1 tablespoon all-purpose flour
1 teaspoon Dijon mustard
2 cups hot cooked noodles
  Snipped parsley (optional)

1. Trim fat from chops. Stir together sage, marjoram, pepper and salt. Rub on both sides of chops. Spray large nonstick skillet with cooking spray; heat over medium heat. Place chops in skillet. Cook 5 minutes, turning once, or until chops are just barely pink. Remove chops from skillet; keep warm.

2. Add onion and garlic to skillet; cook and stir 2 minutes. Add mushrooms and broth. Bring to a boil. Reduce heat and simmer, covered, 3 to 4 minutes or until mushrooms are tender.

3. Whisk together sour cream, flour and mustard in medium bowl. Whisk in about 3 tablespoons broth from skillet. Stir sour cream mixture into skillet. Cook, stirring constantly, until mixture comes to a boil. Serve over pork chops and noodles. Sprinkle with parsley, if desired.   *Makes 4 servings*

Nutrients per Serving (¼ of total recipe):
Calories: 315, Calories from Fat: 29%, Total Fat: 10g, Saturated Fat: 3g, Cholesterol: 67mg, Sodium: 296mg, Carbohydrate: 30g, Dietary Fiber: 2g, Protein: 25g

Dietary Exchanges: 1½ Starch, 1 Vegetable, 3 Lean Meat

Browned Pork Chop with Gravy

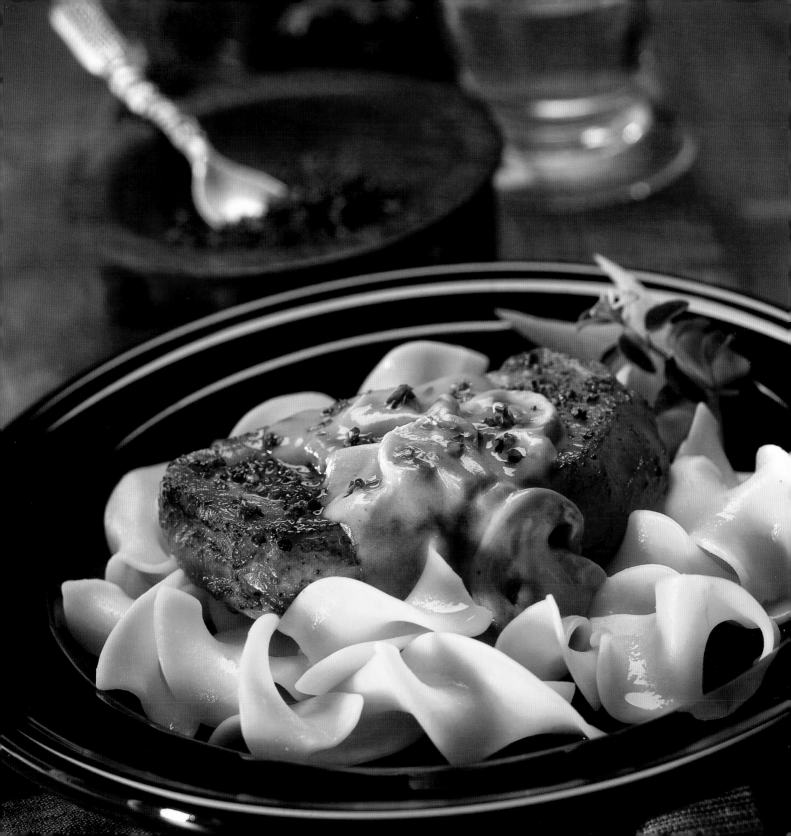

20 Minute Garlic Rosemary Chicken & Brown Rice Dinner

    1 tablespoon oil
    4 small boneless skinless chicken breast halves (about 1 pound)
    ¾ teaspoon garlic powder, divided
    ¾ teaspoon dried rosemary leaves, crushed, divided
    1 can (10½ ounces) ⅓-less-sodium chicken broth (1⅓ cups)
    ⅓ cup water
    2 cups MINUTE® Brown Rice, uncooked

HEAT oil in large nonstick skillet on medium-high heat. Add chicken; sprinkle with ¼ teaspoon each of the garlic powder and rosemary. Cover. Cook 4 minutes on each side or until cooked through. Remove chicken from skillet.

ADD broth and water to skillet; stir. Bring to boil.

STIR in rice and remaining ½ teaspoon each garlic powder and rosemary. Top with chicken; cover. Cook on low heat 5 minutes. Remove from heat. Let stand 5 minutes.   *Makes 4 servings*

Prep/Cook Time: 20 minutes

Nutrients per Serving (¼ of total recipe):
Calories: 340, Calories from Fat: 19%, Total Fat: 7g, Saturated Fat: 1g, Cholesterol: 70mg, Sodium: 290mg, Carbohydrate: 36g, Dietary Fiber: 2g, Protein: 31g

Dietary Exchanges: 2½ Starch, 3 Lean Meat, ½ Fat

Light Orange Chicken

1 can (10¾ ounces) reduced-fat condensed cream of celery soup, undiluted
½ cup fat-free (skim) milk
¼ cup finely chopped onion
2 tablespoons orange marmalade
1 clove garlic, minced
¼ teaspoon dried rosemary leaves
  Vegetable cooking spray
4 boneless skinless chicken breast halves
1 cup julienned carrots
1 cup julienned zucchini

1. Combine soup, milk, onion, marmalade, garlic and rosemary in medium bowl; set aside.

2. Spray large nonstick skillet with cooking spray. Heat over medium heat 1 minute. Add chicken; brown 5 minutes on each side. Remove from skillet.

3. Add carrots and zucchini to skillet; sauté 2 to 3 minutes. Stir in soup mixture. Return chicken to skillet. Reduce heat to low; cover and simmer 5 to 8 minutes or until chicken is no longer pink in center. *Makes 4 servings*

Nutrients per Serving (¼ of total recipe):
Calories: 243, Calories from Fat: 19%, Total Fat: 5g, Saturated Fat: 2g, Cholesterol: 73mg, Sodium: 660mg, Carbohydrate: 20g, Dietary Fiber: 3g, Protein: 29g

Dietary Exchanges: 1 Starch, 1 Vegetable, 3 Lean Meat

Sizzling Skillets

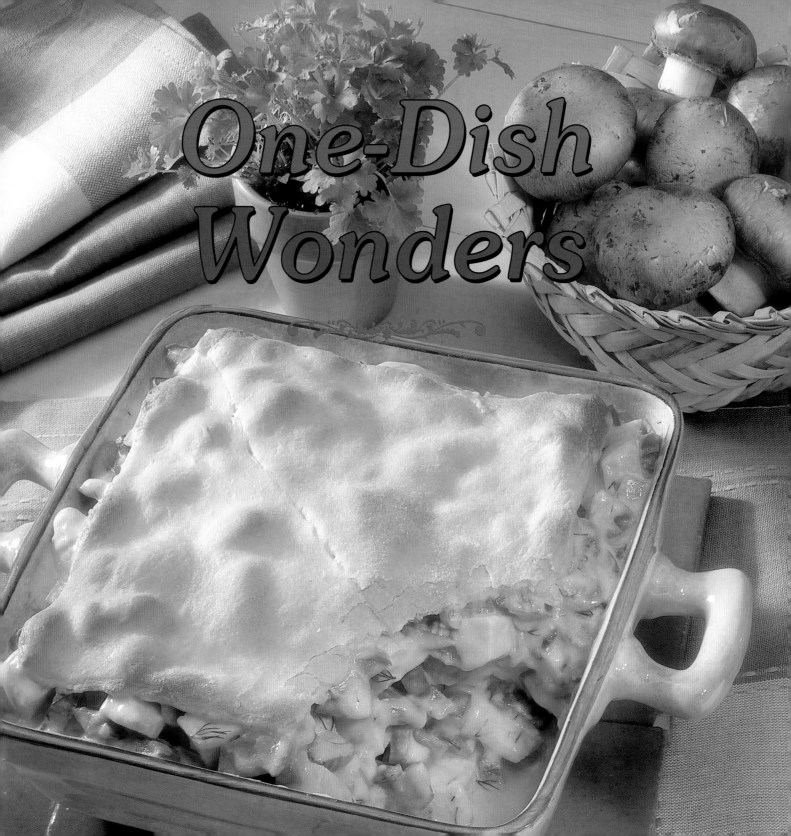

One-Dish Wonders

Chicken Pot Pie

2 teaspoons margarine
½ cup plus 2 tablespoons fat-free reduced-sodium chicken broth, divided
2 cups sliced mushrooms
1 cup diced red bell pepper
½ cup chopped onion
½ cup chopped celery
2 tablespoons all-purpose flour
½ cup fat-free half-and-half
2 cups cubed cooked chicken breasts
1 teaspoon minced fresh dill
½ teaspoon salt
¼ teaspoon black pepper
2 reduced-fat refrigerated crescent rolls

1. Heat margarine and 2 tablespoons chicken broth in medium saucepan until margarine is melted. Add mushrooms, bell pepper, onion and celery. Cook 7 to 10 minutes or until vegetables are tender, stirring frequently.

2. Stir in flour; cook 1 minute. Stir in remaining ½ cup chicken broth; cook and stir until liquid thickens. Reduce heat and stir in half-and-half. Add chicken, dill, salt and black pepper.

3. Preheat oven to 375°F. Spoon mixture into greased 1-quart casserole. Roll out crescent rolls and place on top of chicken mixture. Bake pot pie 20 minutes or until topping is golden and filling is bubbly.

Makes 4 servings

Nutrients per Serving (1 cup):
Calories: 286, Calories from Fat: 27%, Total Fat: 8g, Saturated Fat: 2g, Cholesterol: 54mg, Sodium: 740mg, Carbohydrate: 25g, Dietary Fiber: 2g, Protein: 26g

Dietary Exchanges: 1 Starch, 2 Vegetable, 3 Lean Meat

Chicken Pot Pie

Creamy "Crab" Fettuccine

1 pound imitation crabmeat sticks

6 ounces uncooked fettuccine

3 tablespoons margarine or butter, divided

1 small onion, chopped

2 ribs celery, chopped

½ medium red bell pepper, chopped

2 cloves garlic, minced

1 cup reduced-fat sour cream

1 cup reduced-fat mayonnaise

1 cup (4 ounces) shredded sharp Cheddar cheese

2 tablespoons chopped fresh parsley

¼ teaspoon salt

⅛ teaspoon black pepper

½ cup cornflake crumbs

1. Preheat oven to 350°F. Spray 2-quart square baking dish with nonstick cooking spray. Cut crabmeat into small. Cook pasta according to package directions, omitting salt, until al dente. Drain; set aside.

2. Meanwhile, melt 1 tablespoon margarine in large skillet over medium-high heat. Add onion, celery, bell pepper and garlic; cook and stir 2 minutes or until vegetables are tender.

3. Combine sour cream, mayonnaise, cheese, parsley, salt and black pepper in large bowl. Add crabmeat, pasta and vegetable mixture, stirring gently to combine. Pour into prepared dish.

4. Melt remaining 2 tablespoons margarine. Combine with cornflake crumbs in small bowl; sprinkle evenly over casserole. Bake, uncovered, 30 minutes or until hot and bubbly.   *Makes 6 servings*

Nutrients per Serving (⅙ of total recipe):
Calories: 482, Calories from Fat: 55%, Total Fat: 29g, Saturated Fat: 9g, Cholesterol: 61mg, Sodium: 1,268mg, Carbohydrate: 34g, Dietary Fiber: 2g, Protein: 20g

Dietary Exchanges: 2 Starch, 2 Lean Meat, 5 Fat

Creamy "Crab" Fettuccine

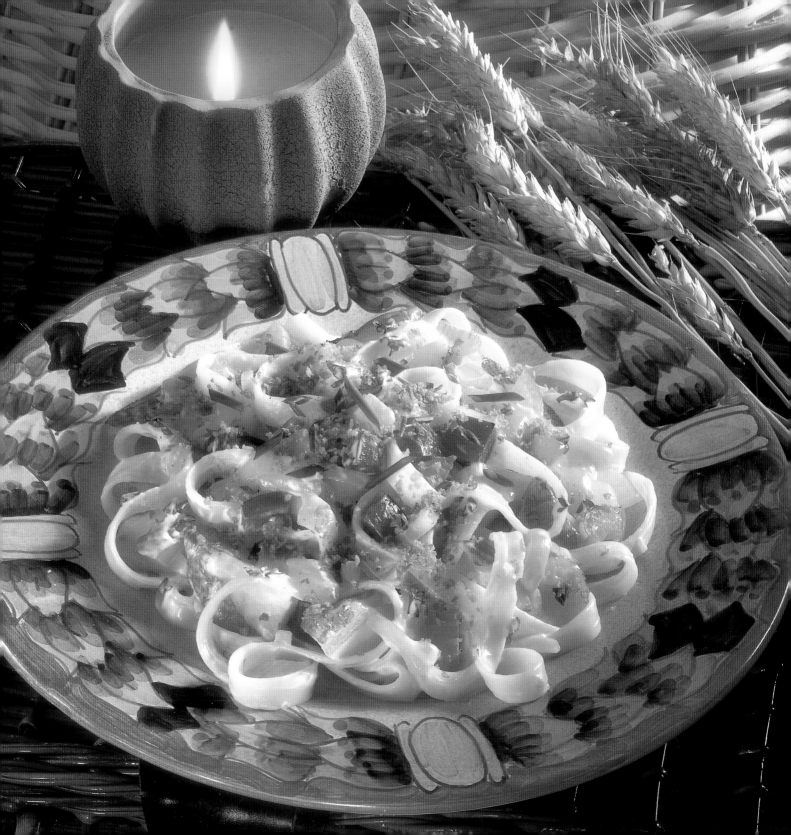

Broccoli Lasagna

1 tablespoon CRISCO® Oil* plus additional for oiling

1 cup chopped onion

3 cloves garlic, minced

1 can (14½ ounces) no-salt-added tomatoes, undrained, chopped

1 can (8 ounces) no-salt-added tomato sauce

1 can (6 ounces) no-salt-added tomato paste

1 cup thinly sliced fresh mushrooms

¼ cup chopped fresh parsley

1 tablespoon red wine vinegar

1 teaspoon *each* dried oregano leaves and dried basil leaves

1 bay leaf

½ teaspoon salt

¼ teaspoon crushed red pepper

1½ cups lowfat cottage cheese

1 cup (4 ounces) shredded low-moisture part-skim mozzarella cheese, divided

6 lasagna noodles, cooked (without salt or fat) and well drained

3 cups chopped broccoli, cooked and well drained

1 tablespoon grated Parmesan cheese

Use your favorite Crisco Oil product.

1. Heat oven to 350°F. Oil 11¾×7½×2-inch baking dish lightly. Heat 1 tablespoon oil in large saucepan on medium heat. Add onion and garlic. Cook and stir until tender. Stir in tomatoes, tomato sauce, tomato paste, mushrooms, parsley, vinegar, oregano, basil, bay leaf, salt and crushed red pepper. Bring to a boil. Reduce heat to low. Cover. Simmer 30 minutes, stirring occasionally. Remove bay leaf.

2. Combine cottage cheese and ½ cup mozzarella cheese in small bowl. Stir well.

continued on page 232

Broccoli Lasagna

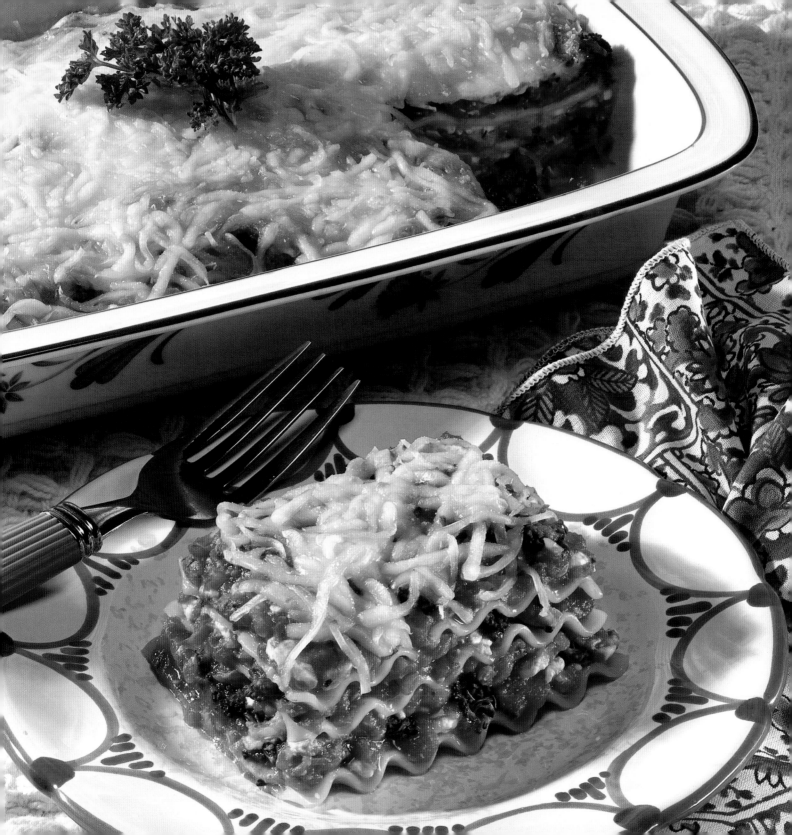

3. Place 2 lasagna noodles in bottom of baking dish. Layer with one cup broccoli, one-third of the tomato sauce and one-third of the cottage cheese mixture. Repeat layers. Cover with foil. Bake at 350°F for 25 minutes. Uncover. Sprinkle with remaining ½ cup mozzarella cheese and Parmesan cheese. Bake, uncovered, 10 minutes or until cheese melts. *Do not overbake.* Let stand 10 minutes before serving. *Makes 8 servings*

Nutrients per Serving (⅛ of total recipe):
Calories: 201, Calories from Fat: 24%, Total Fat: 5g, Saturated Fat: 2g, Cholesterol: 12mg, Sodium: 439mg, Carbohydrate: 25g, Dietary Fiber: 4g, Protein: 14g

Dietary Exchanges: 1 Starch, 2 Vegetable, 1 Lean Meat, ½ Fat

recipe tip

Since lasagna noodles are so large, be sure to cook them in plenty of water to keep them from clumping. Stir the noodles frequently to allow them to cook more evenly and prevent them from sticking to the pan. Leave the pan uncovered and keep the water boiling continuously until the noodles are of the desired doneness. Pasta that is to be baked, such as these lasagna noodles, should be slightly undercooked. The noodles will be easier to handle, and they won't become too soft with baking.

One-Dish Wonders

Shrimp Jambalaya

1 can (28 ounces) diced tomatoes, undrained
1 medium onion, chopped
1 medium red bell pepper, chopped
1 rib celery, chopped (about ½ cup)
2 tablespoons minced garlic
2 teaspoons dried parsley flakes
2 teaspoons dried oregano leaves
1 teaspoon red pepper sauce
½ teaspoon dried thyme leaves
2 pounds large shrimp, cooked, peeled and deveined
2 cups uncooked rice
2 cups fat-free low-sodium chicken broth

Slow Cooker Directions

1. Combine tomatoes with juice, onion, bell pepper, celery, garlic, parsley, oregano, red pepper sauce and thyme in slow cooker. Cover and cook on LOW 8 hours or on HIGH 4 hours. Stir in shrimp. Cover and cook on LOW 20 minutes.

2. Meanwhile, prepare rice according to package directions, substituting broth for water. Serve jambalaya over hot cooked rice. *Makes 8 servings*

Favorite recipe from **Lucy Cannek, Elmhurst, IL**

Nutrients per Serving (⅛ of total recipe):
Calories: 333, Calories from Fat: 8%, Total Fat: 3g, Saturated Fat: 1g, Cholesterol: 179mg, Sodium: 564mg, Carbohydrate: 45g, Dietary Fiber: 2g, Protein: 29g

Dietary Exchanges: 2¼ Starch, 2¼ Vegetable, 3 Lean Meat

One-Dish Wonders

Chicken & Vegetable Tortilla Roll-Ups

1 pound boneless skinless chicken breasts, cooked
1 cup chopped broccoli
1 cup diced carrots
1 can (10¾ ounces) condensed cream of celery soup, undiluted
¼ cup reduced-fat (2%) milk
1 tablespoon dry sherry
½ cup grated Parmesan cheese
6 (10-inch) flour tortillas

1. Preheat oven to 350°F. Cut chicken into 1-inch pieces; set aside.

2. Combine broccoli and carrots in 1-quart microwavable dish. Cover and microwave at HIGH 2 to 3 minutes or until vegetables are crisp-tender; set aside.

3. Combine soup, milk and sherry in small saucepan; cook and stir over medium heat 5 minutes. Stir in Parmesan cheese, chicken, broccoli and carrots. Cook 2 minutes or until cheese is melted. Remove from heat.

4. Spoon ¼ cup chicken mixture onto each tortilla. Roll up and place seam-side-down in 13×9-inch baking dish coated with nonstick cooking spray. Bake, covered, 20 minutes or until heated through.

Makes 6 servings

Nutrients per Serving (1 Roll-Up):
Calories: 285, Calories from Fat: 27%, Total Fat: 8g, Saturated Fat: 3g, Cholesterol: 51mg, Sodium: 714mg, Carbohydrate: 25g, Dietary Fiber: 3g, Protein: 25g

Dietary Exchanges: 2 Starch, 2 Lean Meat, ½ Fat

Chicken & Vegetable Tortilla Roll-Ups

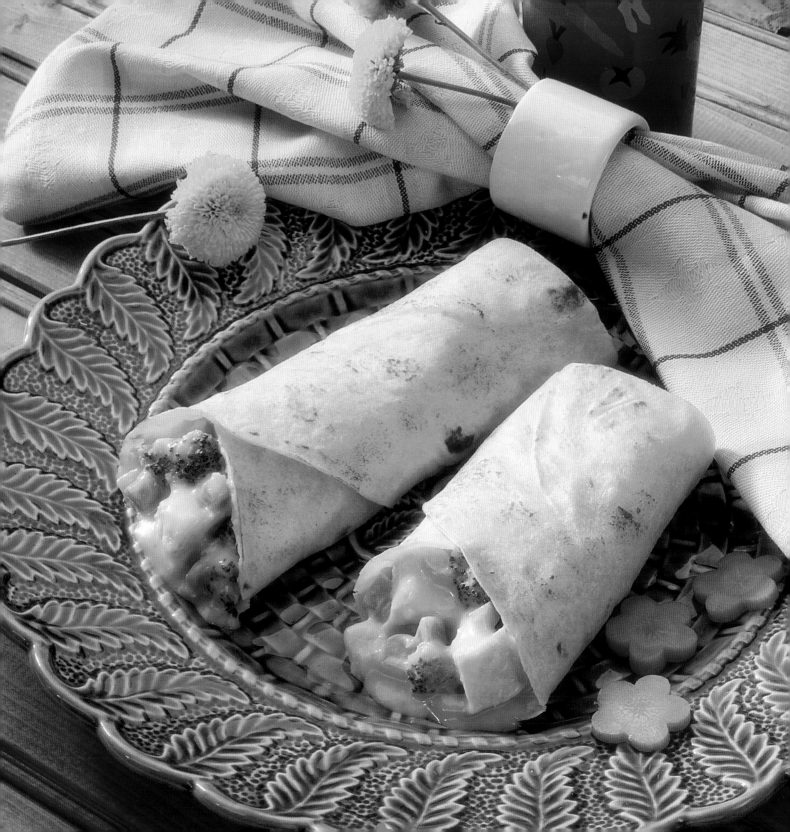

Cannelloni with Tomato-Eggplant Sauce

1 package (10 ounces) fresh spinach

1 cup fat-free ricotta cheese

4 egg whites, beaten

¼ cup (1 ounce) grated Parmesan cheese

2 tablespoons finely chopped fresh parsley

½ teaspoon salt (optional)

8 manicotti (about 4 ounces), cooked (without salt or fat) and cooled

   Tomato-Eggplant Sauce (page 238)

1 cup (4 ounces) shredded reduced-fat mozzarella cheese

1. Preheat oven to 350°F.

2. Wash spinach; do not pat dry. Place spinach in saucepan; cook, covered, over medium-high heat 3 to 5 minutes or until spinach is wilted. Cool slightly and drain; chop finely.

3. Combine ricotta cheese, spinach, egg whites, Parmesan cheese, parsley and salt, if desired, in large bowl; mix well. Spoon mixture into manicotti shells; arrange in 13×9-inch baking pan. Spoon Tomato-Eggplant Sauce over manicotti; sprinkle with mozzarella cheese. Bake, uncovered, 25 to 30 minutes or until hot and bubbly.   *Makes 4 servings*

continued on page 238

Cannelloni with
Tomato-Eggplant Sauce

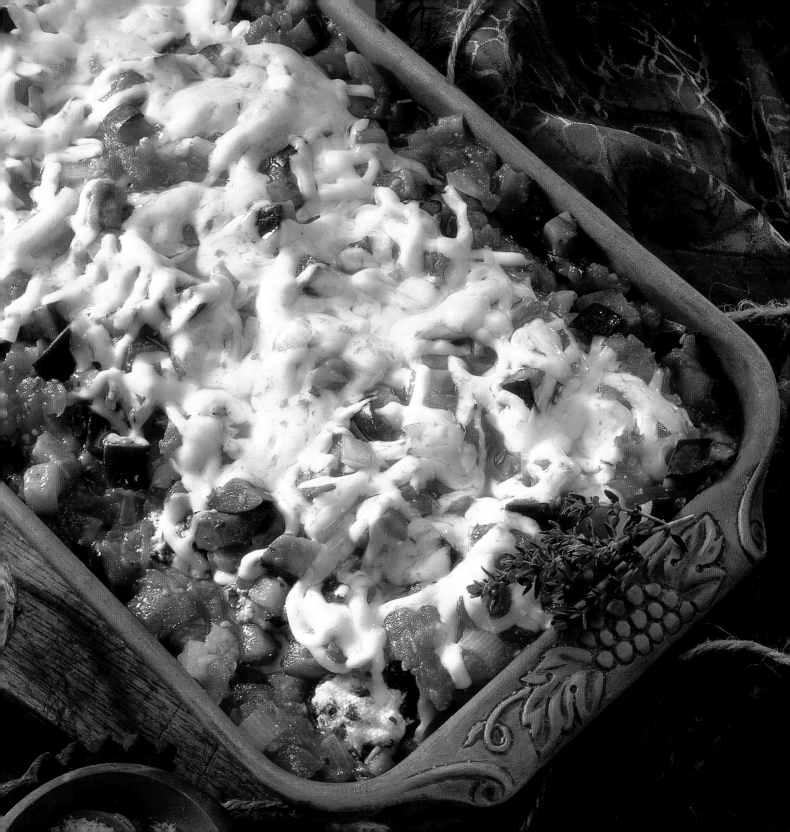

Tomato-Eggplant Sauce

Olive oil-flavored nonstick cooking spray
1 small eggplant, coarsely chopped
½ cup chopped onion
2 cloves garlic, minced
½ teaspoon dried tarragon leaves
¼ teaspoon dried thyme leaves
1 can (16 ounces) no-salt-added whole tomatoes, undrained, coarsely chopped
Salt (optional)
Black pepper (optional)

1. Spray large skillet with cooking spray; heat over medium heat until hot. Add eggplant, onion, garlic, tarragon and thyme; cook and stir about 5 minutes or until vegetables are tender.

2. Stir in tomatoes with juice; bring to a boil. Reduce heat and simmer, uncovered, 3 to 4 minutes. Season to taste with salt and pepper, if desired. *Makes about 2½ cups*

Nutrients per Serving (2 filled manicotti):
Calories: 338, Calories from Fat: 19%, Total Fat: 7g, Saturated Fat: 4g, Cholesterol: 26mg, Sodium: 632mg, Carbohydrate: 40g, Dietary Fiber: 3g, Protein: 30g

Dietary Exchanges: 1½ Starch, 3 Vegetable, 3 Lean Meat

Turkey Breast with Barley-Cranberry Stuffing

2 cups fat-free reduced-sodium chicken broth

1 cup quick-cooking barley, uncooked

½ cup chopped onion

½ cup dried cranberries

2 tablespoons slivered almonds, toasted

½ teaspoon rubbed sage

½ teaspoon garlic-pepper seasoning

Nonstick cooking spray

1 fresh or frozen bone-in turkey breast half (1¾ to 2 pounds), thawed and skinned

⅓ cup finely chopped fresh parsley

Slow Cooker Directions

1. Combine broth, barley, onion, cranberries, almonds, sage and garlic-pepper seasoning in slow cooker.

2. Spray large nonstick skillet with cooking spray. Heat over medium heat until hot. Brown turkey breast on all sides; add to slow cooker. Cover and cook on LOW 3 to 4 hours or until internal temperature reaches 170°F when tested with meat thermometer inserted into thickest part of breast, not touching bone.

3. Transfer turkey to cutting board; cover with foil and let stand 10 to 15 minutes before carving. Internal temperature will rise 5° to 10°F during stand time. Stir parsley into sauce mixture in slow cooker. Spoon sauce over turkey.

Makes 6 servings

Nutrients per Serving (⅙ of total recipe):
Calories: 298, Calories from Fat: 13%, Total Fat: 5g, Saturated Fat: 1g, Cholesterol: 55mg, Sodium: 114mg, Carbohydrate: 33g, Dietary Fiber: 6g, Protein: 31g

Dietary Exchanges: 2 Starch, 3 Lean Meat

Impossibly Easy Salmon Pie

1 can (7½ ounces) salmon packed in water, drained and deboned
½ cup grated Parmesan cheese
¼ cup sliced green onions
1 jar (2 ounces) chopped pimiento, drained
½ cup 1% low-fat cottage cheese
1 tablespoon lemon juice
1½ cups low-fat (1%) milk
¾ cup reduced-fat baking and pancake mix
2 whole eggs
2 egg whites *or* ¼ cup egg substitute
¼ teaspoon salt
¼ teaspoon dried dill weed
¼ teaspoon paprika (optional)

1. Preheat oven to 375°F. Spray 9-inch pie plate with nonstick cooking spray. Combine salmon, Parmesan cheese, onions and pimiento in prepared pie plate; set aside.

2. Combine cottage cheese and lemon juice in blender or food processor container; blend until smooth. Add milk, baking mix, whole eggs, egg whites, salt and dill; blend 15 seconds. Pour over salmon mixture. Sprinkle with paprika, if desired.

3. Bake 35 to 40 minutes or until lightly golden and knife inserted halfway between center and edge comes out clean. Cool 5 minutes before serving. Garnish as desired. *Makes 8 servings*

Nutrients per Serving (⅛ of pie):
Calories: 192, Calories from Fat: 27%, Total Fat: 6g, Saturated Fat: 2g, Cholesterol: 75mg, Sodium: 656mg, Carbohydrate: 19g, Dietary Fiber: 0g, Protein: 16g

Dietary Exchanges: 1 Starch, 2 Lean Meat

Impossibly Easy Salmon Pie

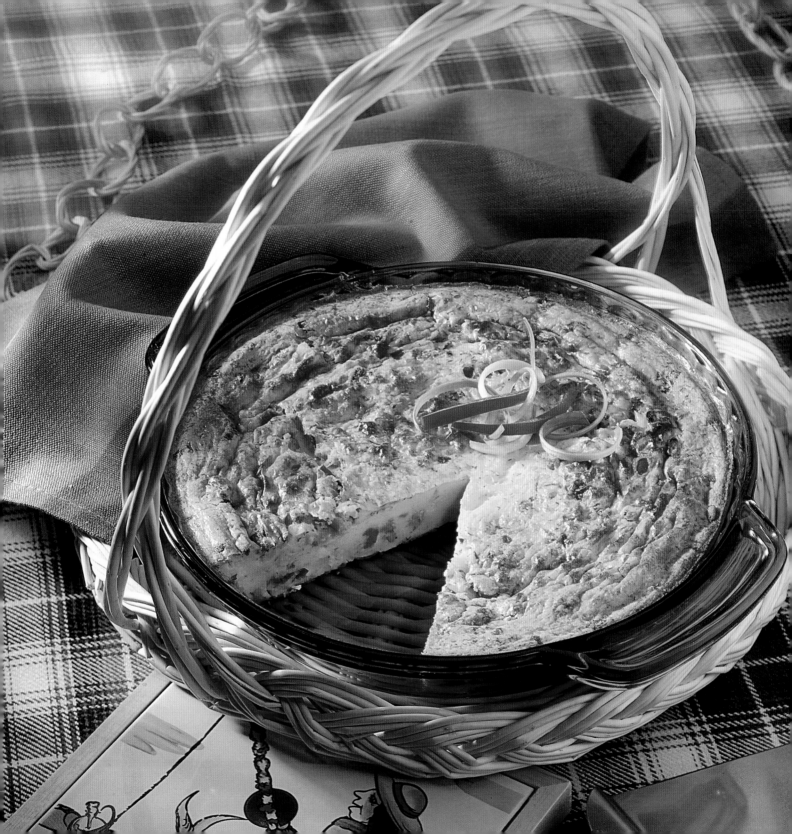

Broccoli, Chicken **and Rice Casserole**

1 box UNCLE BEN'S CHEF'S RECIPE™ Broccoli Rice Au Gratin Supreme
2 cups boiling water
4 boneless, skinless chicken breasts (about 1 pound)
¼ teaspoon garlic powder
2 cups frozen broccoli
1 cup (4 ounces) reduced-fat shredded Cheddar cheese

1. Heat oven to 425°F. In 13×9-inch baking pan, combine rice and contents of seasoning packet. Add boiling water; mix well. Add chicken; sprinkle with garlic powder. Cover and bake 30 minutes.

2. Add broccoli and cheese; continue to bake, covered, 8 to 10 minutes or until chicken is no longer pink in center.   *Makes 4 servings*

Nutrients per Serving (¼ of total recipe):
Calories: 353, Calories from Fat: 24%, Total Fat: 10g, Saturated Fat: 5g, Cholesterol: 87mg, Sodium: 778mg, Carbohydrate: 31g, Dietary Fiber: 3g, Protein: 37g

Dietary Exchanges: 1½ Starch, 1 Vegetable, 4 Lean Meat

recipe tip ....
One 10-ounce package of frozen chopped broccoli is equal to 1½ cups cooked broccoli.

Broccoli, Chicken and Rice Casserole

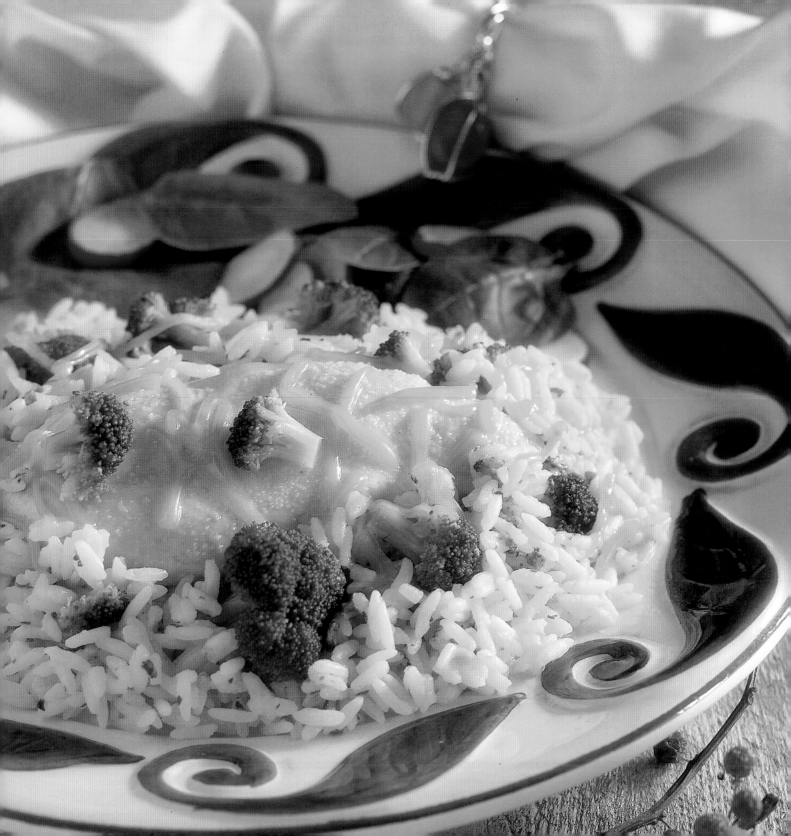

Fresh Vegetable Lasagna

8 ounces uncooked lasagna noodles

1 package (10 ounces) frozen chopped spinach, thawed and well drained

1 cup shredded carrots

½ cup sliced green onions

½ cup sliced red bell pepper

¼ cup chopped fresh parsley

½ teaspoon black pepper

1½ cups 1% low-fat cottage cheese

1 cup buttermilk

½ cup plain nonfat yogurt

2 egg whites

1 cup sliced mushrooms

1 can (14 ounces) artichoke hearts, drained and chopped

2 cups (8 ounces) shredded part-skim mozzarella cheese

¼ cup freshly grated Parmesan cheese

1. Cook pasta according to package directions, omitting salt. Rinse under cold water; drain well.

2. Preheat oven to 375°F. Pat spinach with paper towels to remove excess moisture. Combine spinach, carrots, green onions, bell pepper, parsley and black pepper in large bowl. Combine cottage cheese, buttermilk, yogurt and egg whites in food processor or blender; process until smooth.

3. Spray 13×9-inch baking pan with nonstick cooking spray. Arrange a third of lasagna noodles in bottom of pan. Spread with half each of cottage cheese mixture, vegetable mixture, mushrooms, artichokes and mozzarella. Repeat layers, ending with noodles. Sprinkle with Parmesan. Cover and bake 30 minutes. Remove cover; continue baking 20 minutes or until bubbly and heated through. Let stand 10 minutes before serving. *Makes 8 servings*

Nutrients per Serving (⅛ of total recipe):
Calories: 287, Calories from Fat: 22%, Total Fat: 7g, Saturated Fat: 4g, Cholesterol: 22mg, Sodium: 568mg, Carbohydrate: 33g, Dietary Fiber: 3g, Protein: 23g

Dietary Exchanges: 1 Starch, 3 Vegetable, 2 Lean Meat, ½ Fat

One-Dish Wonders

Chicken Ricotta Enchiladas

⅛ teaspoon garlic powder
⅛ teaspoon black pepper
1 pound chicken tenders
   Nonstick cooking spray
1 cup reduced-fat ricotta cheese
2 tablespoons finely chopped green onion
8 (6-inch) corn tortillas
¼ cup fat-free reduced-sodium chicken broth
1 large tomato, chopped
½ cup chipotle salsa or other salsa
½ cup (2 ounces) shredded reduced-fat mozzarella cheese
   Fresh parsley or cilantro for garnish (optional)

1. Preheat oven to 450°F. Combine garlic powder and pepper in small bowl; sprinkle evenly over chicken. Spray large nonstick skillet with cooking spray; heat over medium-high heat. Add chicken; cook, without stirring, 4 minutes or until golden. Turn chicken; cook 4 minutes more or until no longer pink in center.

2. Combine ricotta and green onion in small bowl; mix well. Spray 13×9×2-inch baking dish with cooking spray; set aside.

3. Spray large skillet with cooking spray; heat over medium heat. Heat tortillas one at a time just until soft, about 15 seconds per side.

4. Spread ricotta mixture across middle of warm tortillas; place chicken on top. Roll up tortillas; place seam-side-down in baking dish. Drizzle chicken broth evenly over top. Combine tomato and salsa. Spoon over enchiladas; top with cheese. Cover with foil; bake 15 minutes or until enchiladas are heated through and cheese is melted. Garnish with parsley or cilantro, if desired.   *Makes 4 servings*

Nutrients per Serving (¼ of total recipe):
Calories: 367, Calories from Fat: 21%, Total Fat: 8g, Saturated Fat: 3g, Cholesterol: 77mg, Sodium: 763mg, Carbohydrate: 32g, Dietary Fiber: 1g, Protein: 39g

Dietary Exchanges: 1½ Starch, 1 Vegetable, 4 Lean Meat

Vegetable Strata

2 slices white bread, cubed
¼ cup shredded reduced-fat Swiss cheese
½ cup sliced carrots
½ cup sliced mushrooms
¼ cup chopped onion
1 clove garlic, crushed
1 teaspoon FLEISCHMANN'S® Original Margarine
½ cup chopped tomato
½ cup snow peas
1 cup EGG BEATERS® Healthy Real Egg Product
¾ cup skim milk

Place bread cubes evenly on bottom of greased 1½-quart casserole dish. Sprinkle with cheese; set aside.

In medium nonstick skillet, over medium heat, sauté carrots, mushrooms, onion and garlic in margarine until tender. Stir in tomato and snow peas; cook 1 to 2 minutes more. Spoon over cheese.

In small bowl, combine Egg Beaters® and milk; pour over vegetable mixture. Bake at 375°F for 45 to 50 minutes or until knife inserted in center comes out clean. Let stand 10 minutes before serving.

Makes 6 servings

Prep Time: 15 minutes
Cook Time: 55 minutes

Nutrients per Serving (⅙ of total recipe):
Calories: 83, Calories from Fat: 13%, Total Fat: 1g, Saturated Fat: <1g, Cholesterol: 3mg, Sodium: 161mg, Carbohydrate: 10g, Dietary Fiber: 1g, Protein: 8g

Dietary Exchanges: 2 Vegetable, ½ Lean Meat

Vegetable Strata

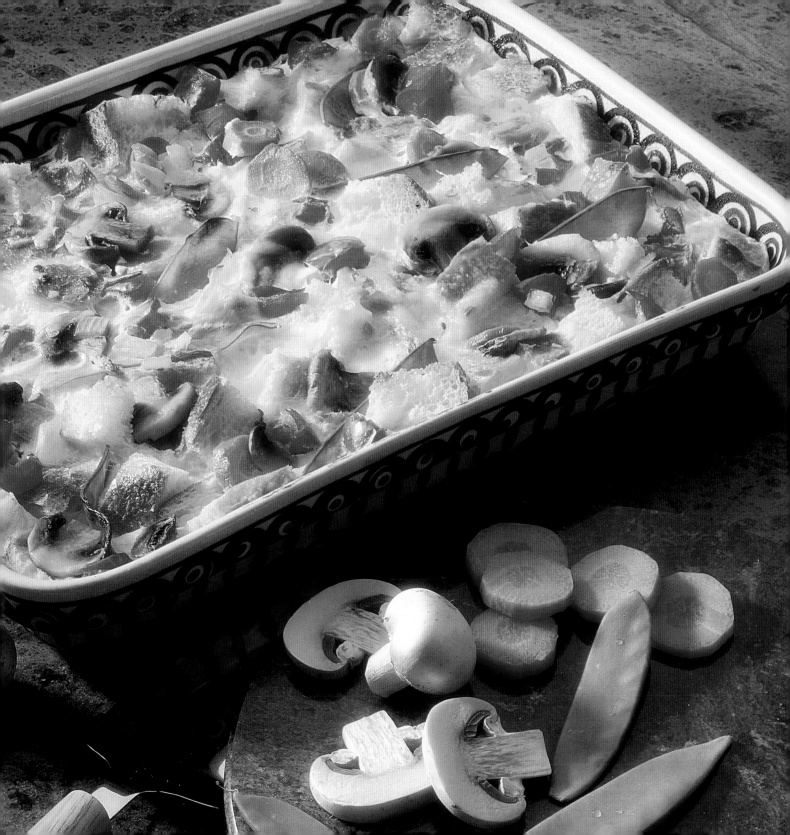

Turkey & Zucchini Enchiladas with Tomatillo-Green Chile Sauce

1¼ pounds turkey leg

1 tablespoon olive oil

1 small onion, thinly sliced

1 tablespoon minced garlic

1 pound zucchini, quartered lengthwise and sliced thinly crosswise

1½ teaspoons cumin

½ teaspoon dried oregano leaves

¾ cup (3 ounces) shredded reduced-fat Monterey Jack cheese

12 (6-inch) corn tortillas

Tomatillo-Green Chile Sauce (recipe follows)

½ cup crumbled feta cheese

6 sprigs fresh cilantro for garnish

1. Place turkey in large saucepan; cover with water. Bring to a boil over high heat. Reduce heat to medium-low. Cover and simmer 1½ to 2 hours or until meat pulls apart easily when tested with fork. Drain; discard skin and bone. Cut meat into small pieces. Place in medium bowl; set aside.

2. Preheat oven to 350°F. Heat oil over medium-high heat in large skillet. Add onion; cook and stir 3 to 4 minutes or until tender. Reduce heat to medium. Add garlic; cook and stir 3 to 4 minutes or until onion is golden. Add zucchini, 2 tablespoons water, cumin and oregano. Cover; cook and stir over medium heat 10 minutes or until zucchini is tender. Add to turkey. Stir in Monterey Jack cheese.

3. Heat large nonstick skillet over medium-high heat. Place 1 inch water in medium bowl. Dip 1 tortilla in water; shake off excess. Place tortilla in hot skillet. Cook 10 to 15 seconds on each side or until tortilla is hot and pliable. Repeat with remaining tortillas.

continued on page 250

Turkey & Zucchini Enchiladas with Tomatillo-Green Chile Sauce

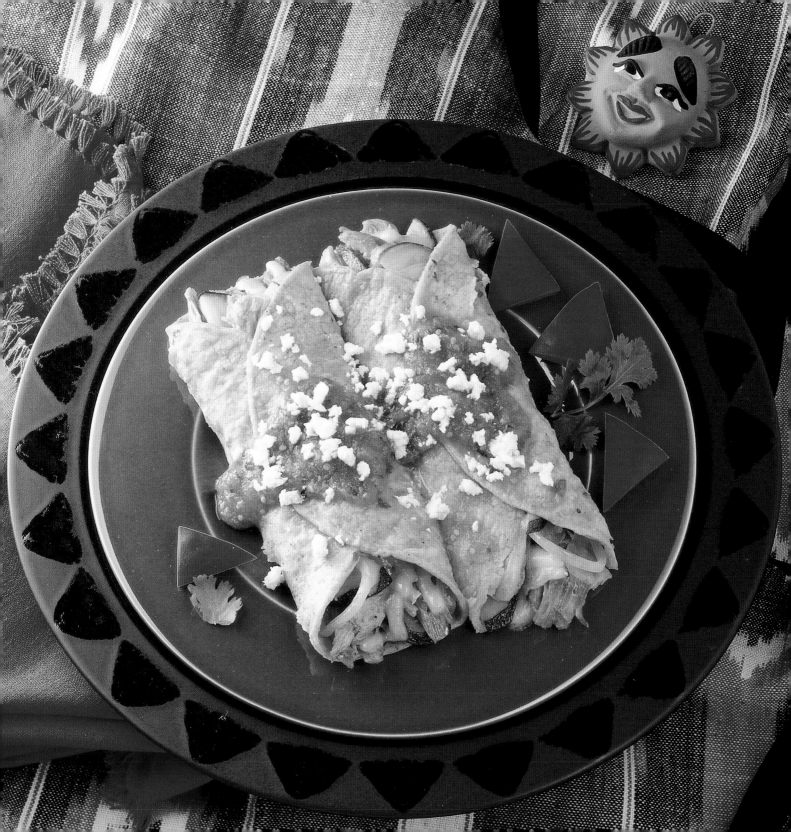

4. Spray bottom of 13×9-inch baking pan with nonstick cooking spray. Spoon ¼ cup filling down center of each tortilla; fold sides to enclose. Place seam-side-down in pan. Brush tops with ½ cup Tomatillo-Green Chile Sauce. Cover; bake 30 to 40 minutes or until heated through. Top with remaining Chile Sauce and feta cheese. Garnish with cilantro. *Makes 6 servings*

Tomatillo-Green Chile Sauce

¾ **pound fresh tomatillos** *or* **2 cans (18 ounces each) whole tomatillos, drained**
1 **can (4 ounces) diced mild green chilies, drained**
½ **cup reduced-sodium chicken broth**
1 **teaspoon dried oregano leaves, crushed**
½ **teaspoon ground cumin**
2 **tablespoons chopped fresh cilantro (optional)**

1. Place tomatillos in large saucepan; cover with water. Bring to a boil over high heat. Reduce heat to medium-high and simmer gently 20 to 30 minutes or until tomatillos are tender.

2. Place tomatillos, chilies, broth (omit if using canned tomatillos), oregano and cumin in food processor or blender; process until smooth. Return mixture to pan. Cover; heat over medium heat until bubbling. Stir in cilantro, if desired. *Makes about 3 cups*

Nutrients per Serving (⅙ of total recipe):
Calories: 377, Calories from Fat: 28%, Total Fat: 12g, Saturated Fat: 3g, Cholesterol: 48mg, Sodium: 284mg, Carbohydrate: 41g, Dietary Fiber: 5g, Protein: 29g

Dietary Exchanges: 2 Starch, 2 Vegetable, 2½ Lean Meat, 1 Fat

Crustless Salmon & Broccoli Quiche

¾ cup cholesterol-free egg substitute
¼ cup plain nonfat yogurt
¼ cup chopped green onions with tops
2 teaspoons all-purpose flour
1 teaspoon dried basil leaves
⅛ teaspoon salt
⅛ teaspoon black pepper
¾ cup frozen broccoli florets, thawed and drained
⅓ cup (3 ounces) drained and flaked water-packed boneless, skinless canned
    salmon
2 tablespoons grated Parmesan cheese
1 plum tomato, thinly sliced
¼ cup fresh bread crumbs

1. Preheat oven to 375°F. Spray 6-cup rectangular casserole or 9-inch pie plate with nonstick cooking spray.

2. Combine egg substitute, yogurt, green onions, flour, basil, salt and pepper in medium bowl until well blended. Stir in broccoli, salmon and Parmesan cheese. Spread evenly in prepared casserole. Top with tomato slices. Sprinkle bread crumbs over top.

3. Bake 20 to 25 minutes or until knife inserted into center comes out clean. Let stand 5 minutes before serving.   *Makes 2 servings*

Nutrients per Serving (½ of total recipe):
Calories: 227, Calories from Fat: 22%, Total Fat: 6g, Saturated Fat: 2g, Cholesterol: 25mg, Sodium: 717mg, Carbohydrate: 20g, Dietary Fiber: 5g, Protein: 25g

Dietary Exchanges: 1 Starch, 1 Vegetable, 2 Lean Meat, ½ Fat

One-Dish Wonders

Easy Chicken Chalupas

1 roasted chicken (about 2 pounds)
12 flour tortillas
2 cups pre-shredded reduced-fat Cheddar cheese
1 cup mild green chile salsa
1 cup mild red chile salsa

1. Preheat oven to 350°F. Spray ovenproof dish with cooking spray.

2. Remove chicken meat from bones and shred. Discard bones and skin.

3. Lay 1 or 2 tortillas in bottom of baking dish, overlapping slightly. Layer tortillas with chicken, cheese and salsas. Repeat layers until baking dish is full. Finish with cheese and salsas.

4. Bake casserole 25 minutes or until bubbly and hot. *Makes 6 servings*

Nutrients per Serving (⅙ of total recipe):
Calories: 646, Calories from Fat: 47%, Total Fat: 34g, Saturated Fat: 12g, Cholesterol: 123mg, Sodium: 948mg, Carbohydrate: 42g, Dietary Fiber: 3g, Protein: 42g

Dietary Exchanges: 3 Starch, 5 Lean Meat, 3 Fat

recipe tip

Serve this easy main dish with some custom toppings on the side. Low-fat sour cream, chopped cilantro, sliced black olives, sliced green onions and sliced avocado taste great with these chalupas!

Easy Chicken Chalupas

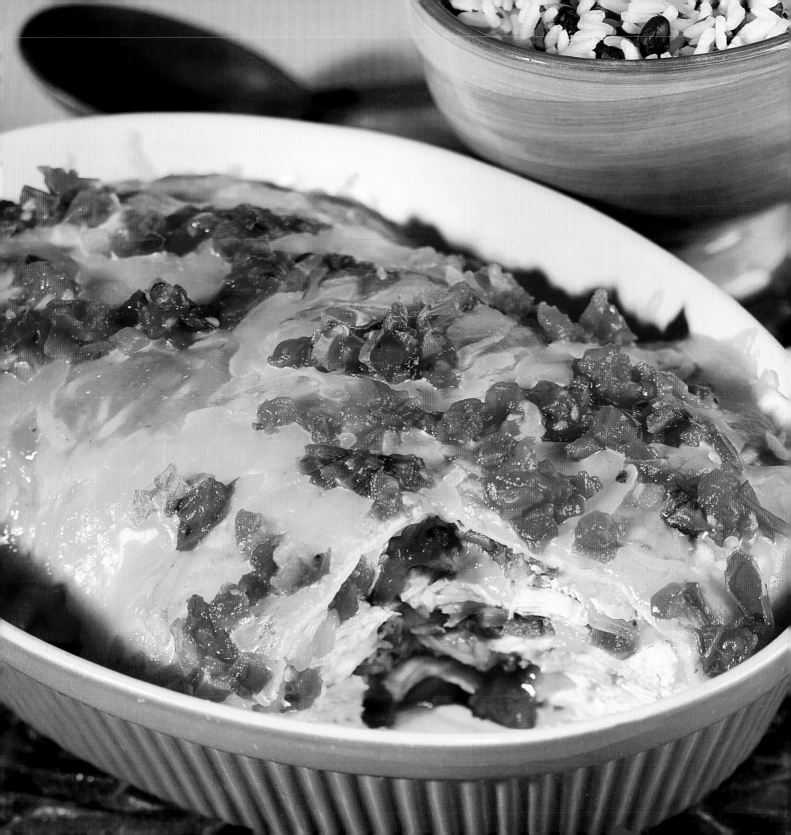

Chili Spaghetti Casserole

8 ounces uncooked spaghetti

1 pound lean ground beef

1 medium onion, chopped

¼ teaspoon salt

⅛ teaspoon black pepper

1 can (15 ounces) vegetarian chili with beans

1 can (14½ ounces) Italian-style stewed tomatoes

1½ cups (6 ounces) shredded sharp Cheddar cheese, divided

½ cup reduced-fat sour cream

1½ teaspoons chili powder

¼ teaspoon garlic powder

1. Preheat oven to 350°F. Spray 13×9-inch baking dish with nonstick cooking spray.

2. Cook pasta according to package directions, omitting salt, until al dente. Drain and place in prepared dish.

3. Meanwhile, place beef and onion in large skillet; season with salt and pepper. Brown beef over medium-high heat until beef is no longer pink, stirring to separate meat. Drain fat. Stir in chili, tomatoes, 1 cup cheese, sour cream, chili powder and garlic powder.

4. Add chili mixture to pasta; stir until pasta is well coated. Sprinkle with remaining ½ cup cheese.

5. Cover tightly with foil and bake 30 minutes or until hot and bubbly. Let stand 5 minutes before serving. *Makes 8 servings*

Nutrients per Serving (⅛ of casserole):
Calories: 393, Calories from Fat: 41%, Total Fat: 18g, Saturated Fat: 9g, Cholesterol: 65mg, Sodium: 442mg, Carbohydrate: 33g, Dietary Fiber: 5g, Protein: 24g

Dietary Exchanges: 2 Starch, 1 Vegetable, 3 Lean Meat, 1½ Fat

Easy Tex-Mex Bake

8 ounces uncooked thin mostaccioli
Nonstick cooking spray
1 pound ground turkey breast
⅔ cup bottled medium or mild salsa
1 package (10 ounces) frozen corn, thawed and drained
1 container (16 ounces) 1% low-fat cottage cheese
1 egg
1 tablespoon minced fresh cilantro
½ teaspoon white pepper
¼ teaspoon ground cumin
½ cup (2 ounces) shredded Monterey Jack cheese

1. Cook pasta according to package directions, omitting salt. Drain and rinse well; set aside.

2. Spray large nonstick skillet with cooking spray. Add turkey; cook until no longer pink, about 5 minutes. Stir in salsa and corn. Remove from heat.

3. Preheat oven to 350°F. Combine cottage cheese, egg, cilantro, white pepper and cumin in small bowl.

4. Spoon ½ turkey mixture into bottom of 11×7-inch baking dish. Top with pasta. Spoon cottage cheese mixture over pasta. Top with remaining turkey mixture. Sprinkle Monterey Jack cheese over casserole.

5. Bake 25 to 30 minutes or until heated through. *Makes 6 servings*

Nutrients per Serving (⅙ of total recipe):
Calories: 365, Calories from Fat: 15%, Total Fat: 6g, Saturated Fat: 3g, Cholesterol: 99mg, Sodium: 800mg, Carbohydrate: 39g, Dietary Fiber: 4g, Protein: 38g

Dietary Exchanges: 2 Starch, 4 Lean Meat

One-Dish Wonders

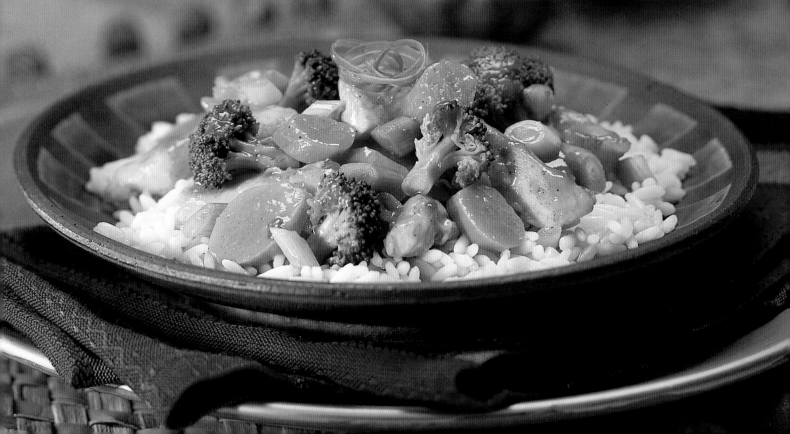

Especially Eastern

Thai Curry **Stir-Fry**

½ cup fat-free reduced-sodium chicken broth

2 teaspoons cornstarch

2 teaspoons reduced-sodium soy sauce

1½ teaspoons curry powder

⅛ teaspoon red pepper flakes

Nonstick olive oil cooking spray

3 green onions, sliced

2 cloves garlic, minced

2 cups broccoli florets

⅔ cup sliced carrot

1½ teaspoons olive oil

6 ounces boneless skinless chicken breast, cut into bite-size pieces

⅔ cup hot cooked rice, prepared without salt

1. Stir together broth, cornstarch, soy sauce, curry powder and red pepper flakes. Set aside.

2. Spray nonstick wok or large nonstick skillet with cooking spray. Heat over medium-high heat. Add onions and garlic; stir-fry 1 minute. Remove from wok.

3. Add broccoli and carrot to wok; stir-fry 2 to 3 minutes or until crisp-tender. Remove from wok.

4. Add oil to hot wok. Add chicken and stir-fry 2 to 3 minutes or until no longer pink. Stir broth mixture. Add to wok. Cook and stir until broth mixture comes to a boil and thickens slightly. Return all vegetables to wok. Heat through.

5. Serve chicken mixture with rice. Garnish as desired. *Makes 2 servings*

Nutrients per Serving (½ of total recipe):
Calories: 273, Calories from Fat: 20%, Total Fat: 6g, Saturated Fat: 1g, Cholesterol: 57mg, Sodium: 308mg, Carbohydrate: 27g, Dietary Fiber: 5g, Protein: 28g

Dietary Exchanges: 1 Starch, 2 Vegetable, 3 Lean Meat

Thai Curry Stir-Fry

Wonton Soup

¼ pound lean ground pork

2 ounces medium-size raw shrimp, peeled, deveined and minced

2 tablespoons minced green onions and tops

4 teaspoons KIKKOMAN® Soy Sauce, divided

½ teaspoon cornstarch

¼ teaspoon grated fresh gingerroot

24 wonton wrappers

4 cups water

3 cans (about 14 ounces each) chicken broth

¼ cup dry sherry

½ pound bok choy cabbage

2 tablespoons chopped green onions and tops

½ teaspoon Oriental sesame oil

Combine pork, shrimp, minced green onions, 2 teaspoons soy sauce, cornstarch and ginger in medium bowl; mix well. Arrange several wonton wrappers on clean surface; cover remaining wrappers to prevent drying out. Place 1 teaspoonful pork mixture in center of each wrapper. Fold wrapper over filling to form a triangle. Gently fold center point down and moisten left corner with water. Twist and overlap opposite corner over moistened corner; press firmly to seal. Repeat with remaining wrappers. Bring water to boil in large saucepan. Add wontons. Boil gently 3 minutes; remove with slotted spoon. Discard water. Pour broth and sherry into same saucepan. Cut bok choy crosswise into ½-inch slices, separating stems from leaves. Add stems to broth mixture; bring to boil. Add cooked wontons; simmer 1 minute. Add bok choy leaves and chopped green onions; simmer 1 minute longer. Remove from heat; stir in remaining 2 teaspoons soy sauce and sesame oil. Serve immediately. *Makes 6 servings*

Nutrients per Serving (⅙ of total recipe):
Calories: 203, Calories from Fat: 30%, Total Fat: 7g, Saturated Fat: 2g, Cholesterol: 31mg, Sodium: 1265mg, Carbohydrate: 22g, Dietary Fiber: 1g, Protein: 11g

Dietary Exchanges: 1 Starch, 1 Vegetable, 1 Lean Meat, 1 Fat

Wonton Soup

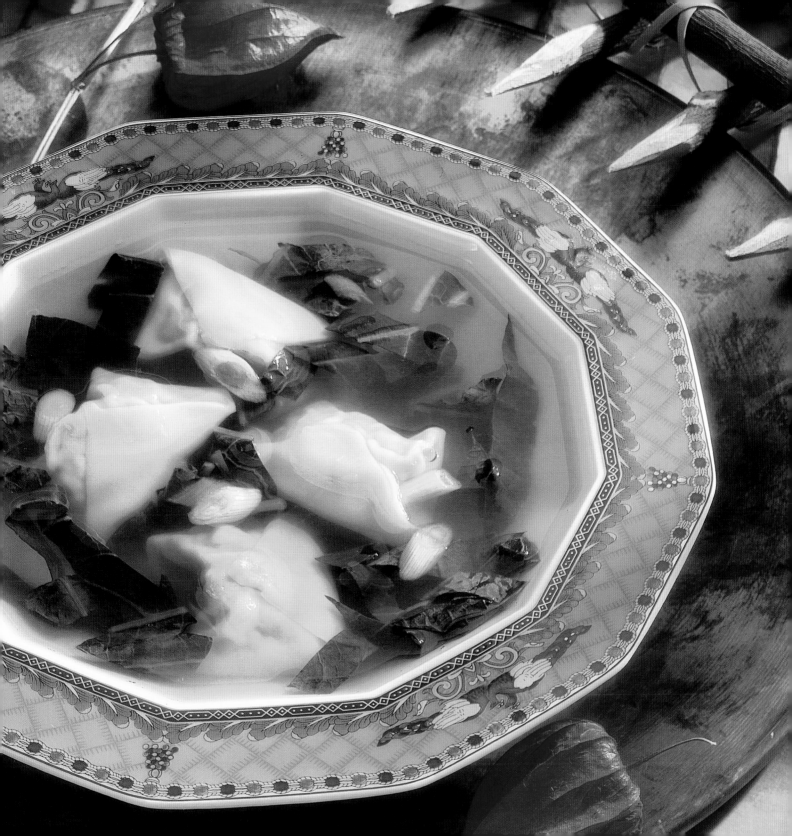

Vegetarian **Fried Rice**

4 dried mushrooms

4 cups long-grain rice, cooked without added salt or fat

3 eggs

¾ teaspoon salt, divided

2½ tablespoons vegetable oil, divided

1 teaspoon minced fresh ginger

1 clove garlic, minced

3 green onions with tops, thinly sliced

4 ounces bean curd, cut into ¼-inch cubes and deep-fried

1 tablespoon soy sauce

¼ teaspoon sugar

1 cup bean sprouts, coarsely chopped

½ cup thawed frozen peas

1. Place mushrooms in small bowl; cover with hot water. Let stand 30 minutes; drain, reserving liquid. Squeeze out excess water from mushrooms. Remove stems; discard. Chop caps.

2. Rub rice with wet hands so all the grains are separated.

3. Beat eggs with ¼ teaspoon salt in medium bowl. Heat ½ tablespoon oil in wok or large skillet over medium heat. Add eggs; cook and stir until soft curds form.

4. Remove wok from heat; cut eggs into small pieces with spoon. Remove from wok; set aside.

5. Heat remaining 2 tablespoons oil in wok over high heat. Add ginger, garlic and onions; stir-fry 10 seconds. Add mushrooms, ¼ cup reserved mushroom liquid, bean curd, soy sauce and sugar. Cook until most of the liquid evaporates, about 4 minutes. Add bean sprouts and peas; cook 30 seconds.

6. Stir in rice and remaining ½ teaspoon salt; heat thoroughly. Stir in eggs just before serving.

Makes 4 servings

Nutrients per Serving (¼ of total recipe):
Calories: 501, Calories from Fat: 35%, Total Fat: 19g, Saturated Fat: 3g, Cholesterol: 159mg, Sodium: 757mg, Carbohydrate: 57g, Dietary Fiber: 3g, Protein: 24g

Dietary Exchanges: 3 Starch, 2 Vegetable, 1 Lean Meat, 4 Fat

Oriental Pork Stir-Fry

1½ pounds pork tenderloin
2 teaspoons vegetable oil
1 teaspoon grated fresh ginger
1 clove garlic, minced
2 medium green bell peppers, cut into thin strips
1 (8-ounce) can sliced water chestnuts, drained
3 tablespoons soy sauce
1 tablespoon cornstarch
1½ cups cherry tomato halves

Partially freeze pork; cut pork into 3×½×⅛-inch strips. Preheat nonstick skillet over high heat; add oil. Stir-fry ginger and garlic in hot oil 30 seconds; remove from skillet. Add pork to skillet; stir-fry 5 minutes or until browned. Remove from skillet. Stir-fry remaining pork 5 minutes or until browned; remove from skillet. Add peppers and water chestnuts; stir-fry 3 to 4 minutes. Combine soy sauce and cornstarch; stir into vegetable mixture. Stir in pork; heat through. Add tomato halves, stirring to combine. Serve immediately.

Makes 6 servings

Prep Time: 20 minutes

Favorite recipe from **National Pork Board**

Nutrients per Serving (⅙ of total recipe):
Calories: 187, Calories from Fat: 25%, Total Fat: 5g, Saturated Fat: 2g, Cholesterol: 73mg, Sodium: 525mg, Carbohydrate: 11g, Dietary Fiber: 2g, Protein: 26g

Dietary Exchanges: 1 Vegetable, 3 Lean Meat

Grilled Oriental Shrimp Kabobs

3 tablespoons soy sauce or reduced-sodium soy sauce

1 tablespoon regular or seasoned rice vinegar

1 tablespoon dark sesame oil

2 cloves garlic, minced

¼ teaspoon red pepper flakes

1 pound uncooked large shrimp, peeled and deveined

1. For marinade, combine soy sauce, vinegar, oil, garlic and pepper flakes in small bowl; mix well. Cover; refrigerate up to 3 days.

2. Combine marinade and shrimp in resealable plastic food storage bag. Seal bag securely. Refrigerate at least 30 minutes or up to 2 hours, turning bag once.

3. Spray grid of grill with nonstick cooking spray. Prepare grill for direct cooking.

4. Drain shrimp, reserving marinade. Thread shrimp onto 12-inch-long skewers. Place skewers on prepared grid; brush with half of reserved marinade.

5. Grill skewers on covered grill over medium coals 5 minutes. Turn skewers over; brush with remaining half of marinade. Grill 3 to 5 minutes or until shrimp are opaque. Discard any remaining marinade.

Makes 4 servings

Serving Suggestion: Serve with fried rice and fresh pineapple spears.

Make-Ahead Time: up to 3 days in refrigerator
Final Prep and Cook Time: 20 minutes

Nutrients per Serving (¼ of total recipe):
Calories: 129, Calories from Fat: 32%, Total Fat: 4g, Saturated Fat: <1g, Cholesterol: 173mg, Sodium: 596mg, Carbohydrate: 1g, Dietary Fiber: <1g, Protein: 20g

Dietary Exchanges: 2½ Lean Meat

Grilled Oriental Shrimp Kabobs

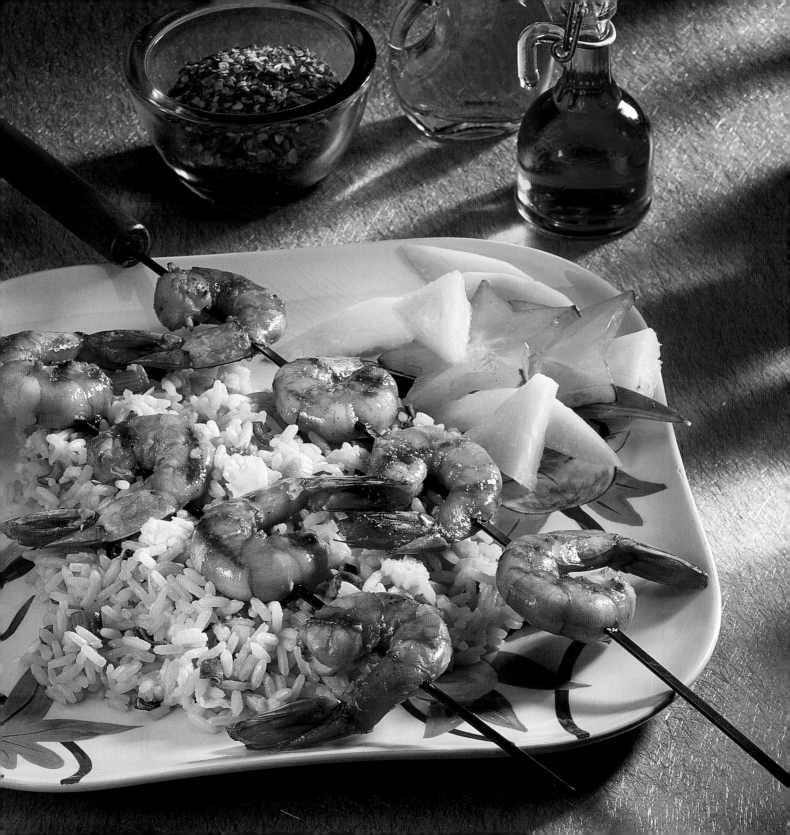

Japanese Noodle Soup

1 package (8½ ounces) Japanese udon noodles
1 teaspoon vegetable oil
1 medium red bell pepper, cut into thin strips
1 medium carrot, diagonally sliced
2 green onions, thinly sliced
2 cans (about 14 ounces each) fat-free reduced-sodium beef broth
1 cup water
1 teaspoon reduced-sodium soy sauce
½ teaspoon grated fresh ginger
½ teaspoon black pepper
2 cups thinly sliced fresh shiitake mushrooms, stems removed
4 ounces daikon (Japanese radish), peeled and cut into thin strips
4 ounces firm tofu, drained and cut into ½-inch cubes

1. Cook noodles according to package directions, omitting salt; drain. Rinse; set aside.

2. Heat oil in large nonstick saucepan until hot. Add bell pepper, carrot and green onions; cook until slightly softened, about 3 minutes. Stir in beef broth, water, soy sauce, ginger and black pepper; bring to a boil. Add mushrooms, daikon and tofu; reduce heat and simmer 5 minutes.

3. Place noodles in soup tureen; ladle soup over noodles. *Makes 6 servings*

Nutrients per Serving (⅙ of total recipe):
Calories: 144, Calories from Fat: 16%, Total Fat: 3g, Saturated Fat: <1g, Cholesterol: 0mg, Sodium: 107mg, Carbohydrate: 24g, Dietary Fiber: 3g, Protein: 9g

Dietary Exchanges: 1½ Starch, ½ Vegetable, ½ Fat

Angel Hair Noodles with Peanut Sauce

¼ cup Texas peanuts, puréed
2 tablespoons low-fat chicken broth or water
1 tablespoon soy sauce
1 tablespoon rice vinegar
10 ounces dried bean thread noodles
½ tablespoon vegetable oil
1 pound chicken breast, boned, skinned and thinly sliced
½ cucumber, peeled, seeded and cut into matchstick pieces
2 medium carrots, shredded

To make sauce, combine peanut purée, chicken broth, soy sauce and vinegar in small bowl; set aside.

Bring 4 cups water to a boil in medium saucepan. Add noodles, stirring to separate strands. Cook, stirring, 30 seconds or until noodles are slightly soft. Drain in colander and rinse under cold running water. Drain well; cut noodles in half and set aside.

Heat wok or wide skillet over high heat. Add oil, swirling to coat sides. Add chicken and stir-fry 1 minute or until opaque. Add cucumber, carrots and sauce; cook, stirring to mix well. Remove from heat. Add noodles and toss until evenly coated. Sprinkle with extra peanuts, if desired.

Makes 6 servings

Favorite recipe from **Texas Peanut Producers Board**

Nutrients per Serving (⅙ of total recipe):
Calories: 306, Calories from Fat: 16%, Total Fat: 5g, Saturated Fat: 1g, Cholesterol: 44mg, Sodium: 214mg, Carbohydrate: 44g, Dietary Fiber: 2g, Protein: 20g

Dietary Exchanges: 3 Starch, 2 Lean Meat

Beef Teriyaki Stir-Fry

1 cup uncooked rice
1 pound beef sirloin, thinly sliced
½ cup teriyaki marinade, divided
2 tablespoons vegetable oil, divided
1 medium onion, halved and sliced
2 cups frozen green beans, rinsed and drained

1. Cook rice according to package directions, omitting salt.

2. Combine beef and ¼ cup marinade in medium bowl; set aside.

3. Heat ½ tablespoon oil in wok or large skillet over medium-high heat until hot. Add onion; stir-fry 3 to 4 minutes or until crisp-tender. Remove from wok to medium bowl.

4. Heat ½ tablespoon oil in wok. Stir-fry beans 3 minutes or until crisp-tender and hot. Drain off excess liquid. Add beans to onions in bowl.

5. Heat remaining 1 tablespoon oil in wok. Drain beef, discarding marinade. Stir-fry beef about 3 minutes or until browned. Stir in vegetables and remaining ¼ cup marinade; cook and stir 1 minute or until heated through. Serve with rice.   *Makes 4 servings*

Prep and Cook Time: 22 minutes

Nutrients per Serving (¼ of total recipe):
Calories: 428, Calories from Fat: 24%, Total Fat: 11g, Saturated Fat: 2g, Cholesterol: 53mg, Sodium: 1300mg, Carbohydrate: 48g, Dietary Fiber: 3g, Protein: 31g

Dietary Exchanges: 3 Starch, 1 Vegetable, 3 Lean Meat, ½ Fat

Beef Teriyaki Stir-Fry

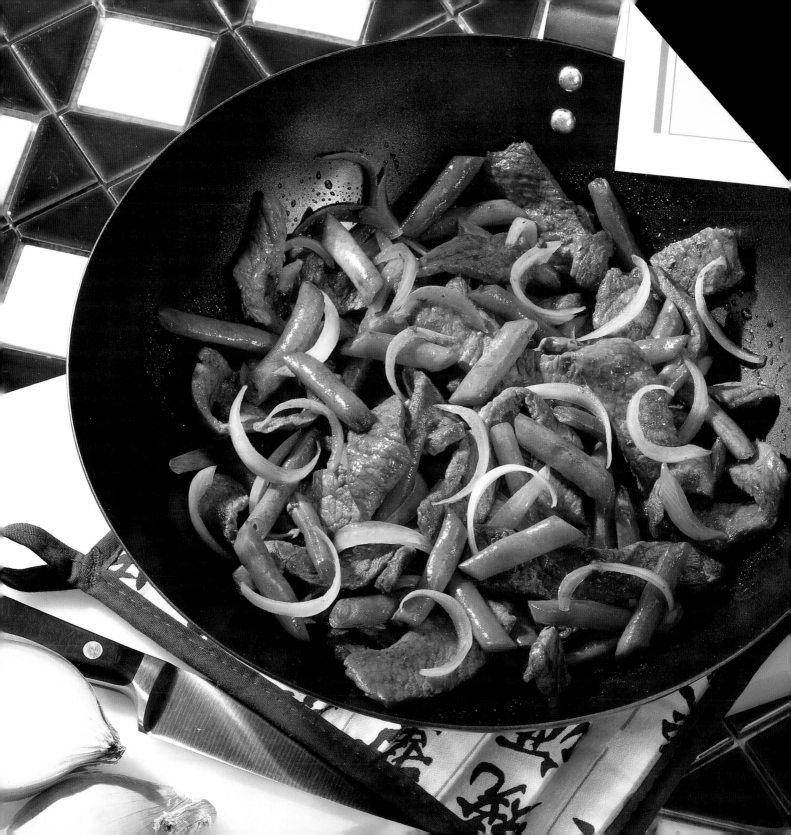

Grilled Chinese Salmon

3 tablespoons soy sauce
2 tablespoons dry sherry
2 cloves garlic, minced
1 pound salmon steaks or fillets
2 tablespoons finely chopped fresh cilantro

1. Combine soy sauce, sherry and garlic in shallow dish. Add salmon; turn to coat. Cover and refrigerate at least 30 minutes or up to 2 hours.

2. Drain salmon; reserve marinade. Arrange steaks (arrange fillets skin-side-down) on oiled rack of broiler pan or oiled grid over hot coals. Broil or grill 5 to 6 inches from heat 10 minutes. Baste with reserved marinade after 5 minutes of broiling; discard any remaining marinade. Sprinkle with cilantro.

Makes 4 servings

Nutrients per Serving (¼ of total recipe):
Calories: 223, Calories from Fat: 49%, Total Fat: 12g, Saturated Fat: 3g, Cholesterol: 74mg, Sodium: 744mg, Carbohydrate: 1g, Dietary Fiber: <1g, Protein: 24g

Dietary Exchanges: 3 Lean Meat, 1 Fat

recipe tip
By substituting reduced-sodium soy sauce for the regular soy sauce in this recipe, you'll be cutting the amount of sodium by nearly half!

Grilled Chinese Salmon

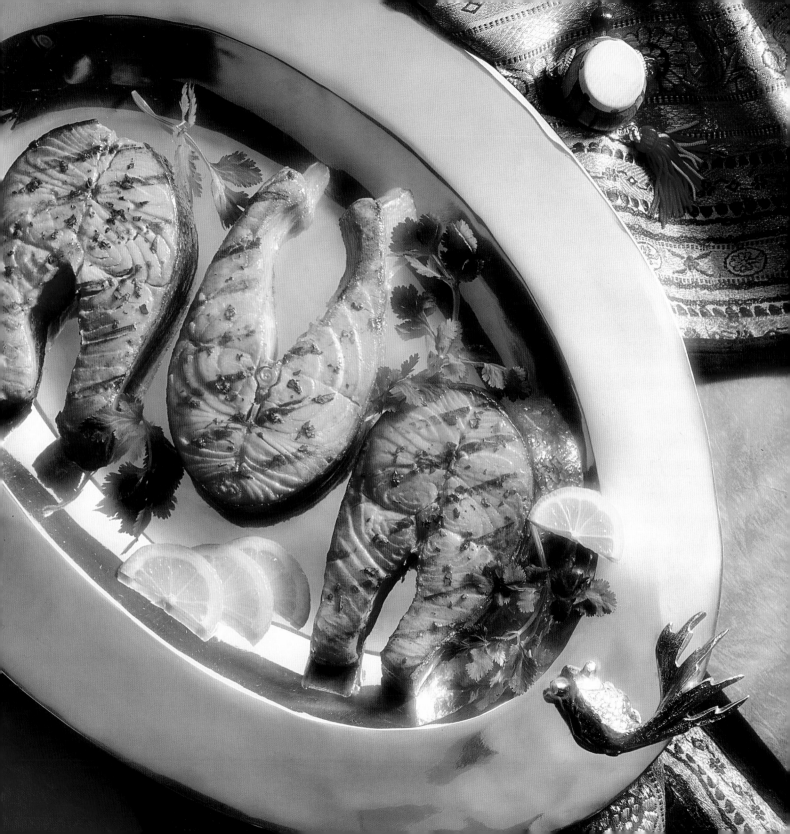

Chicken Stir-Fry

4 boneless skinless chicken breast halves (about 1½ pounds)
2 tablespoons vegetable oil
2 tablespoons orange juice
2 tablespoons light soy sauce
1 tablespoon cornstarch
1 bag (16 ounces) BIRDS EYE® frozen Farm Fresh Mixtures Broccoli, Carrots
    & Water Chestnuts

- Cut chicken into ½-inch-thick strips.

- In wok or large skillet, heat oil over medium-high heat.

- Add chicken; cook 5 minutes, stirring occasionally.

- Meanwhile, in small bowl, combine orange juice, soy sauce and cornstarch; blend well and set aside.

- Add vegetables to chicken; cook 5 minutes more or until chicken is no longer pink in center, stirring occasionally.

- Stir in soy sauce mixture; cook 1 minute or until heated through.

Makes 4 servings

Serving Suggestion: Serve over hot cooked rice.

Birds Eye® Idea: When cooking rice, add one teaspoon lemon juice to each quart of water you use, so grains will stay white and separate.

Prep Time: 5 minutes
Cook Time: 12 minutes

Nutrients per Serving (¼ of total recipe):
Calories: 300, Calories from Fat: 28%, Total Fat: 9g, Saturated Fat: 1g, Cholesterol: 99mg, Sodium: 399mg, Carbohydrate: 9g, Dietary Fiber: 3g, Protein: 41g

Dietary Exchanges: 1 Vegetable, 5 Lean Meat

Chicken Stir-Fry

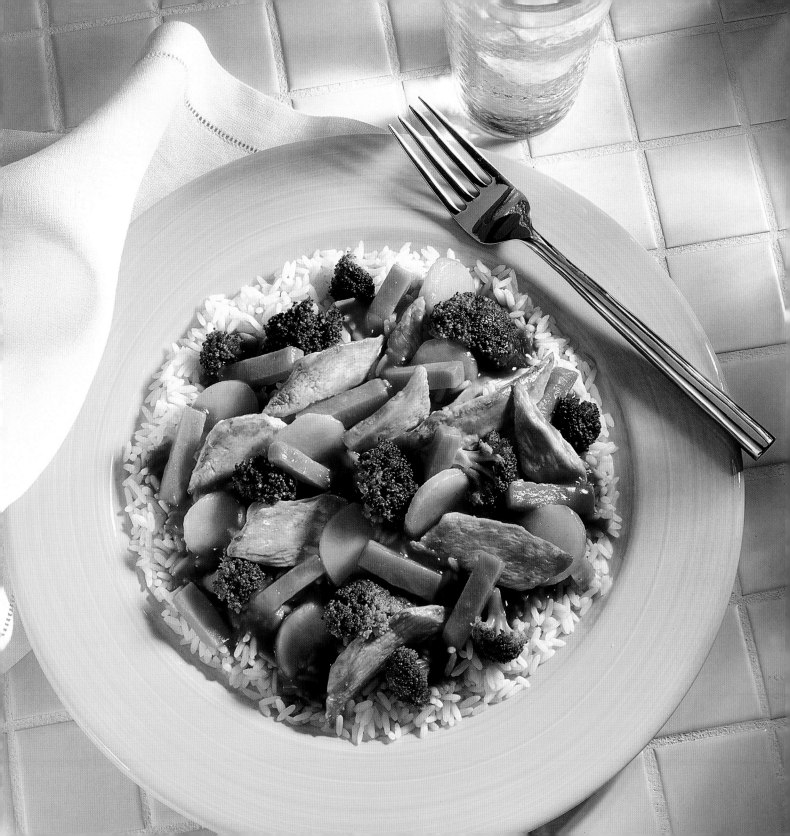

Sesame Fish in Parchment

2 tablespoons KIKKOMAN® Lite Soy Sauce
½ teaspoon grated fresh lemon peel
½ teaspoon Oriental sesame oil
  Parchment paper
4 small white fish steaks (halibut, sea bass or salmon), about ¾ inch thick
1 tablespoon chopped fresh cilantro
1½ teaspoons sesame seed, toasted

Combine lite soy sauce, lemon peel and sesame oil in small bowl; set aside. Cut parchment paper into four 13-inch-square pieces; fold squares in half. Unfold parchment and place 1 fish steak near crease of each square. Spoon equal amount soy sauce mixture over fish. Combine cilantro and sesame seed in small bowl; sprinkle equally over fish. Fold parchment over fish; roll and crimp edges together tightly. Place packages on large baking sheet. Bake in 425°F oven 15 minutes, or until fish flakes easily when tested with fork. Transfer packages to serving plates. Just before serving, cut a cross on top of each package with sharp knife or scissors and pull back paper. *Makes 4 servings*

Nutrients per Serving (1 fish steak):
Calories: 141, Calories from Fat: 25%, Total Fat: 4g, Saturated Fat: 1g, Cholesterol: 36mg, Sodium: 349mg, Carbohydrate: 1g, Dietary Fiber: <1g, Protein: 24g

Dietary Exchanges: 3 Lean Meat

recipe tip

When storing fresh fish, wrap it tightly in plastic wrap. If possible, place the package on ice and store it in the coldest part of the refrigerator. Be sure the melting ice drains away from the fish, since flesh that comes in contact with moisture may become discolored. Fresh fish should be used within one day.

Chicken Chop Suey

1 package (1 ounce) dried black Chinese mushrooms
3 tablespoons reduced-sodium soy sauce
1 tablespoon cornstarch
1 pound boneless skinless chicken breasts or thighs
2 cloves garlic, minced
1 tablespoon peanut or vegetable oil
½ cup thinly sliced celery
½ cup sliced water chestnuts
½ cup bamboo shoots
1 cup chicken broth
   Hot cooked white rice or chow mein noodles (optional)
   Thinly sliced green onions (optional)

1. Place mushrooms in small bowl; cover with warm water. Soak 20 minutes to soften. Drain; squeeze out excess water. Discard stems; quarter caps.

2. Blend soy sauce with cornstarch in cup until smooth.

3. Cut chicken into 1-inch pieces; toss with garlic in small bowl. Heat wok or large skillet over medium-high heat; add oil. Add chicken mixture and celery; stir-fry 2 minutes. Add water chestnuts and bamboo shoots; stir-fry 1 minute. Add broth and mushrooms; cook and stir 3 minutes or until chicken is no longer pink. Stir soy sauce mixture and add to wok. Cook and stir 1 to 2 minutes or until sauce boils and thickens. Serve over rice, and garnish with green onions, if desired.

Makes 4 servings

Nutrients per Serving (¼ of total recipe without rice):
Calories: 208, Calories from Fat: 28%, Total Fat: 6g, Saturated Fat: 1g, Cholesterol: 58mg, Sodium: 657mg, Carbohydrate: 11g, Dietary Fiber: 1g, Protein: 25g

Dietary Exchanges: 2 Vegetable, 3 Lean Meat

Beef **and Broccoli**

1 pound lean beef tenderloin
2 teaspoons minced fresh ginger
2 cloves garlic, minced
½ teaspoon vegetable oil
3 cups broccoli florets
¼ cup water
2 tablespoons teriyaki sauce
2 cups hot cooked white rice
Red bell pepper, cut into thin strips (optional)

1. Cut beef across the grain into ⅛-inch slices; cut each slice into 1½-inch pieces. Toss beef with ginger and garlic in medium bowl.

2. Heat oil in wok or large nonstick skillet over medium heat. Add beef mixture; stir-fry 3 to 4 minutes or until beef is barely pink in center. Remove and reserve.

3. Add broccoli and water to wok; cover and steam 3 to 5 minutes or until broccoli is crisp-tender.

4. Return beef and any accumulated juices to wok. Add teriyaki sauce. Cook until heated through.

5. Serve over rice. Garnish with bell pepper strips, if desired. *Makes 4 servings*

Nutrients per Serving (¼ of total recipe):
Calories: 392, Calories from Fat: 26%, Total Fat: 11g, Saturated Fat: 4g, Cholesterol: 95mg, Sodium: 393mg, Carbohydrate: 34g, Dietary Fiber: 3g, Protein: 37g

Dietary Exchanges: 2 Starch, 1 Vegetable, 4 Lean Meat

Beef and Broccoli

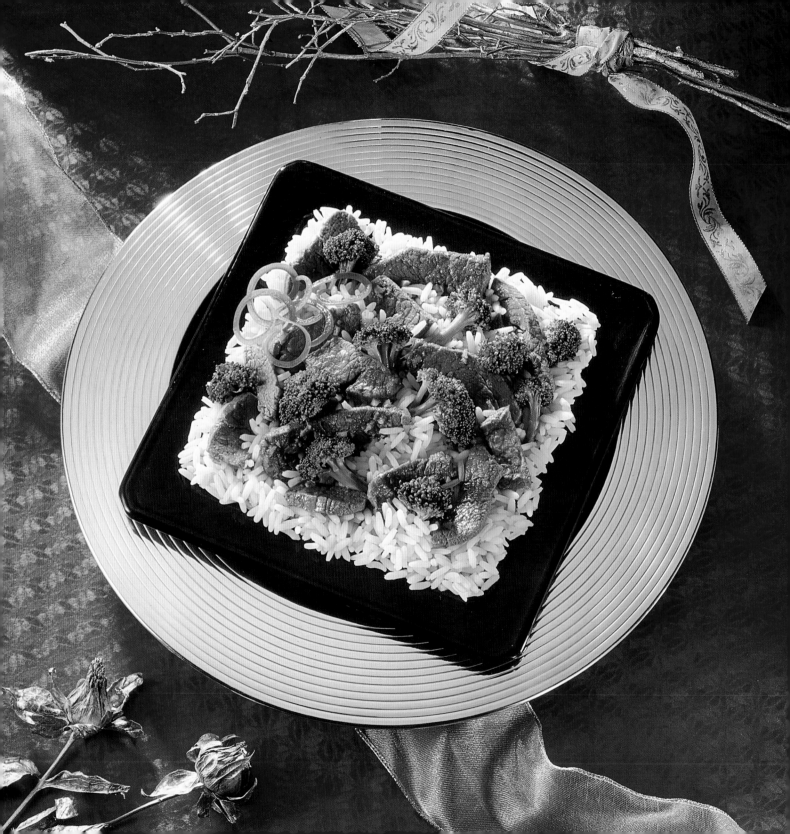

Asian Noodle Soup

4 ounces dried Chinese egg noodles

3 cans (14 ounces each) ⅓-less-salt chicken broth

2 slices fresh gingerroot

2 cloves garlic, peeled and cut into halves

½ cup fresh snow peas, cut into 1-inch pieces

3 tablespoons chopped green onions

1 tablespoon chopped fresh cilantro

1½ teaspoons hot chili oil

½ teaspoon dark sesame oil

   Red chili pepper strips for garnish (optional)

1. Cook noodles according to package directions, omitting salt. Drain and set aside.

2. Combine chicken broth, gingerroot and garlic in large saucepan; bring to a boil over high heat. Reduce heat to low; simmer about 15 minutes. Remove gingerroot and garlic with slotted spoon and discard.

3. Add snow peas, green onions, cilantro, chili oil and sesame oil to broth; simmer 3 to 5 minutes. Stir in noodles; serve immediately. Garnish with red chili pepper strips, if desired. *Makes 4 servings*

Nutrients per Serving (¼ of total recipe):
Calories: 118, Calories from Fat: 30%, Total Fat: 4g, Saturated Fat: <1g, Cholesterol: 4mg, Sodium: 152mg, Carbohydrate: 17g, Dietary Fiber: 3g, Protein: 4g

Dietary Exchanges: ½ Starch, 1½ Vegetable, 1 Fat

Asian Noodle Soup

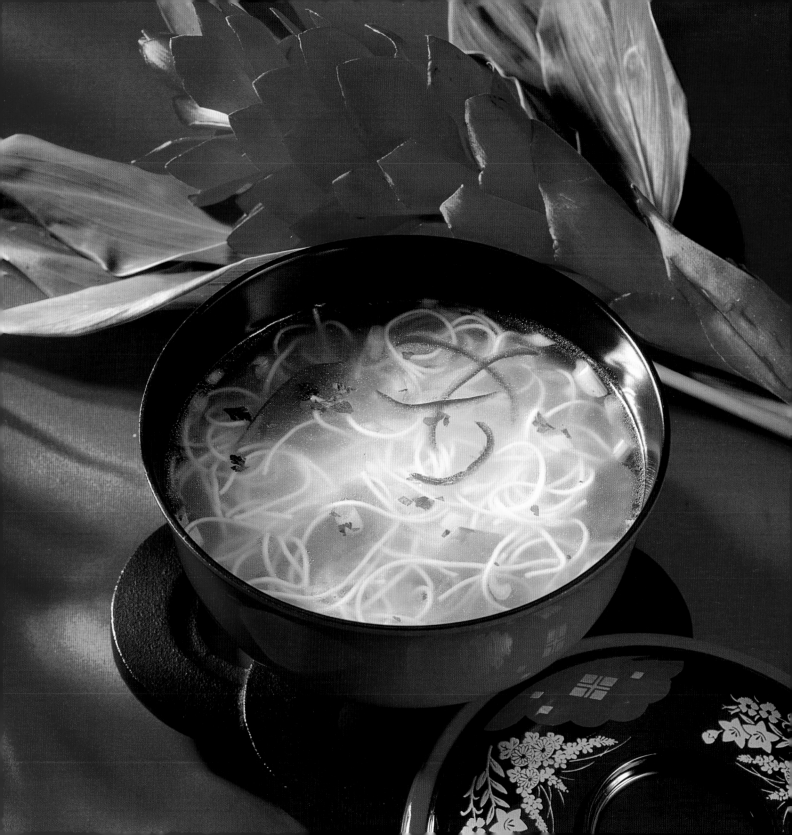

Oriental Chicken **Kabobs**

1 pound boneless skinless chicken breasts

2 small zucchini or yellow squash, cut into 1-inch slices

8 large fresh mushrooms

1 cup red, yellow or green bell pepper pieces

2 tablespoons low-sodium soy sauce

2 tablespoons dry sherry

1 teaspoon dark sesame oil

2 cloves garlic, minced

2 large green onions, cut into 1-inch pieces

1. Cut chicken into 1½-inch pieces; place in large plastic bag. Add zucchini, mushrooms and bell pepper to bag. Combine soy sauce, sherry, oil and garlic in cup; pour over chicken and vegetables. Close bag securely; turn to coat. Marinate in refrigerator at least 30 minutes or up to 4 hours.

2. Soak 4 (12-inch) skewers in water 20 minutes.

3. Drain chicken and vegetables; reserve marinade. Alternately thread chicken and vegetables with onions onto skewers.

4. Place on rack of broiler pan. Brush with half of reserved marinade. Broil 5 to 6 inches from heat 5 minutes. Turn kabobs over; brush with remaining marinade. Broil 5 minutes or until chicken is no longer pink. Garnish with green onion brushes, if desired.   *Makes 4 servings*

Nutrients per Serving (1 kabob):
Calories: 135, Calories from Fat: 21%, Total Fat: 3g, Saturated Fat: 1g, Cholesterol: 46mg, Sodium: 307mg, Carbohydrate: 6g, Dietary Fiber: 2g, Protein: 19g

Dietary Exchanges: 1 Vegetable, 2 Lean Meat

Oriental Chicken Kabobs

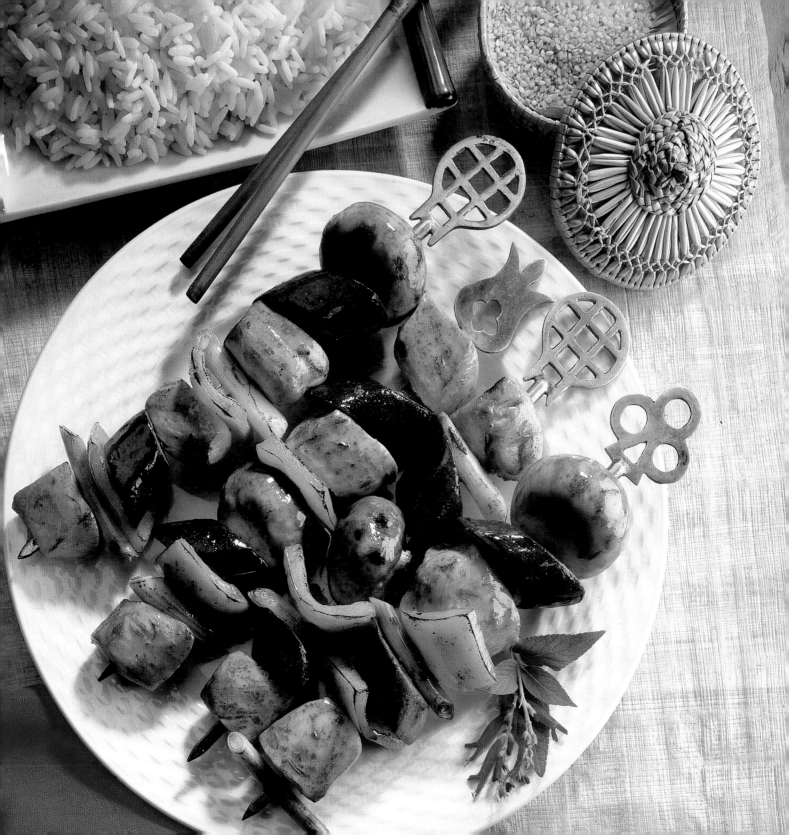

Thai Chicken Stir-Fry with Peanut Sauce

Peanut Sauce (recipe follows)
¾ pound boneless skinless chicken breasts
Nonstick cooking spray
1 small onion, thinly sliced
2 tablespoons water
1 large red bell pepper, diced
1 package (10 ounces) fresh spinach leaves, washed and torn
3 cups hot cooked white rice
3 tablespoons chopped fresh basil, mint or cilantro leaves

1. Prepare Peanut Sauce. Slice chicken breasts crosswise into thin strips.

2. Spray large nonstick skillet with cooking spray; heat over high heat. Add chicken; stir-fry 4 minutes or until no longer pink in center. Remove chicken; set aside. Add onion and water to same skillet; stir-fry 4 to 5 minutes or until water cooks away and onion is crisp-tender and golden. Stir in Peanut Sauce. Add bell pepper and chicken; bring to a boil. Cook and stir until slightly thickened and heated through.

3. Meanwhile, place steaming rack in large Dutch oven. Add water just to base of rack. Bring water to a boil over high heat. Place spinach on steaming rack. Turn spinach with tongs until bright green and beginning to wilt. Divide rice evenly among 4 plates. Place spinach on top of rice. Spoon chicken mixture over spinach. Sprinkle with basil. *Makes 4 servings*

Peanut Sauce

¼ cup reduced-fat creamy peanut butter

1 tablespoon brown sugar

2 teaspoons dark sesame oil

¼ teaspoon paprika

¼ teaspoon coconut extract (optional)

½ cup fat-free reduced-sodium chicken broth

2 tablespoons reduced-sodium soy sauce

3 tablespoons lime juice

Stir together peanut butter, sugar, sesame oil, paprika and coconut extract, if desired, in small bowl until blended. Add chicken broth, soy sauce and lime juice; stir until smooth. *Makes about 1 cup*

Nutrients per Serving (¼ of stir-fry with sauce):
Calories: 436, Calories from Fat: 23%, Total Fat: 11g, Saturated Fat: 2g, Cholesterol: 52mg, Sodium: 385mg, Carbohydrate: 54g, Dietary Fiber: 4g, Protein: 31g

Dietary Exchanges: 3 Starch, 2 Vegetable, 3 Lean Meat

recipe tip

Peanut butter, when included in a low-fat, heart-healthy eating plan, may help lower blood cholesterol and reduce the risk of heart disease.

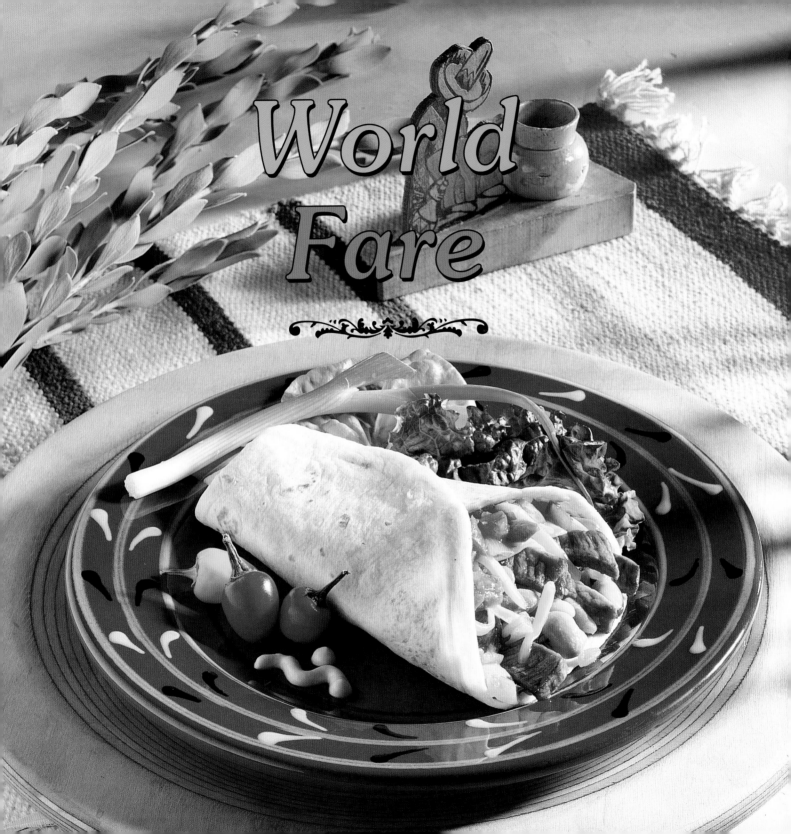

World Fare

Beef & Bean Burritos

Nonstick cooking spray
½ pound beef round steak, cut into ½-inch pieces
3 cloves garlic, minced
1 can (about 15 ounces) pinto beans, rinsed and drained
1 can (4 ounces) diced mild green chilies, drained
¼ cup finely chopped fresh cilantro
6 (6-inch) flour tortillas
½ cup (2 ounces) shredded reduced-fat Cheddar cheese
Salsa (optional)
Nonfat sour cream (optional)

1. Spray nonstick skillet with cooking spray; heat over medium heat until hot. Add steak and garlic; cook and stir 5 minutes or until steak is cooked to desired doneness.

2. Stir beans, chilies and cilantro into skillet; cook and stir 5 minutes or until heated through.

3. Spoon steak mixture evenly down center of each tortilla; sprinkle cheese evenly over top. Fold bottom end of tortilla over filling; roll to enclose. Garnish with salsa and nonfat sour cream, if desired.

Makes 6 servings

Nutrients per Serving (⅙ of total recipe):
Calories: 278, Calories from Fat: 22%, Total Fat: 7g, Saturated Fat: 2g, Cholesterol: 31mg, Sodium: 956mg, Carbohydrate: 36g, Dietary Fiber: 1g, Protein: 19g

Dietary Exchanges: 2 Starch, 1 Vegetable, 1½ Lean Meat, ½ Fat

Beef & Bean Burrito

Chicken Scaloppine with **Lemon-Caper Sauce**

1 pound boneless skinless chicken breasts

3 tablespoons all-purpose flour, divided

¼ teaspoon black pepper

¼ teaspoon chili powder

½ cup fat-free reduced-sodium chicken broth

1 tablespoon lemon juice

1 tablespoon drained capers

Nonstick cooking spray

½ teaspoon olive oil

1. Place chicken breasts, one at a time, between sheets of waxed paper. Pound to ¼-inch thickness. Combine 2 tablespoons flour, pepper and chili powder in shallow plate. Dip chicken pieces in flour mixture to lightly coat both sides.

2. Combine broth, lemon juice, remaining 1 tablespoon flour and capers in small bowl.

3. Spray large skillet with cooking spray; heat over medium-high heat. Place chicken in hot pan in single layer; cook 1½ minutes. Turn over; cook 1 to 1½ minutes or until chicken is no longer pink in center. Repeat with remaining chicken (brush pan with ¼ teaspoon oil each time you add pieces, to prevent sticking). If cooking more than 2 batches, reduce heat to medium to prevent burning chicken. Remove chicken from skillet.

4. Stir broth mixture and pour into skillet. Boil 1 to 2 minutes or until thickened. Serve immediately over chicken.

Makes 4 servings

Nutrients per Serving (¼ of total recipe):
Calories: 144, Calories from Fat: 26%, Total Fat: 4g, Saturated Fat: 1g, Cholesterol: 58mg, Sodium: 67mg, Carbohydrate: 4g, Dietary Fiber: <1g, Protein: 22g

Dietary Exchanges: 2½ Lean Meat

*Chicken Scaloppine with
Lemon-Caper Sauce*

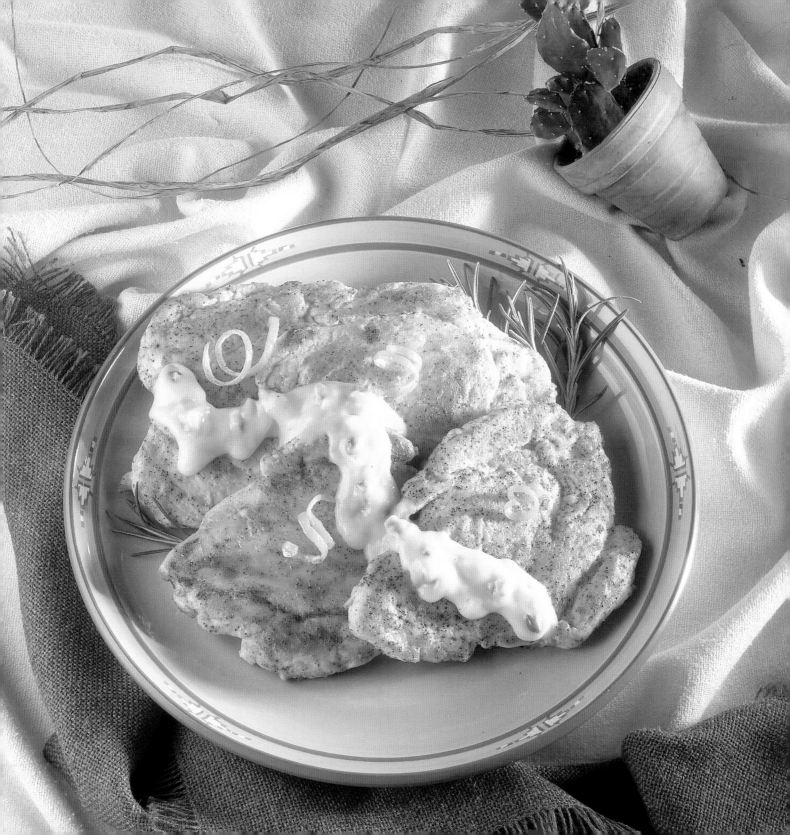

Quick Tuscan Bean, Tomato and Spinach Soup

2 cans (14½ ounces each) diced tomatoes with onions, undrained

1 can (14½ ounces) fat-free reduced-sodium chicken broth

2 teaspoons sugar

2 teaspoons dried basil leaves

¾ teaspoon reduced-sodium Worcestershire sauce

1 can (15 ounces) small white beans, rinsed and drained

3 ounces fresh baby spinach leaves or chopped spinach leaves, stems removed

2 teaspoons extra-virgin olive oil

1. Combine tomatoes with juice, chicken broth, sugar, basil and Worcestershire sauce in Dutch oven or large saucepan; bring to a boil over high heat. Reduce heat and simmer, uncovered, 10 minutes.

2. Stir in beans and spinach and cook 5 minutes longer or until spinach is tender.

3. Remove from heat; stir in oil just before serving.

Makes 4 servings

Nutrients per Serving (1½ cups):
Calories: 148, Calories from Fat: 20%, Total Fat: 4g, Saturated Fat: 1g, Cholesterol: 0mg, Sodium: 1218mg, Carbohydrate: 26g, Dietary Fiber: 7g, Protein: 9g

Dietary Exchanges: 1½ Starch, 1 Lean Meat

recipe tip ....

This soup is packed with phytochemicals in the tomatoes, spinach, and even beans. Phytochemicals are components of plant foods shown to help prevent heart disease, cancer, Alzheimer's and more.

Quick Tuscan Bean, Tomato and Spinach Soup

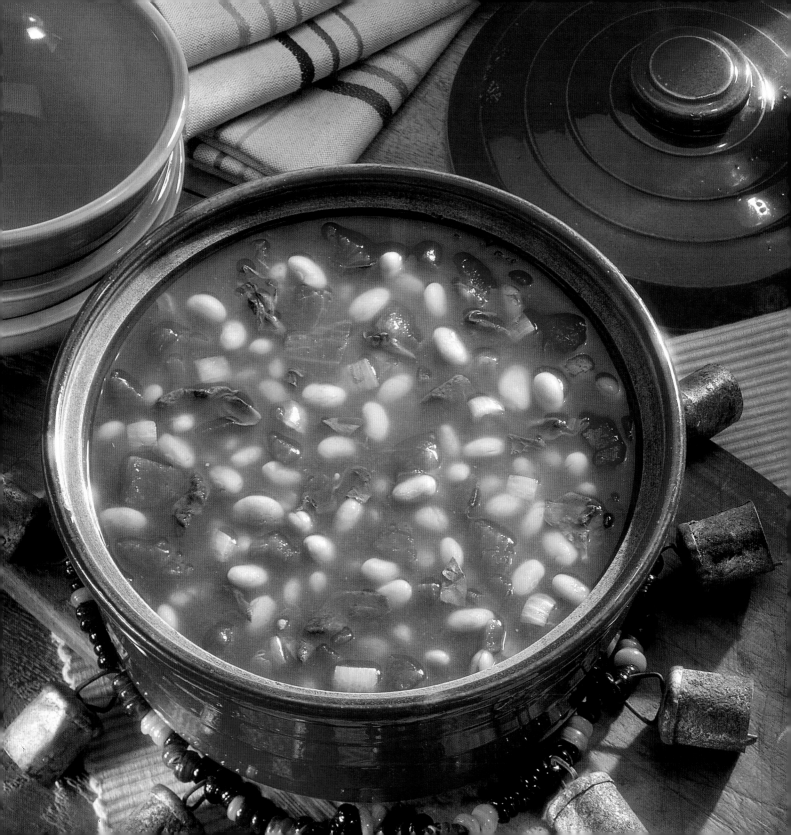

Spanish Braised Chicken
with Green Olives and Rice

2 pounds bone-in skinless chicken thighs

1 teaspoon paprika

   Nonstick cooking spray

¾ cup dry sherry

1 can (about 14 ounces) fat-free reduced-sodium chicken broth plus water to
   measure 2¼ cups

¾ cup sliced pimiento-stuffed green olives

1½ teaspoons dried sage leaves

1½ cups long-grain white rice

1. Sprinkle chicken thighs with paprika. Spray large nonstick skillet with cooking spray; heat over medium-high heat. Add thighs; cook, without stirring, 3 to 4 minutes or until golden. Turn chicken; cook 3 to 4 minutes.

2. Add sherry to skillet. Slide metal spatula under chicken and scrape cooked bits from bottom of skillet. Add chicken broth, olives and sage; bring to a boil. Reduce heat to low; cover and simmer 10 minutes. Pour rice into liquid around chicken; gently stir to distribute evenly in skillet. Return to a boil; cover and simmer 18 minutes or until liquid is absorbed and rice is tender.   *Makes 6 servings*

Nutrients per Serving (⅙ of total recipe):
Calories: 376, Calories from Fat: 25%, Total Fat: 10g, Saturated Fat: 2g, Cholesterol: 62mg, Sodium: 522mg, Carbohydrate: 40g, Dietary Fiber: 1g, Protein: 21g

Dietary Exchanges: 2½ Starch, 2 Lean Meat, 1 Fat

World Fare

Irish Stew

1 cup fat-free reduced-sodium chicken broth

1 teaspoon dried marjoram leaves

1 teaspoon dried parsley leaves

¾ teaspoon salt

½ teaspoon garlic powder

¼ teaspoon black pepper

1¼ pounds white potatoes, peeled and cut into 1-inch pieces

1 pound lean lamb stew meat, cut into 1-inch cubes

8 ounces frozen cut green beans

2 small leeks, cut lengthwise into halves then crosswise into slices

1½ cups coarsely chopped carrots

Slow Cooker Directions

Combine broth, marjoram, parsley, salt, garlic powder and pepper in large bowl; mix well. Pour mixture into slow cooker. Add potatoes, lamb, green beans, leeks and carrots. Cover and cook on LOW 7 to 9 hours.

Makes 6 servings

Nutrients per Serving (⅙ of total recipe):
Calories: 256, Calories from Fat: 20%, Total Fat: 32g, Saturated Fat: 2g, Cholesterol: 52mg, Sodium: 388mg, Carbohydrate: 32g, Dietary Fiber: 5g, Protein: 20g

Dietary Exchanges: 1 Starch, 3 Vegetable, 2 Lean Meat

recipe tip

Leeks are notorious for collecting soil and grit between their leaf layers. After halving the leeks in this recipe, rinse them thoroughly under cold running water to remove any embedded soil. For really stubborn dirt, soak the leeks in a bowl of water for 15 minutes, changing the water until it is clear and the leeks are free of dirt.

World Fare

Italian-Style **Brisket**

¾ cup fat-free reduced-sodium beef broth or water, divided
½ cup chopped onion
1 clove garlic, minced
1 can (14½ ounces) no-salt-added diced tomatoes, undrained
¼ cup dry red wine
¾ teaspoon dried oregano leaves
¼ teaspoon dried thyme leaves
¼ teaspoon black pepper
1¼ pounds well-trimmed beef brisket
3 cups sliced mushrooms
3 cups halved and thinly sliced zucchini
3 cups cooked egg noodles

1. Heat ¼ cup beef broth in Dutch oven. Add onion and garlic; cover and simmer 5 minutes. Stir in tomatoes with juice, remaining ½ cup beef broth, red wine, oregano, thyme and pepper. Bring to a boil.

2. Reduce heat to low; add beef brisket. Cover and simmer 1½ hours, basting occasionally with tomato mixture.

3. Add mushrooms and zucchini; simmer, covered, 30 to 45 minutes or until beef is tender.

4. Remove beef. Simmer vegetable mixture 5 to 10 minutes to thicken slightly. Cut beef across the grain into 12 thin slices.

Makes 6 servings

Nutrients per Serving (⅙ of total recipe):
Calories: 283, Calories from Fat: 20%, Total Fat: 6g, Saturated Fat: 2g, Cholesterol: 81mg, Sodium: 107mg, Carbohydrate: 28g, Dietary Fiber: 3g, Protein: 27g

Dietary Exchanges: 1 Starch, 2 Vegetable, 3 Lean Meat

Italian-Style Brisket

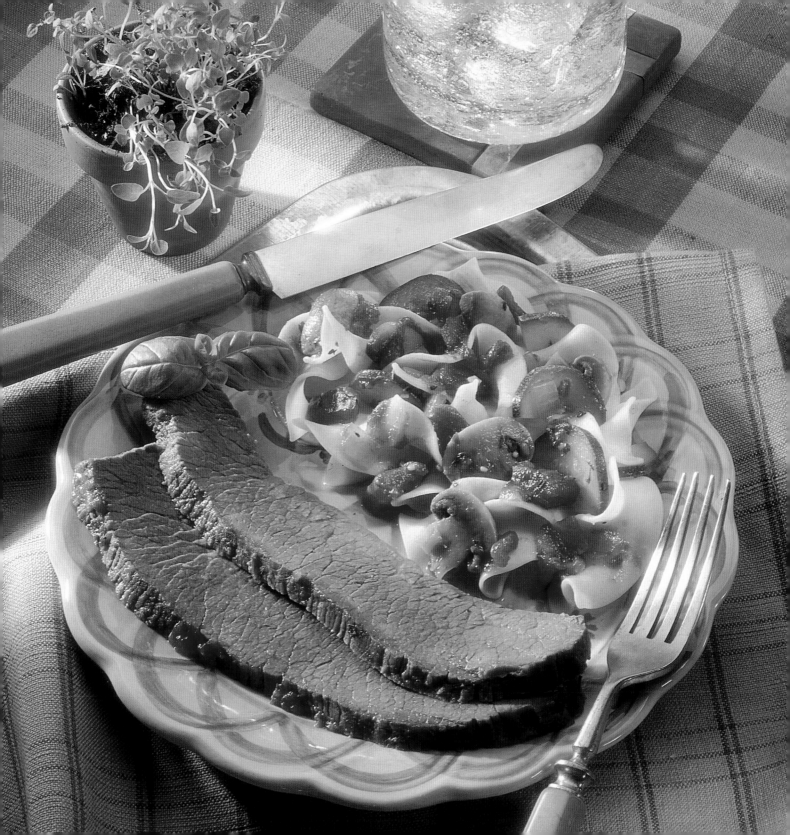

Marinated Chicken and Pesto Pizza

8 ounces chicken tenders
¼ cup prepared fat-free Italian salad dressing
 Nonstick cooking spray
½ cup sun-dried tomatoes
1 cup chopped plum tomatoes
1 tablespoon prepared pesto
1 teaspoon salt-free Italian herb blend
¼ teaspoon red pepper flakes
1 (12-inch) prepared pizza crust
1 cup (4 ounces) shredded part-skim mozzarella cheese

1. Cut chicken tenders into 2×½-inch strips. Place in resealable plastic food storage bag. Pour Italian dressing over chicken. Seal bag and turn to coat. Marinate at room temperature 15 minutes, turning several times. Remove chicken from marinade; discard marinade. Spray large nonstick skillet with cooking spray; heat over medium heat until hot. Add chicken; cook and stir 5 minutes or until no longer pink in center.

2. Meanwhile, cover sun-dried tomatoes with boiling water in small bowl; let stand 10 minutes. Drain; cut tomatoes into ¼-inch strips.

3. Preheat oven to 450°F. Combine plum tomatoes, pesto, herb blend and pepper in small bowl. Spread on pizza crust. Add chicken and sun-dried tomatoes; sprinkle with cheese.

4. Bake 8 to 10 minutes or until cheese melts and pizza is heated through. *Makes 6 servings*

Nutrients per Serving (⅙ of pizza):
Calories: 322, Calories from Fat: 29%, Total Fat: 10g, Saturated Fat: 1g, Cholesterol: 30mg, Sodium: 512mg, Carbohydrate: 38g, Dietary Fiber: 3g, Protein: 16g

Dietary Exchanges: 2½ Starch, 1 Vegetable, 1½ Lean Meat, ½ Fat

Marinated Chicken and Pesto Pizza

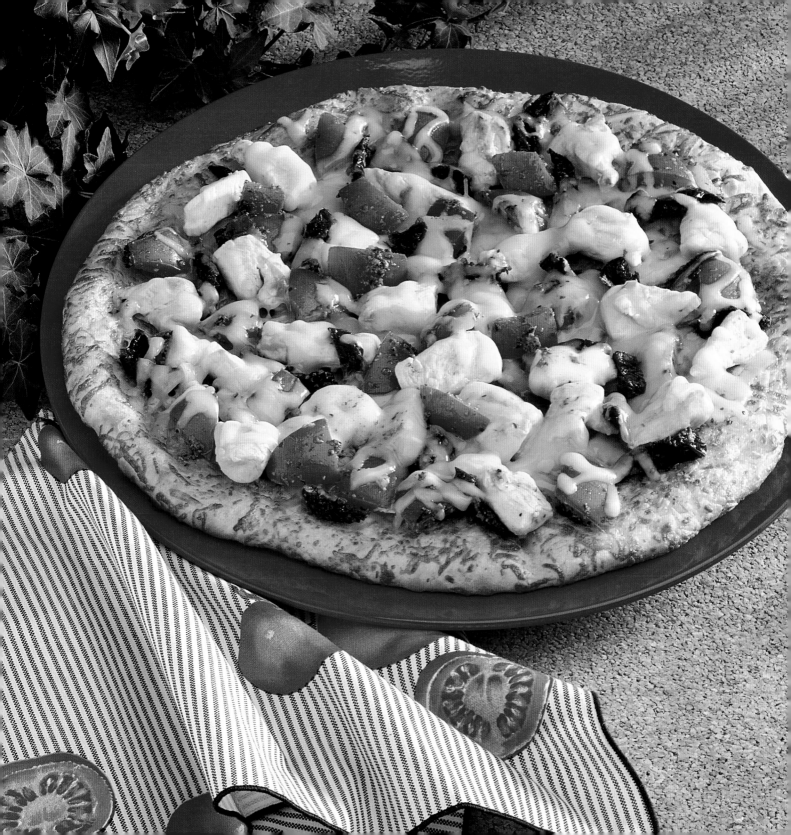

Linguine with **White Clam Sauce**

2 tablespoons CRISCO® Oil*

2 cloves garlic, minced

2 cans (6½ ounces *each*) chopped clams, undrained

½ cup chopped fresh parsley

¼ cup dry white wine or clam juice

1 teaspoon dried basil leaves

1 pound linguine, cooked (without salt or fat) and well drained

Use your favorite Crisco Oil product.

1. Heat oil and garlic in medium skillet on medium heat.

2. Drain clams, reserving liquid. Add reserved liquid and parsley to skillet. Reduce heat to low. Simmer 3 minutes, stirring occasionally.

3. Add clams, wine and basil. Simmer 5 minutes, stirring occasionally. Add to hot linguine. Toss lightly to coat. *Makes 8 servings*

Nutrients per Serving (⅛ of total recipe):
Calories: 266, Calories from Fat: 20%, Total Fat: 6g, Saturated Fat: <1g, Cholesterol: 31mg, Sodium: 166mg, Carbohydrate: 33g, Dietary Fiber: 2g, Protein: 18g

Dietary Exchanges: 2 Starch, 2 Lean Meat

recipe tip ....
Canned clams can often be found near the pasta section in supermarkets.

Turkey Stuffed Chiles Rellenos

1 package (1½ pounds) BUTTERBALL® 99% Fat Free Fresh Ground Turkey Breast
1 envelope (1¼ ounces) taco seasoning mix
⅓ cup water
6 large poblano chilies, stems on, slit lengthwise and seeded
1 cup (4 ounces) shredded reduced-fat Cheddar cheese
1½ cups tomato salsa

Spray large nonstick skillet with nonstick cooking spray; heat over medium heat until hot. Brown turkey in skillet over medium-high heat 6 to 8 minutes or until no longer pink, stirring to separate meat. Add taco seasoning and water. Bring to a boil. Reduce heat to low; simmer 5 minutes, stirring occasionally. In separate pan, cook chilies in boiling water 5 minutes; remove and drain. Combine turkey mixture and Cheddar cheese. Fill chilies with mixture. Pour salsa into 11×7-inch baking dish. Place stuffed chilies slit side up in baking dish. Bake, uncovered, in preheated 400°F oven 15 minutes. Serve hot with additional salsa and sour cream, if desired. *Makes 6 servings*

Preparation Time: 30 minutes

Nutrients per Serving (1 stuffed chili):
Calories: 244, Calories from Fat: 19%, Total Fat: 5g, Saturated Fat: 3g, Cholesterol: 75mg, Sodium: 848mg, Carbohydrate: 15g, Dietary Fiber: 1g, Protein: 35g

Dietary Exchanges: 2 Vegetable, 4 Lean Meat

World Fare

Black Bean Pancakes & Salsa

1 cup GUILTLESS GOURMET® Black Bean Dip (Spicy or Mild)

2 egg whites

½ cup unbleached all-purpose flour

½ cup skim milk

1 tablespoon canola oil

Nonstick cooking spray

½ cup fat free sour cream

½ cup GUILTLESS GOURMET® Roasted Red Pepper Salsa

Yellow tomatoes and fresh mint leaves (optional)

For pancake batter, place bean dip, egg whites, flour, milk and oil in blender or food processor; blend until smooth. Refrigerate 2 hours or overnight.

Preheat oven to 350°F. Coat large nonstick skillet with cooking spray; heat over medium heat until hot. For each pancake, spoon 2 tablespoons batter into skillet; cook until bubbles form and break on pancake surface. Turn pancakes over; cook until lightly browned on other side. Place on baking sheet; keep warm in oven. Repeat to make 16 small pancakes. (If batter becomes too thick, thin with more milk.) Serve hot with sour cream and salsa. Garnish with tomatoes and mint, if desired.

Makes 4 servings

Nutrients per Serving (4 pancakes plus 1 ounce sour cream):
Calories: 192, Calories from Fat: 18%, Total Fat: 4g, Saturated Fat: 0g, Cholesterol: 0mg, Sodium: 746mg, Carbohydrate: 27g, Dietary Fiber: 2g, Protein: 12g

Dietary Exchanges: 1½ Starch, 1 Lean Meat

World Fare

Black Bean Pancakes & Salsa

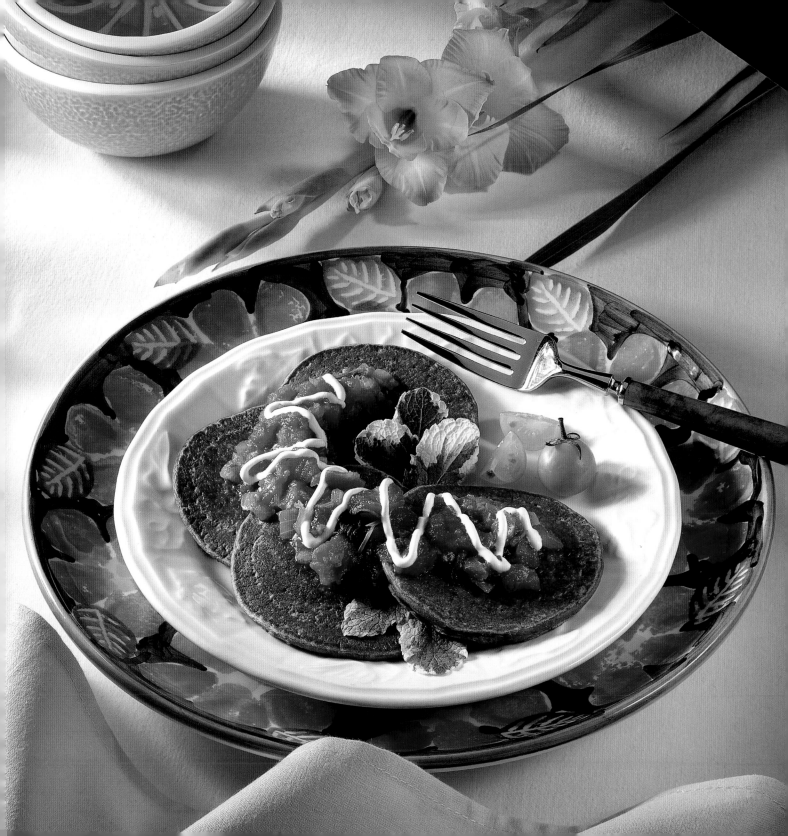

Spicy Lasagna Roll-Ups

Nonstick cooking spray
1 pound ground turkey breast or extra-lean ground beef
½ cup chopped onion
2 cloves garlic, minced
1 teaspoon dried Italian seasoning
¼ teaspoon red pepper flakes
1 can (10¾ ounces) reduced-fat condensed tomato soup, undiluted
1 cup chopped zucchini
¾ cup water
1 (15-ounce) container fat-free ricotta cheese
½ cup shredded part-skim mozzarella cheese
1 egg
4 lasagna noodles, cooked without added salt or fat

1. Preheat oven to 350°F. Spray large nonstick skillet with cooking spray; heat over medium heat until hot. Add turkey, onion, garlic, Italian seasoning and red pepper flakes; cook and stir until turkey is no longer pink and onion is tender. Add soup, zucchini and water; simmer 5 minutes. Pour soup mixture into shallow 2-quart baking dish.

2. Combine ricotta and mozzarella cheeses and egg in medium bowl; mix well. Lay lasagna noodles on flat surface; spread ½ cup cheese mixture onto each noodle. Roll up noodles, enclosing filling; place rolls seam-side-down over soup mixture.

3. Cover and bake 30 minutes; uncover and continue baking an additional 10 minutes or until sauce is bubbly. Place lasagna rolls on serving dish; spoon sauce over rolls. *Makes 4 servings*

Nutrients per Serving (1 Roll-Up):
Calories: 562, Calories from Fat: 17%, Total Fat: 11g, Saturated Fat: 4g, Cholesterol: 121mg, Sodium: 642mg, Carbohydrate: 67g, Dietary Fiber: 3g, Protein: 50g

Dietary Exchanges: 4 Starch, 2 Vegetable, 4 Lean Meat

Spicy Lasagna Roll-Ups

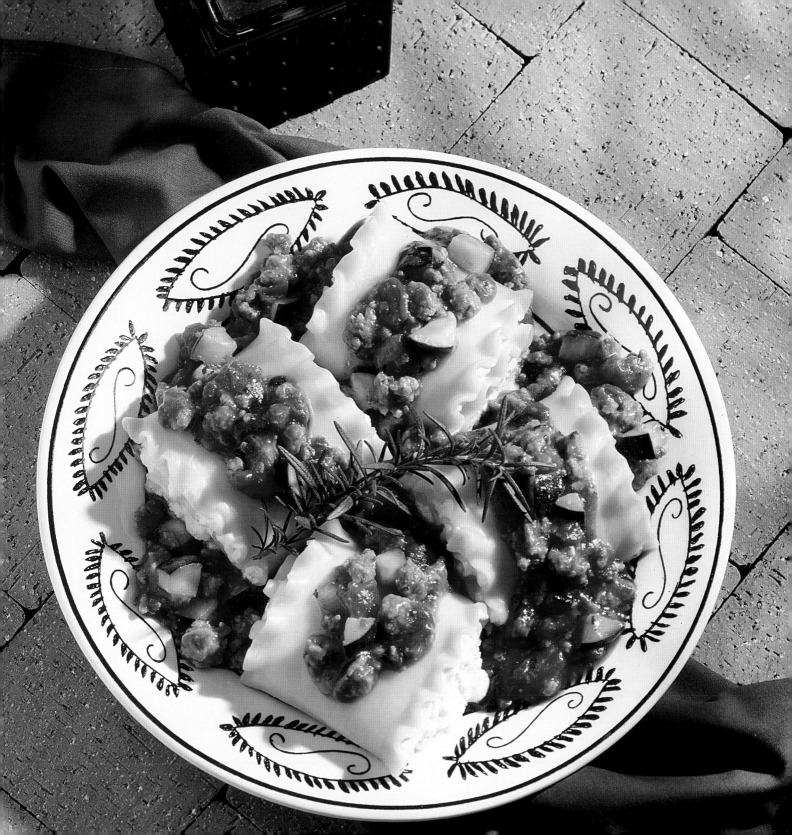

Moroccan Lentil & Vegetable Soup

1 tablespoon olive oil

1 cup chopped onion

4 medium cloves garlic, minced

½ cup dry lentils, sorted, rinsed and drained

1½ teaspoons ground coriander

1½ teaspoons ground cumin

½ teaspoon black pepper

½ teaspoon ground cinnamon

3¾ cups fat-free reduced-sodium chicken broth

½ cup chopped celery

½ cup chopped sun-dried tomatoes (not packed in oil)

1 medium yellow summer squash, chopped

½ cup chopped green bell pepper

½ cup chopped fresh parsley

1 cup chopped plum tomatoes

¼ cup chopped fresh cilantro or basil

1. Heat oil in medium saucepan over medium heat. Add onion and garlic; cook 4 to 5 minutes or until onion is tender, stirring occasionally. Stir in lentils, coriander, cumin, black pepper and cinnamon; cook 2 minutes. Add chicken broth, celery and sun-dried tomatoes; bring to a boil over high heat. Reduce heat to low; simmer, covered, 25 minutes.

2. Stir in squash, bell pepper and parsley. Continue cooking, covered, 10 minutes or until lentils are tender. Top with plum tomatoes and cilantro just before serving. *Makes 6 servings*

Nutrients per Serving (⅙ of total recipe):
Calories: 131, Calories from Fat: 20%, Total Fat: 3g, Saturated Fat: <1g, Cholesterol: 0mg, Sodium: 264mg, Carbohydrate: 20g, Dietary Fiber: 2g, Protein: 8g

Dietary Exchanges: 1 Starch, 1 Vegetable, ½ Fat

Moroccan Lentil & Vegetable Soup

World Fare

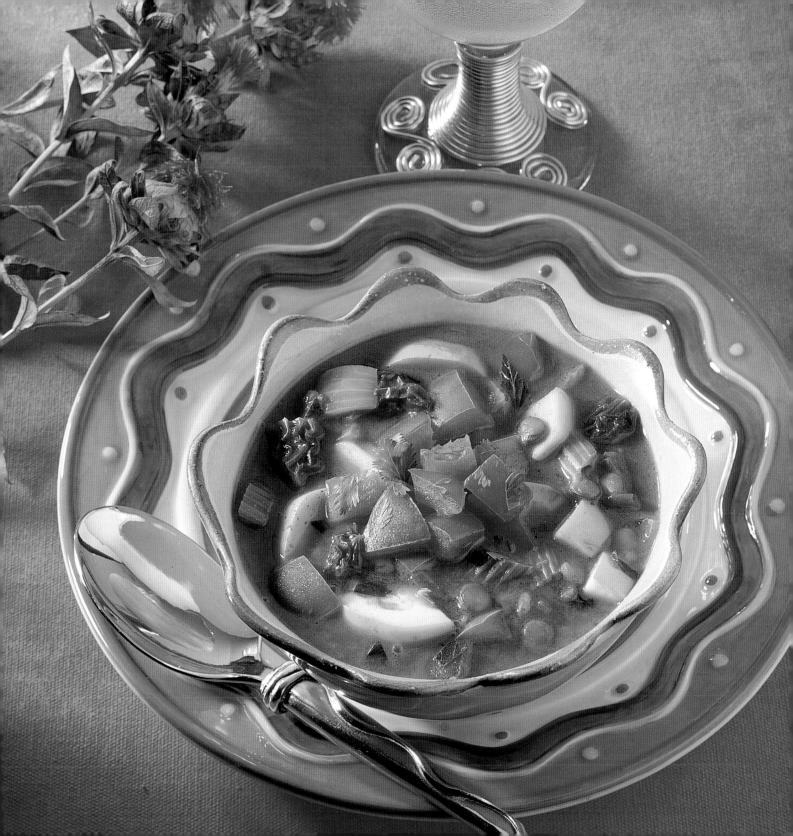

Tortilla "Pizza"

1 can (10 ounces) chunk white chicken in water, drained
1 can (14½ ounces) Mexican-style stewed tomatoes, drained
1 green onion, minced
2 teaspoons cumin, divided
½ teaspoon garlic powder
1 cup fat-free refried beans
¼ cup chopped fresh cilantro, divided
2 large or 4 small flour tortillas
1 cup (4 ounces) shredded Monterey Jack cheese with jalapeño peppers

1. Preheat broiler. Combine chicken and tomatoes in medium bowl. Add green onion, 1 teaspoon cumin and garlic powder. Mix well; set aside.

2. Mix refried beans, remaining 1 teaspoon cumin and 2 tablespoons cilantro in small bowl. Set aside.

3. Place tortillas on baking sheet. Broil 30 seconds to 1 minute per side or until crisp but not browned. Remove from oven. *Decrease oven temperature to 400°F.* Spread each tortilla evenly with bean mixture. Spoon chicken mixture over beans; top with cheese. Bake 5 minutes.

4. Reset oven temperature to broil. Broil tortillas 2 to 3 minutes or until cheese melts. Do not let tortilla edges burn. Remove from oven; top with remaining cilantro. Serve immediately. (If using large tortillas, cut each in half.)

Makes 4 servings

Serving Suggestion: Serve with a green salad tossed with avocado pieces and lemon vinaigrette.

Prep and Cook Time: 19 minutes

Nutrients per Serving (¼ of total recipe):
Calories: 339, Calories from Fat: 44%, Total Fat: 16g, Saturated Fat: 8g, Cholesterol: 69mg, Sodium: 913mg, Carbohydrate: 21g, Dietary Fiber: 3g, Protein: 25g

Dietary Exchanges: 1 Starch, 1 Vegetable, 3 Lean Meat, 2 Fat

Chicken **Provençal**

3 tablespoons low-fat plain yogurt

2 tablespoons mayonnaise

½ small clove garlic, minced

1 (3-pound) broiler-fryer chicken, cut up and skinned

½ teaspoon dried thyme

Salt (optional)

Black pepper (optional)

1 tablespoon vegetable oil

1 can (14½ ounces) DEL MONTE® Original Recipe Stewed Tomatoes

1 can (8 ounces) DEL MONTE® Tomato Sauce

2 small zucchini, sliced

1. Combine yogurt, mayonnaise and garlic in small bowl; set aside.

2. Sprinkle chicken with thyme. Season with salt and pepper, if desired. In large skillet, brown chicken in oil over medium-high heat; drain.

3. Add tomatoes and tomato sauce; cover and simmer about 20 minutes or until chicken is no longer pink, stirring occasionally. Add zucchini during last 5 minutes. Serve with garlic sauce.

Makes 6 servings

Prep Time: 5 minutes
Cook Time: 30 minutes

Nutrients per Serving (⅙ of total recipe):
Calories: 357, Calories from Fat: 42%, Total Fat: 17g, Saturated Fat: 5g, Cholesterol: 161mg, Sodium: 621mg, Carbohydrate: 10g, Dietary Fiber: 3g, Protein: 43g

Dietary Exchanges: 1½ Vegetable, 6 Lean Meat

World Fare

Chili Beef & Red Pepper Fajitas
with Chipotle Salsa

   6 ounces top sirloin steak, thinly sliced

½ lime

1½ teaspoons chili powder

½ teaspoon ground cumin

½ cup diced plum tomatoes

¼ cup mild picante sauce

½ canned chipotle chili pepper in adobo sauce (optional)

   Nonstick cooking spray

½ cup sliced onion

½ medium red bell pepper, cut into thin strips

 2 (10-inch) fat-free flour tortillas, warmed

¼ cup nonfat sour cream

 2 tablespoons chopped fresh cilantro leaves (optional)

Place steak on plate. Squeeze lime over top; sprinkle with chili powder and cumin. Toss to coat well; let stand 10 minutes. Meanwhile, combine tomatoes and picante sauce in small bowl. If using chipotle, mash completely on small plate. Stir into tomato mixture. Coat 12-inch skillet with cooking spray. Heat over high heat. Add onion and pepper; cook and stir 3 minutes or until beginning to blacken on edges; remove. Lightly spray skillet with cooking spray. Add beef; cook and stir 1 minute. Return onion and pepper; cook 1 minute. Place ½ beef mixture in center of each tortilla; top with ¼ cup salsa, 2 tablespoons sour cream and cilantro, if desired. Fold or serve open-faced. *Makes 2 servings*

Nutrients per Serving (½ of total recipe):
Calories: 245, Calories from Fat: 16%, Total Fat: 4g, Saturated Fat: 2g, Cholesterol: 45mg, Sodium: 530mg, Carbohydrate: 31g, Dietary Fiber: 9g, Protein: 21g

Dietary Exchanges: 1 Starch, 2 Vegetable, 2 Lean Meat

Chili Beef & Red Pepper Fajita
with Chipotle Salsa

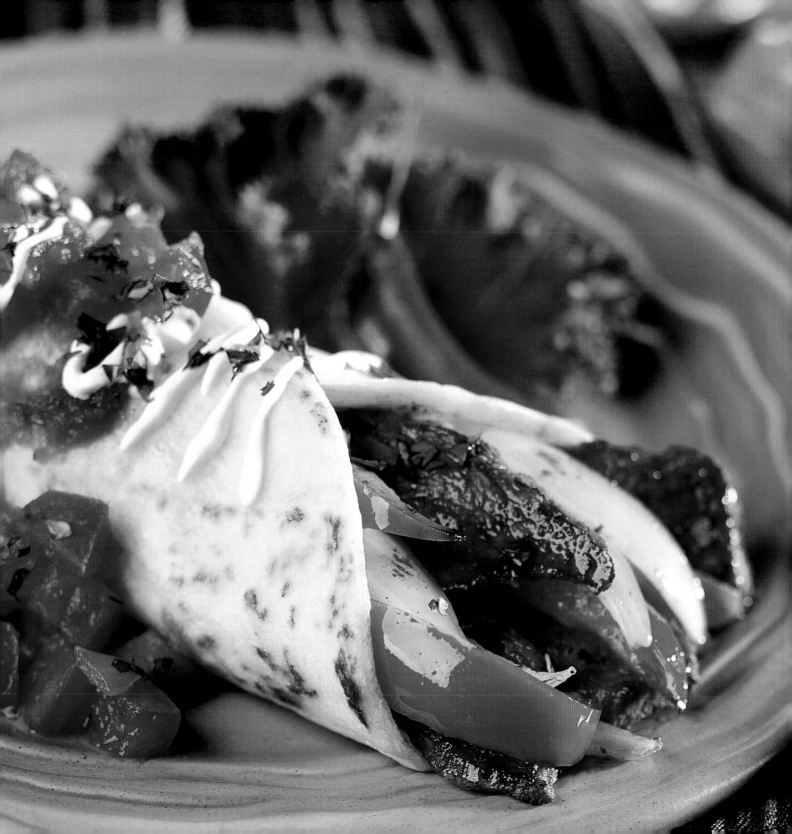

Refreshing Gazpacho

2 cups low-sodium tomato juice

1 can (about 14 ounces) fat-free reduced-sodium beef broth

1 can (10¾ ounces) reduced-fat condensed tomato soup, undiluted

1½ cups peeled and diced cucumbers

1½ cups diced green bell peppers

1 cup shredded carrots

1 cup diced celery

½ cup sliced green onions

⅓ cup chopped fresh parsley

2 cloves garlic, minced

1 tablespoon lime juice

2 teaspoons low-sodium Worcestershire sauce

½ teaspoon salt (optional)

½ teaspoon dried oregano leaves

Fat-free sour cream

Chopped fresh cilantro

Combine tomato juice, beef broth, soup, cucumbers, peppers, carrots, celery, green onions, parsley, garlic, lime juice, Worcestershire, salt, if desired, and oregano in large bowl. Chill at least 2 hours to blend flavors. Top with sour cream and cilantro. *Makes 4 servings*

Nutrients per Serving (¼ of total recipe):
Calories: 136, Calories from Fat: 11%, Total Fat: 2g, Saturated Fat: <1g, Cholesterol: 0mg, Sodium: 423mg, Carbohydrate: 28g, Dietary Fiber: 5g, Protein: 6g

Dietary Exchanges: 1 Starch, 3 Vegetable

Baked Chicken and Garlic Orzo

Nonstick cooking spray
4 chicken breast halves, skinned
¼ cup dry white wine
10 ounces uncooked orzo pasta
1 cup chopped onions
4 cloves garlic, minced
2 tablespoons chopped fresh parsley
1 teaspoon dried oregano leaves
1 can (about 14 ounces) fat-free reduced-sodium chicken broth
¼ cup water
Paprika
1 teaspoon lemon pepper
¼ teaspoon salt
2 teaspoons olive oil
1 lemon, cut into 8 wedges

1. Preheat oven to 350°F. Spray large nonstick skillet with cooking spray. Heat over high heat until hot. Add chicken breast halves. Brown, meat side down, 1 to 2 minutes or until lightly browned. Remove chicken from skillet; set aside.

2. Reduce heat to medium-high; add wine. Stir with flat spatula, scraping brown bits from bottom of pan. Cook 30 seconds or until slightly reduced; set aside.

3. Spray 9-inch square baking pan with nonstick cooking spray. Add pasta, onions, garlic, parsley, oregano, chicken broth, water and wine mixture; stir. Place chicken breasts on top. Sprinkle lightly with paprika and lemon pepper. Bake, uncovered, 1 hour and 10 minutes. Remove chicken. Add salt and olive oil to baking pan; mix well. Place chicken on top. Serve with lemon. *Makes 4 servings*

Nutrients per Serving (¼ of total recipe):
Calories: 483, Calories from Fat: 13%, Total Fat: 7g, Saturated Fat: 1g, Cholesterol: 73mg, Sodium: 231mg, Carbohydrate: 64g, Dietary Fiber: 1g, Protein: 38g

Dietary Exchanges: 4 Starch, 1 Vegetable, 3 Lean Meat

World Fare

Turkey Bolognese Sauce

½ cup *each* chopped onion, chopped carrots and chopped celery
¼ cup chopped green bell pepper
2 ounces Canadian bacon, chopped
2 cloves garlic, minced
1 tablespoon olive oil
½ pound ground turkey breast
½ cup ⅓-less-salt chicken broth
1 can (10 ounces) no-salt-added whole tomatoes, undrained
¼ cup no-salt-added tomato paste
1 bay leaf
¼ teaspoon grated nutmeg
⅛ teaspoon black pepper
½ pound fresh mushrooms, sliced
½ cup low fat (1%) milk

1. Place onion, carrots, celery, bell pepper, bacon and garlic in large saucepan. Add oil; cook and stir over medium heat 5 minutes or until vegetables are tender. Add turkey; cook and stir until completely browned. Add broth, tomatoes, tomato paste, bay leaf, nutmeg and black pepper. Bring to a boil over high heat; cover and reduce heat to medium. Simmer 45 minutes, stirring occasionally. Uncover; simmer 15 minutes.

2. Add mushrooms; simmer 10 minutes. Stir in milk; simmer 5 minutes. Remove bay leaf before serving. *Makes 8 servings*

Note: This sauce tastes great served over hot cooked pasta.

Nutrients per Serving (⅛ of sauce without pasta):
Calories: 94, Calories from Fat: 27%, Total Fat: 3g, Saturated Fat: 1g, Cholesterol: 17mg, Sodium: 145mg, Carbohydrate: 9g, Dietary Fiber: 2g, Protein: 9g

Dietary Exchanges: 1½ Vegetable, 1 Lean Meat

Turkey Bolognese Sauce

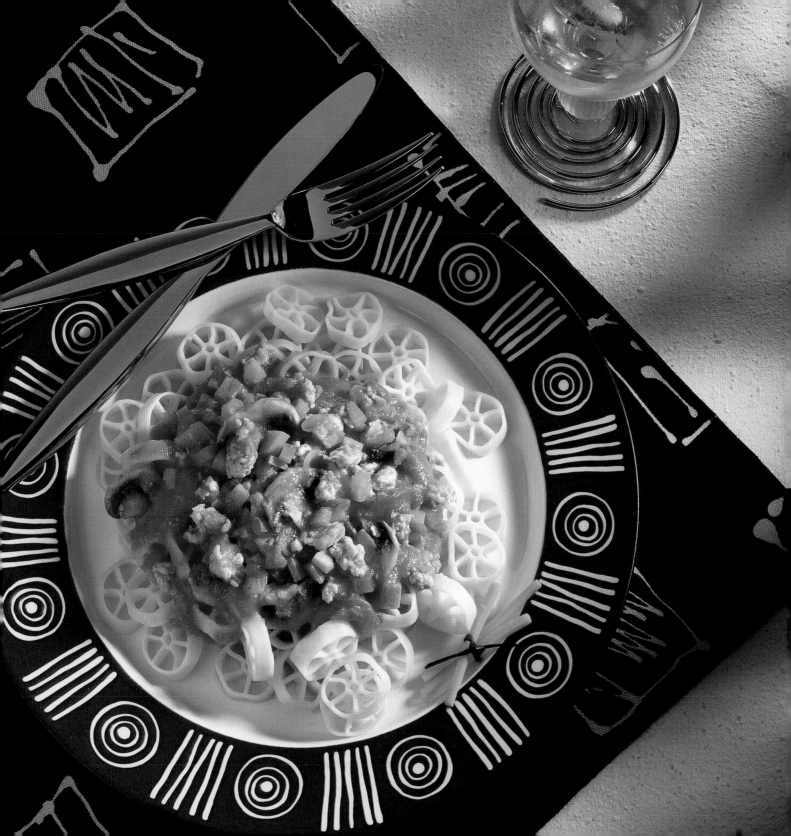

Seafood Paella

1 tablespoon olive oil

4 cloves garlic, minced

4½ cups finely chopped onions

2 cups uncooked long-grain white rice

2 cups *each* clam juice and dry white wine

3 tablespoons fresh lemon juice

½ teaspoon paprika

¼ cup boiling water

½ teaspoon saffron or ground turmeric

1½ cups peeled and diced plum tomatoes

½ cup chopped fresh parsley

1 jar (8 ounces) roasted red peppers, drained and thinly sliced, divided

1 pound bay scallops

1½ cups frozen peas, thawed

10 clams, scrubbed

10 mussels, scrubbed

1 cup water

20 large shrimp (1 pound), shelled and deveined

Preheat oven to 375°F. Heat oil in large ovenproof skillet or paella pan over medium-low heat. Add garlic; cook just until it sizzles. Add onions and rice; cook and stir 10 minutes or until onions are soft. Stir in clam juice, wine, lemon juice and paprika; mix well. Combine boiling water and saffron in small bowl; stir until saffron is dissolved. Stir into onion mixture. Stir in tomatoes, parsley and half the red peppers. Bring to a boil over medium heat. Remove from heat; cover. Place on lowest shelf of oven. Bake 1 hour or until liquid is absorbed. Remove; stir in scallops and peas. Turn off oven; return paella.

continued on page 312

Seafood Paella

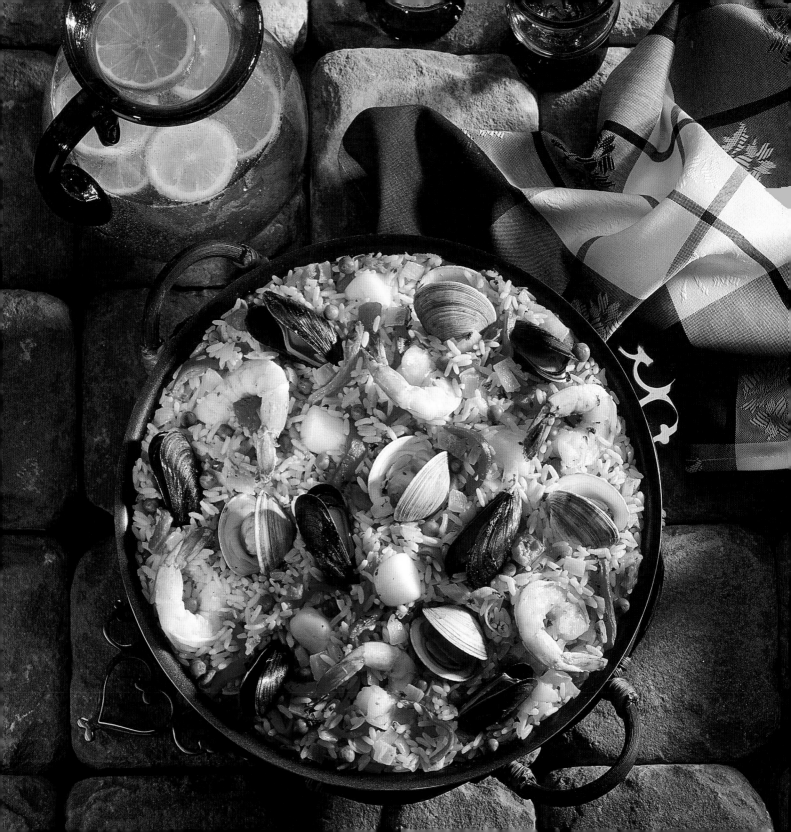

In Dutch oven, steam clams and mussels 4 to 6 minutes in 1 cup water, removing each as shell opens. (Discard unopened clams or mussels.) Steam shrimp 2 to 3 minutes just until shrimp turn pink and opaque. Remove paella; arrange shellfish on top. Garnish with red peppers.   *Makes 10 servings*

Nutrients per Serving (¹⁄₁₀ of total recipe):
Calories: 357, Calories from Fat: 9%, Total Fat: 4g, Saturated Fat: 1g, Cholesterol: 98mg, Sodium: 281mg, Carbohydrate: 46g, Dietary Fiber: 3g, Protein: 27g

Dietary Exchanges: 2½ Starch, 2½ Vegetable, 2 Lean Meat

Fettuccine **Alfredo**

          2 teaspoons margarine
          3 cloves garlic, finely chopped
        4½ teaspoons all-purpose flour
        1½ cups fat-free (skim) milk
          ½ cup grated Parmesan cheese
        3½ teaspoons Neufchâtel cheese
          ¼ teaspoon white pepper
          4 ounces hot cooked fettuccine
          ¼ cup chopped fresh parsley

Melt margarine in medium saucepan. Add garlic. Cook and stir 1 minute. Stir in flour. Gradually stir in milk. Cook until sauce thickens, stirring constantly. Add cheeses and pepper; cook until melted. Serve on fettuccine; top with parsley.   *Makes 4 servings*

Nutrients per Serving (¼ of total recipe):
Calories: 242, Calories from Fat: 33%, Total Fat: 9g, Saturated Fat: 4g, Cholesterol: 18mg, Sodium: 344mg, Carbohydrate: 27g, Dietary Fiber: 1g, Protein: 14g

Dietary Exchanges: 2 Starch, 1 Lean Meat, 1 Fat

Turkey Enchiladas

1 pound ground turkey (98% fat-free, if available)
1 cup minced onion
½ cup (2 ounces) grated reduced-fat Cheddar cheese
½ cup (4 ounces) diced mild green chilies
½ cup finely chopped green onions
½ cup nonfat yogurt
½ cup (2 ounces) finely chopped California walnuts
   Salt and pepper, if desired
8 flour tortillas (7 to 8 inches)
   Additional 1 to 1½ cups yogurt
   Sprigs fresh cilantro or parsley
   Tomato salsa

For filling, place turkey and onion in large nonstick skillet. Cook over medium heat, breaking turkey into small pieces with spatula until cooked through. Turn into large bowl; let cool slightly. Preheat oven to 350°F. Spray 13×9-inch baking pan with nonstick cooking spray.

Add cheese, chilies, green onions, ½ cup yogurt and walnuts to turkey mixture; combine thoroughly. Season with salt and pepper, if desired. Spoon ½ cup down middle of each tortilla and roll up loosely. Place seam-side down in prepared baking pan.

Tightly cover pan with foil; bake 25 minutes. Remove foil and bake 5 minutes longer. Top each enchilada with spoonful of yogurt and garnish with cilantro. Serve with remaining yogurt and salsa, if desired.

Makes 4 servings

Favorite recipe from **Walnut Marketing Board**

Nutrients per Serving (2 enchiladas):
Calories: 502, Calories from Fat: 32%, Total Fat: 18g, Saturated Fat: 4g, Cholesterol: 51mg, Sodium: 623mg, Carbohydrate: 46g, Dietary Fiber: 5g, Protein: 40g

Dietary Exchanges: 3 Starch, 4 Lean Meat, 1 Fat

Mediterranean **Chicken Kabobs**

2 pounds boneless skinless chicken breasts or tenders, cut into 1-inch pieces

1 small eggplant, peeled and cut into 1-inch pieces

1 medium zucchini, cut crosswise into ½-inch slices

2 medium onions, each cut into 8 wedges

16 medium mushrooms, stems removed

16 cherry tomatoes

1 cup fat-free reduced-sodium chicken broth

⅔ cup balsamic vinegar

3 tablespoons olive oil or vegetable oil

2 tablespoons dried mint leaves

4 teaspoons dried basil leaves

1 tablespoon dried oregano leaves

2 teaspoons grated lemon peel

Chopped fresh parsley (optional)

4 cups hot cooked couscous

1. Alternately thread chicken, eggplant, zucchini, onions, mushrooms and tomatoes onto 16 metal skewers; place in large glass baking dish.

2. Combine chicken broth, vinegar, oil, mint, basil and oregano in small bowl; pour over kabobs. Cover; marinate in refrigerator 2 hours; turn kabobs occasionally. Remove kabobs; discard marinade.

3. Broil kabobs 6 inches from heat source 10 to 15 minutes or until chicken is no longer pink in center, turning kabobs halfway through cooking time. Or, grill kabobs on covered grill over medium-hot coals 10 to 15 minutes or until chicken is no longer pink in center, turning kabobs halfway through cooking time. Stir lemon peel and parsley, if desired, into couscous; serve with kabobs. *Makes 8 servings*

Nutrients per Serving (2 kabobs plus ½ cup couscous):
Calories: 300, Calories from Fat: 16%, Total Fat: 5g, Saturated Fat: 1g, Cholesterol: 69mg, Sodium: 79mg, Carbohydrate: 32g, Dietary Fiber: 4g, Protein: 31g

Dietary Exchanges: 1 Starch, 3 Vegetable, 3 Lean Meat

Mediterranean Chicken Kabobs

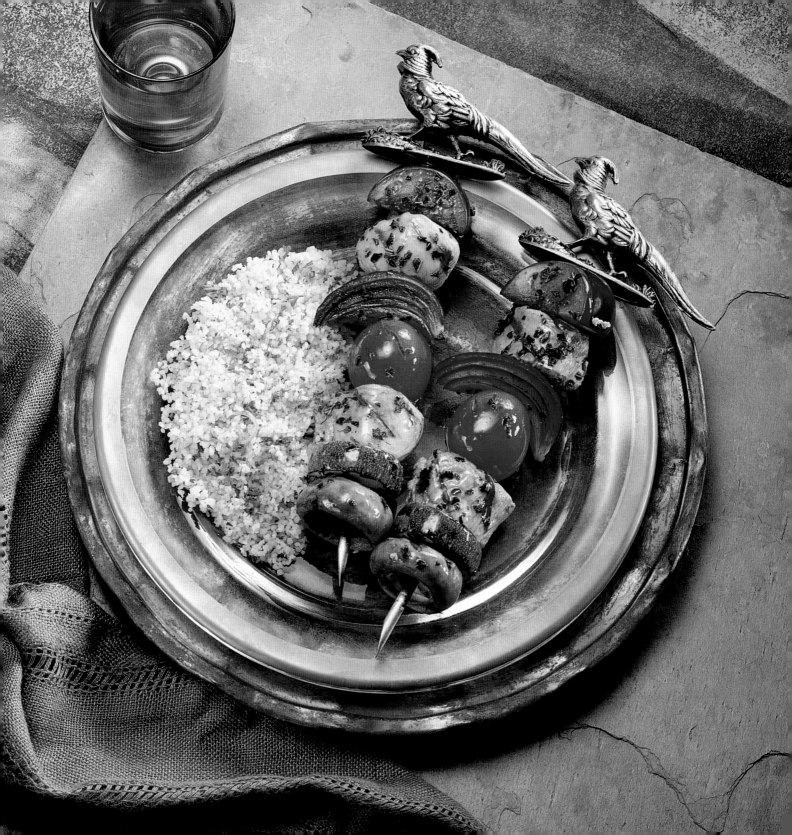

Summer Minestrone

Olive oil-flavored nonstick cooking spray
2 carrots, sliced
1 cup halved green beans
½ cup sliced celery
½ cup thinly sliced leek
2 cloves garlic, minced
1 tablespoon fresh sage *or* ½ teaspoon dried sage leaves
1 tablespoon fresh oregano *or* ½ teaspoon dried oregano leaves
3 cans (14½ ounces each) fat-free reduced-sodium chicken broth
1 medium zucchini, halved lengthwise and cut into ½-inch slices
1 cup quartered mushrooms
8 ounces cherry tomatoes, halved
¼ cup minced fresh parsley
3 ounces uncooked small rotini
Salt and black pepper
8 teaspoons grated Parmesan cheese

1. Spray large saucepan with cooking spray. Heat over medium heat until hot. Add carrots, green beans, celery, leek, garlic, sage and oregano. Cook and stir 3 to 5 minutes. Add chicken broth; bring to a boil. Reduce heat and simmer about 5 minutes or until vegetables are just crisp-tender.

2. Add zucchini, mushrooms, tomatoes and parsley; bring to a boil. Stir in pasta. Reduce heat and simmer, uncovered, about 8 minutes or until pasta and vegetables are tender. Season to taste with salt and pepper. Ladle soup into bowls; sprinkle each with l teaspoon Parmesan cheese.

Makes 8 servings

Nutrients per Serving (1 cup):
Calories: 93, Calories from Fat: 9%, Total Fat: 1g, Saturated Fat: <1g, Cholesterol: 1mg, Sodium: 96mg, Carbohydrate: 15g, Dietary Fiber: 2g, Protein: 7g

Dietary Exchanges: ½ Starch, 2 Vegetable

Rush-Hour Lasagna

Nonstick cooking spray
8 ounces ground round
2 cups no-salt-added spaghetti sauce
1 can (4 ounces) sliced mushrooms, drained
4 cloves garlic, minced
2 tablespoons chopped fresh parsley
1½ teaspoons dried oregano leaves
1½ teaspoons fennel seeds (optional)
6 uncooked lasagna noodles
½ cup nonfat cottage cheese
6 tablespoons grated fat-free Parmesan cheese
¾ cup (3 ounces) grated fat-free mozzarella cheese

1. Preheat oven to 350°F. Spray large nonstick skillet with cooking spray. Heat over high heat until hot. Brown beef in skillet over medium-high heat 6 to 8 minutes or until no longer pink, stirring to separate beef; drain fat. Add spaghetti sauce, mushrooms, garlic, parsley, oregano and fennel, if desired. Bring to a boil. Reduce heat to low; simmer, uncovered, 8 minutes or until slightly thickened.

2. Spray 8-inch square baking pan with nonstick cooking spray. Place 2 noodles on bottom of pan. Spoon one-third sauce over noodles, ¼ cup cottage cheese over sauce and top with 2 tablespoons Parmesan cheese. Repeat layers, ending with noodles. Spread remaining sauce on top of noodles and sprinkle with mozzarella cheese.

3. Cover and bake 30 minutes. Remove cover; continue baking 10 minutes. Remove from oven; top with 2 tablespoons Parmesan cheese. Let stand 10 minutes before serving.   *Makes 4 servings*

Nutrients per Serving (¼ of total recipe):
Calories: 310, Calories from Fat: 28%, Total Fat: 9g, Saturated Fat: 2g, Cholesterol: 32mg, Sodium: 460mg, Carbohydrate: 27g, Dietary Fiber: 5g, Protein: 29g

Dietary Exchanges: 1 Starch, 3 Vegetable, 3 Lean Meat

World Fare

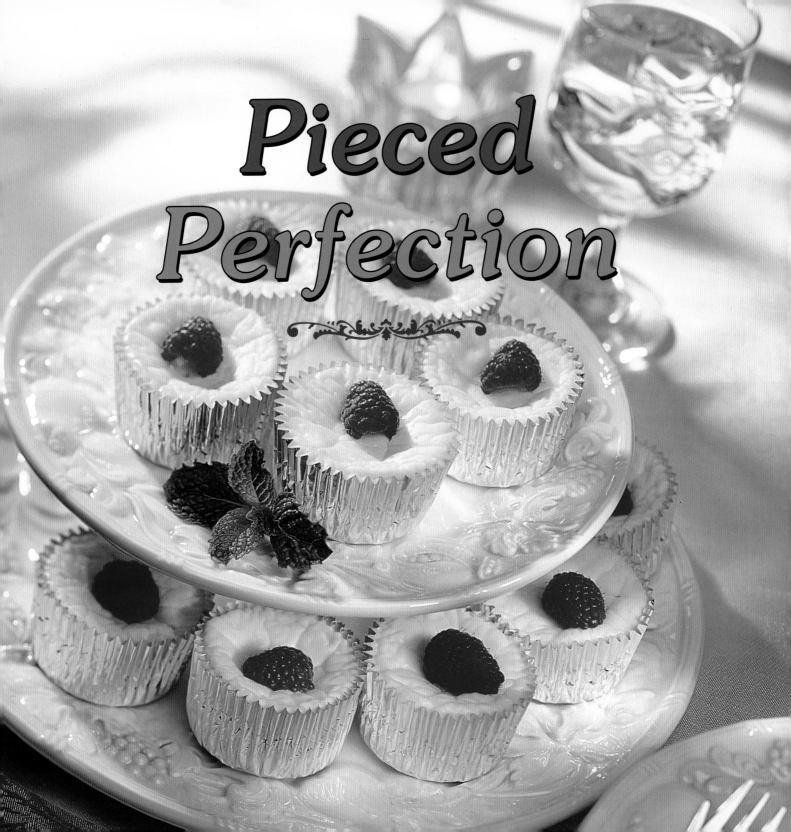

Pieced
Perfection

Raspberry Cheese Tarts

Crust
1¼ cups graham cracker crumbs
5 tablespoons light margarine (50% less fat and calories)
¼ cup SPLENDA® Granular

Filling
4 ounces reduced-fat cream cheese
½ cup plain nonfat yogurt
1 cup SPLENDA® Granular
½ cup egg substitute
1 cup frozen raspberries

Crust
1. Preheat oven to 350°F. In medium bowl, mix together graham cracker crumbs, margarine and ¼ cup SPLENDA®. Press about 1 tablespoon of crust mixture into 10 muffin pan cups lined with paper liners. Set aside.

Filling
2. In small bowl, beat cream cheese with electric mixer on low speed until soft, about 30 seconds. Add yogurt and beat on low speed until smooth, approximately 1 minute. Stir in SPLENDA® and egg substitute until well blended.

3. Place 1½ tablespoons raspberries (4 to 5) into each muffin cup. Divide filling evenly among muffin cups. Bake for 20 minutes or until firm. Refrigerate for 2 hours before serving. Garnish as desired.

Makes 10 servings

Nutrients per Serving (1 tart or 2.6 ounces/82g):
Calories: 140, Calories from Fat: 43%, Total Fat: 6g, Saturated Fat: 2g, Cholesterol: 6mg, Sodium: 255mg, Carbohydrate: 15g, Dietary Fiber: 1g, Protein: 5g

Dietary Exchanges: 1 Starch, 1 Fat

Raspberry Cheese Tarts

Pear-Ginger Upside-Down Cake

2 unpeeled Bosc or Anjou pears, cored and sliced ¼ inch thick
3 tablespoons fresh lemon juice
1 to 2 tablespoons melted butter
1 to 2 tablespoons packed brown sugar
1 cup all-purpose flour
1 teaspoon baking powder
¼ teaspoon baking soda
1 teaspoon ground cinnamon
⅛ teaspoon salt
⅓ cup fat-free (skim) milk
3 tablespoons no-sugar-added apricot spread
1 egg
1 tablespoon minced fresh ginger
1 tablespoon vegetable oil

1. Preheat oven to 375°F. Spray 10-inch deep-dish pie pan with nonstick cooking spray. Toss pears in lemon juice; drain. Brush butter evenly onto bottom of prepared pan; sprinkle sugar over butter. Arrange pears in dish; bake 10 minutes.

2. Meanwhile, combine flour, baking powder, baking soda, cinnamon and salt in small bowl; set aside. Combine milk, apricot spread, egg, ginger and oil in medium bowl; mix well. Add flour mixture; stir until well mixed (batter is very thick). Carefully spread batter evenly over pears to edges of pan. Bake 20 to 25 minutes or until golden brown and toothpick inserted in center comes out clean. Cool 5 minutes; use knife to loosen cake from sides of pan. Place 10-inch plate over top of pan; quickly turn over to transfer cake to plate. Place any pears left in pan on top of cake. Serve warm. *Makes 8 servings*

Nutrients per Serving (⅛ of cake):
Calories: 139, Calories from Fat: 27%, Total Fat: 4g, Saturated Fat: 1g, Cholesterol: 31mg, Sodium: 174mg, Carbohydrate: 23g, Dietary Fiber: 2g, Protein: 3g

Dietary Exchanges: 1½ Starch, ½ Fat

Pear-Ginger Upside-Down Cake

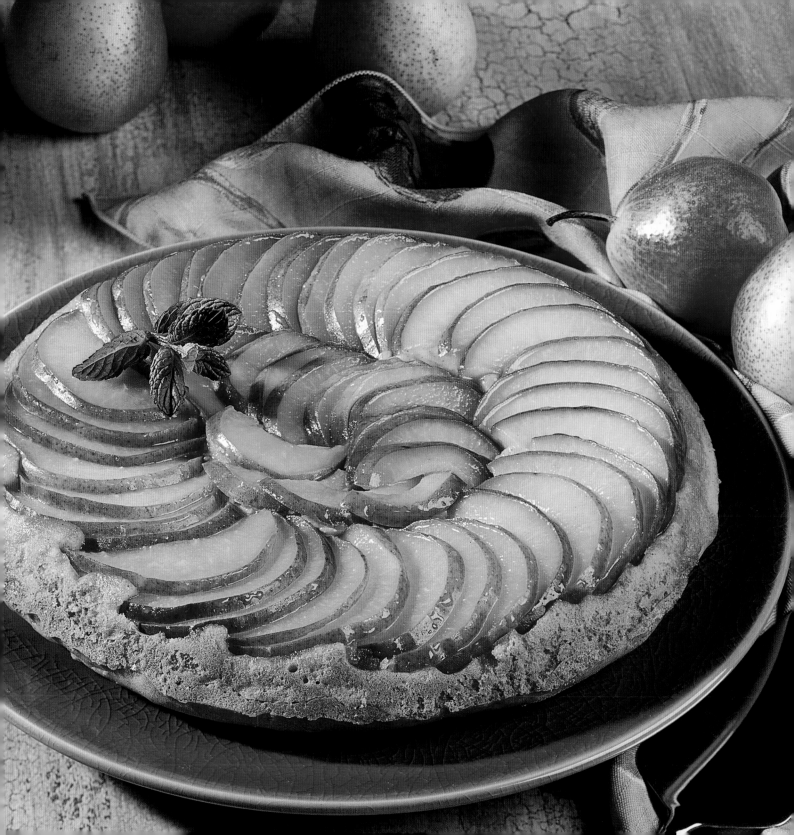

Chocolate Cupcakes

6 tablespoons lower fat margarine (40% oil)
1 cup sugar
1¼ cups all-purpose flour
⅓ cup HERSHEY'S Cocoa
1 teaspoon baking soda
Dash salt
1 cup lowfat buttermilk
½ teaspoon vanilla extract
1 teaspoon powdered sugar

1. Heat oven to 350°F. Line 18 muffin cups (2½ inches in diameter) with paper bake cups.

2. Melt margarine in large saucepan over low heat. Remove from heat; stir in sugar.

3. Stir together flour, cocoa, baking soda and salt in small bowl; add alternately with buttermilk and vanilla to mixture in saucepan. Stir with whisk until well blended. Fill muffin cups ⅔ full with batter.

4. Bake 18 to 20 minutes or until wooden pick inserted in centers comes out clean. Remove from pans to wire racks. Cool completely.

5. Sift powdered sugar over tops of cupcakes. Store, covered, at room temperature.

Makes 18 cupcakes

Nutrients per Serving (1 cupcake):
Calories: 102, Calories from Fat: 19%, Total Fat: 2g, Saturated Fat: <1g, Cholesterol: 1mg, Sodium: 130mg, Carbohydrate: 19g, Dietary Fiber: 1g, Protein: 2g

Dietary Exchanges: 1 Starch, ½ Fat

Key Lime Pie

1 cup graham cracker crumbs

3 tablespoons melted margarine

1 teaspoon EQUAL® FOR RECIPES *or* 3 packets EQUAL® sweetener *or*
  2 tablespoons EQUAL® SPOONFUL™

1 envelope (¼ ounce) unflavored gelatin

1¾ cups skim milk, divided

1 package (8 ounces) reduced-fat cream cheese, softened

⅓ to ½ cup fresh lime juice

3½ teaspoons EQUAL® FOR RECIPES *or* 12 packets EQUAL® sweetener *or* ½ cup
  EQUAL® SPOONFUL™

Lime slices, raspberries and fresh mint sprigs, for garnish (optional)

• Combine graham cracker crumbs, margarine and 1 teaspoon Equal® For Recipes *or* 3 packets Equal® sweetener *or* 2 tablespoons Equal® Spoonful™ in bottom of 7-inch springform pan; pat evenly onto bottom and ½ inch up side of pan.

• Sprinkle gelatin over ½ cup milk in small saucepan; let stand 2 to 3 minutes. Cook over low heat, stirring constantly, until gelatin is dissolved. Beat cream cheese in small bowl until fluffy; beat in remaining 1¼ cups milk and gelatin mixture. Mix in lime juice and 3½ teaspoons Equal® For Recipes *or* 12 packets Equal® sweetener *or* ½ cup Equal® Spoonful™. Refrigerate pie until set, about 2 hours.

• To serve, loosen side of pie from pan with small spatula and remove side of pan. Place pie on serving plate; garnish with lime slices, raspberries and mint, if desired. *Makes 8 servings*

Nutrients per Serving (⅛ of pie):
Calories: 150, Calories from Fat: 52%, Total Fat: 10g, Saturated Fat: 5g, Cholesterol: 16mg, Sodium: 231mg, Carbohydrate: 11g, Dietary Fiber: <1g, Protein: 6g

Dietary Exchanges: 2 Starch, 2½ Fat

Pieced Perfection

Boston Babies

1 package (18¼ ounces) yellow cake mix

3 eggs *or* ¾ cup cholesterol-free egg substitute

⅓ cup unsweetened applesauce

1 package (4-serving size) sugar-free vanilla pudding and pie filling mix

2 cups low-fat (1%) milk or fat-free (skim) milk

⅓ cup sugar

⅓ cup unsweetened cocoa powder

1 tablespoon cornstarch

1½ cups water

1½ teaspoons vanilla

1. Line 24 (2½-inch) muffin cups with paper liners; set aside.

2. Prepare cake mix according to lower-fat package directions, using applesauce. Pour batter into prepared muffin cups. Bake according to package directions; cool completely. Freeze 12 cupcakes for another use.

3. Prepare pudding according to package directions, using 2 cups milk; cover and refrigerate.

4. Combine sugar, cocoa, cornstarch and water in large microwavable bowl; whisk until smooth. Microwave at HIGH 4 to 6 minutes, stirring every 2 minutes, until slightly thickened. Stir in vanilla.

5. To serve, drizzle 2 tablespoons chocolate glaze over each dessert plate. Cut cupcakes in half; place 2 halves on top of chocolate on each dessert plate. Top each with about 2 heaping tablespoonfuls pudding. Garnish, if desired. Serve immediately. *Makes 12 servings*

Nutrients per Serving (1 cupcake plus 2 tablespoons chocolate glaze and 2 tablespoons pudding): Calories: 158, Calories from Fat: 22%, Total Fat: 4g, Saturated Fat: 1g, Cholesterol: 29mg, Sodium: 175mg, Carbohydrate: 28g, Dietary Fiber: <1g, Protein: 3g

Dietary Exchanges: 2 Starch, ½ Fat

Boston Baby

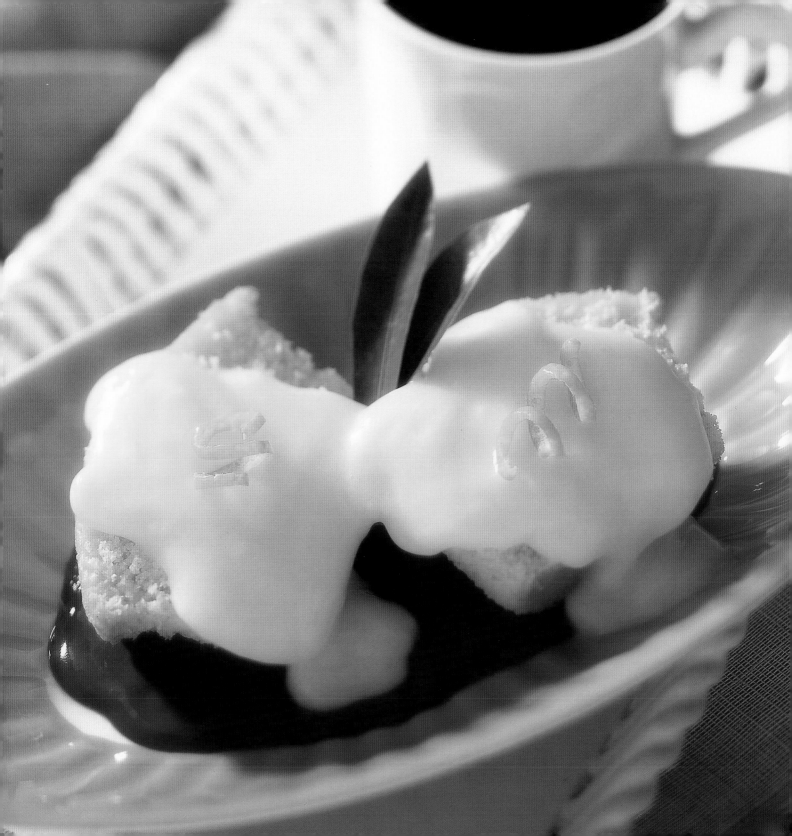

Date Cake Squares

1¼ cups water

1 cup chopped dates

¾ cup chopped pitted prunes

½ cup dark raisins

8 tablespoons margarine, cut into pieces

2 eggs

1 teaspoon vanilla

1 cup all-purpose flour

5½ teaspoons EQUAL® FOR RECIPES *or* 18 packets EQUAL® sweetener *or* ¾ cup
    EQUAL® SPOONFUL™

1 teaspoon baking soda

½ teaspoon ground cinnamon

¼ teaspoon ground nutmeg

¼ teaspoon salt

¼ cup chopped walnuts

• Combine water, dates, prunes and raisins in medium saucepan; heat to boiling. Reduce heat and simmer, uncovered, until fruit is tender and water is absorbed, about 10 minutes. Remove from heat and add margarine, stirring until melted; cool to room temperature.

• Mix eggs and vanilla into fruit mixture; mix in combined flour, Equal®, baking soda, cinnamon, nutmeg and salt. Spread batter evenly in greased 11×7×2-inch baking dish; sprinkle with walnuts.

• Bake in preheated 350°F oven until cake springs back when touched lightly, 30 to 35 minutes. Cool on wire rack; cut evenly into squares. *Makes 2 dozen squares*

Nutrients per Serving (1 square):
Calories: 112, Calories from Fat: 39%, Total Fat: 5g, Saturated Fat: 1g, Cholesterol: 18mg, Sodium: 127mg, Carbohydrate: 15g, Dietary Fiber: 1g, Protein: 3g

Dietary Exchanges: 1 Fruit, 1 Fat

Date Cake Squares

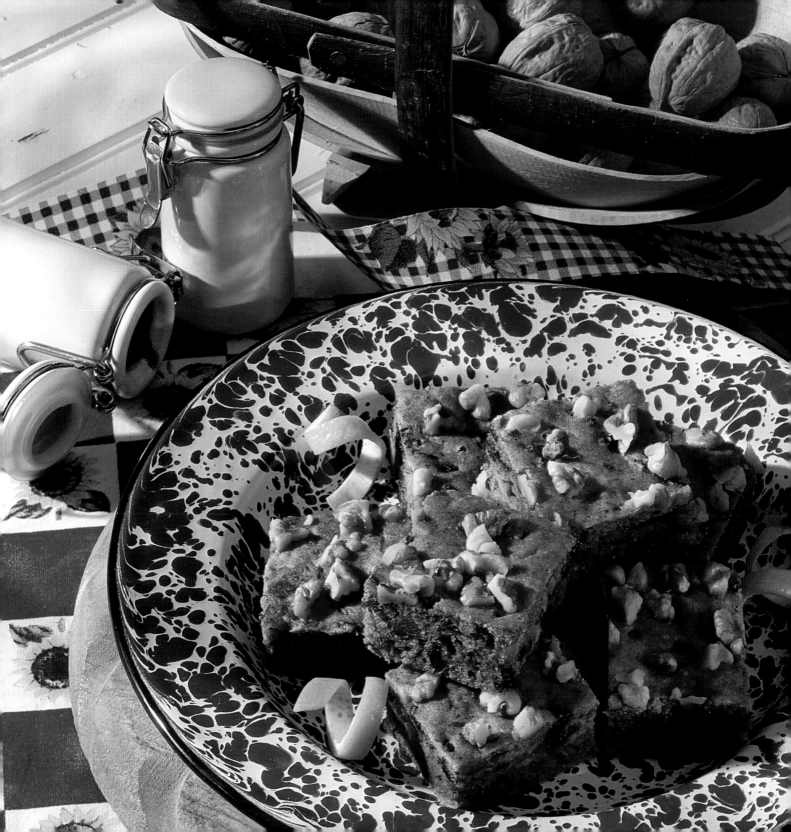

Low Fat Lemon Soufflé Cheesecake

1 whole graham cracker, crushed

⅔ cup boiling water

1 package (4-serving size) JELL-O® Brand Lemon Flavor Sugar Free Low Calorie
    Gelatin Dessert

1 cup BREAKSTONE'S® *or* KNUDSEN® 2% Cottage Cheese

1 container (8 ounces) PHILADELPHIA FREE® Fat Free Cream Cheese

2 cups thawed COOL WHIP FREE® Whipped Topping

SPRINKLE ½ of the crumbs onto side of 8- or 9-inch springform pan or 9-inch pie plate which has been sprayed with no stick cooking spray.

STIR boiling water into gelatin in large bowl at least 2 minutes until completely dissolved. Pour into blender container. Add cheeses; cover. Blend on medium speed until smooth, scraping down sides occasionally.

POUR into large bowl. Gently stir in whipped topping. Pour into prepared pan; smooth top. Sprinkle remaining crumbs around outside edge. Garnish as desired.

REFRIGERATE 4 hours or until set. Remove side of pan just before serving. Store leftover cheesecake in refrigerator. *Makes 8 servings*

Prep Time: 15 minutes plus refrigerating

Nutrients per Serving (⅛ of cheesecake):
Calories: 100, Calories from Fat: 18%, Total Fat: 2g, Saturated Fat: 2g, Cholesterol: 10mg, Sodium: 300mg, Carbohydrate: 11g, Dietary Fiber: 0g, Protein: 9g

Dietary Exchanges: 1 Starch, ½ Lean Meat

Pieced Perfection

Low Fat Lemon Soufflé Cheesecake

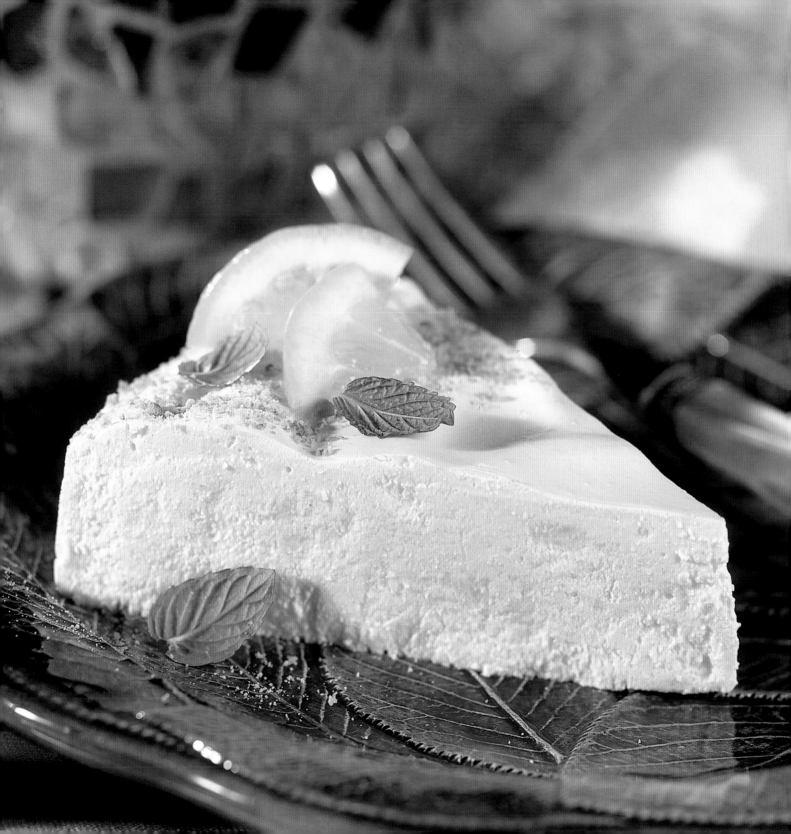

Coconut Custard Pie

Pastry for single crust 9-inch pie
4 eggs
¼ teaspoon salt
2 cups skim milk
½ cup flaked coconut
5½ teaspoons EQUAL® FOR RECIPES *or* 18 packets EQUAL® sweetener *or* ¾ cup
    EQUAL® SPOONFUL™
2 teaspoons coconut extract

• Roll pastry on floured surface into circle 1-inch larger than inverted 9-inch pie pan. Ease pastry into pan; trim and flute edge.

• Beat eggs and salt in large bowl until thick and lemon colored, about 5 minutes. Mix in milk and remaining ingredients. Pour mixture into pastry shell.

• Bake pie in preheated 425°F oven for 15 minutes. Reduce temperature to 350°F and bake until sharp knife inserted halfway between center and edge of pie comes out clean, 20 to 25 minutes. Cool on wire rack. Serve at room temperature, or refrigerate and serve chilled. *Makes 8 servings*

Tip: Never pour a filling into a pie shell until just before baking. Allowing the filling to stand in an unbaked pie shell will lead to a soggy crust.

Nutrients per Serving (⅛ of pie):
Calories: 223, Calories from Fat: 52%, Total Fat: 13g, Saturated Fat: 5g, Cholesterol: 107mg, Sodium: 281mg, Carbohydrate: 19g, Dietary Fiber: 1g, Protein: 7g

Dietary Exchanges: 1 Starch, 1 Lean Meat, 2 Fat

Southern Peanut Butter Cheesecake

½ cup low-fat graham cracker crumbs

8 ounces light cream cheese, cut into cubes

8 ounces fat-free cream cheese, cut into cubes

½ cup fat-free sour cream

½ cup fat-free ricotta or low-fat cottage cheese

⅓ cup peanut butter

½ cup firmly packed dark brown sugar

2 teaspoons vanilla extract

6 egg whites *or* ¾ cup egg substitute

Coat 9-inch springform pan with cooking spray. Sprinkle graham cracker crumbs evenly over bottom of pan. Set aside. Process cream cheese, sour cream and ricotta cheese in a food processor until smooth. Add peanut butter; mix. Slowly add sugar and vanilla extract. Slowly pour eggs through food chute with processor running. Blend until combined. Spoon mixture over graham cracker crumbs. Bake in 300°F oven 50 minutes. Center will be soft, but will firm during chilling. Turn oven off and leave cheesecake in oven 30 minutes more. Remove from oven; let cool to room temperature on wire rack. Cover and chill 8 hours. Serve with assorted fresh berries. *Makes 10 servings*

Favorite recipe from **Peanut Advisory Board**

Nutrients per Serving (¹⁄₁₀ of cheesecake):
Calories: 140, Calories from Fat: 29%, Total Fat: 5g, Saturated Fat: 2g, Cholesterol: 10mg, Sodium: 240mg, Carbohydrate: 14g, Dietary Fiber: 0g, Protein: 13g

Dietary Exchanges: 1 Starch, 1 Lean Meat, ½ Fat

Strawberry Cream Pie

1 package (8 ounces) reduced-fat cream cheese, softened
1¾ teaspoons EQUAL® FOR RECIPES *or* 6 packets EQUAL® sweetener *or* ¼ cup
    EQUAL® SPOONFUL™
1 teaspoon vanilla
    Reduced-fat graham cracker crust (9 inch) or homemade graham cracker crust
1 cup cold water
2 tablespoons cornstarch
1 package (0.3 ounce) sugar-free strawberry gelatin
3½ teaspoons EQUAL® FOR RECIPES *or* 12 packets EQUAL® sweetener *or* ½ cup
    EQUAL® SPOONFUL™
1 pint strawberries, hulled and sliced
8 tablespoons frozen light whipped topping (optional)

• Beat cream cheese, 1¾ teaspoons Equal® for Recipes and vanilla in small bowl until fluffy; spread evenly in bottom of crust. Mix cold water and cornstarch in small saucepan; heat to boiling, whisking constantly until thickened, about 1 minute. Add gelatin and 3½ teaspoons Equal® for Recipes, whisking until gelatin is dissolved. Cool 10 minutes.

• Arrange half of strawberries over cream cheese; spoon half of gelatin mixture over strawberries. Arrange remaining strawberries over pie and spoon remaining gelatin mixture over strawberries.

• Refrigerate until pie is set and chilled, 1 to 2 hours. Serve with whipped topping, if desired.

Makes 8 servings

Nutrients per Serving (⅛ of pie):
Calories: 185, Calories from Fat: 40%, Total Fat: 8g, Saturated Fat: 4g, Cholesterol: 13mg, Sodium: 246mg, Carbohydrate: 22g, Dietary Fiber: 1g, Protein: 4g

Dietary Exchanges: 1 Starch, ½ Fruit, 1½ Fat

Strawberry Cream Pie

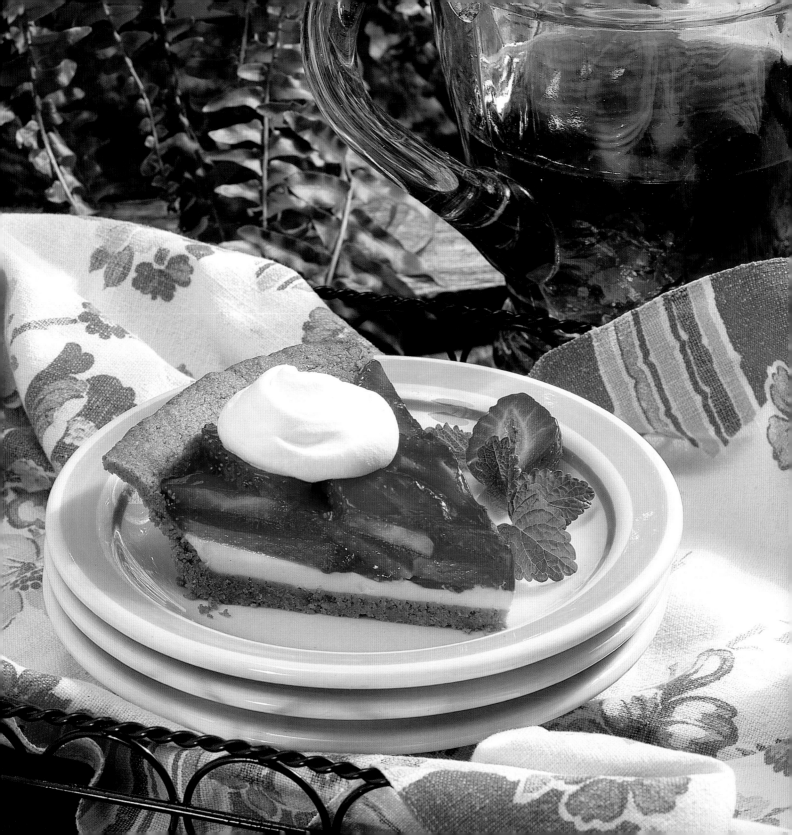

Blueberry Chiffon Cake

3 tablespoons reduced-fat margarine

¾ cup graham cracker crumbs

2 cups fresh or thawed frozen blueberries

½ cup cold water

2 envelopes unflavored gelatin

2 containers (8 ounces each) fat-free cream cheese

1 container (8 ounces) Neufchâtel cheese

¾ cup sugar, divided

⅔ cup nonfat sour cream

½ cup lemon juice

1 tablespoon grated lemon peel

6 egg whites*

*Use only grade A clean, uncracked eggs.

1. Preheat oven to 350°F. Melt margarine in small saucepan over medium heat. Stir in graham cracker crumbs. Press crumb mixture firmly onto bottom and 1 inch up side of 9-inch springform pan. Bake 10 minutes. Remove from oven. Cool 10 minutes. Arrange blueberries in single layer on top of crust. Refrigerate until needed.

2. Place water in small saucepan; sprinkle gelatin over water. Let stand 3 minutes to soften. Heat gelatin mixture over low heat until completely dissolved, stirring constantly.

3. Combine cheeses in large bowl with electric mixer. Beat at medium speed until well blended. Beat in ½ cup sugar until well blended. Beat in sour cream, lemon juice and lemon peel until well blended. Beat in gelatin mixture until well blended.

4. With clean, dry beaters, beat egg whites in medium bowl with electric mixer at medium speed until soft peaks form. Gradually add remaining ¼ cup sugar. Beat at high speed until stiff peaks form. Fold egg whites into cream cheese mixture. Gently spoon mixture into prepared crust. Cover with plastic wrap. Refrigerate 6 hours or until firm. *Makes 16 servings*

Nutrients per Serving (¹⁄₁₆ of cake):
Calories: 165, Calories from Fat: 28%, Total Fat: 5g, Saturated Fat: 2g, Cholesterol: 14mg, Sodium: 342mg, Carbohydrate: 20g, Dietary Fiber: 1g, Protein: 10g

Dietary Exchanges: ½ Starch, 1 Fruit, 1 Lean Meat, ½ Fat

Cherry Cocoa Cake

1 cup water
½ cup cocoa
½ cup margarine
2 cups all-purpose flour
1¾ cups sugar
½ cup low-fat cherry yogurt
1 egg, slightly beaten
1 teaspoon baking soda
1 teaspoon vanilla
½ teaspoon salt
1 tablespoon powdered sugar

In a large saucepan, combine water, cocoa and margarine. Cook over medium heat, stirring frequently, until mixture comes to a full boil. Remove from heat; stir in flour and sugar. Add yogurt, egg, baking soda, vanilla and salt; mix thoroughly.

Pour batter into a 15½×10-inch baking pan coated with nonstick cooking spray. Bake at 375°F for 20 to 25 minutes or until wooden pick inserted in center comes out clean. Cool in pan on wire rack. Sprinkle powdered sugar over top. Cut evenly into squares. *Makes 32 servings*

Favorite recipe from **North Dakota Wheat Commission**

Nutrients per Serving (1 square):
Calories: 105, Calories from Fat: 27%, Total Fat: 3g, Saturated Fat: 1g, Cholesterol: 7mg, Sodium: 113mg, Carbohydrate: 18g, Dietary Fiber: <1g, Protein: 1g

Dietary Exchanges: 1 Starch, ½ Fat

Pumpkin-Fig Cheesecake

12 nonfat fig bar cookies

2 packages (8 ounces each) fat-free cream cheese, softened

1 package (8 ounces) reduced-fat cream cheese, softened

1 can (15 ounces) pumpkin

1 cup SPLENDA® No-Calorie Sweetener, granular form

1 cup cholesterol-free egg substitute

½ cup nonfat evaporated milk

1 tablespoon vanilla extract

2 teaspoons pumpkin pie spice mix

¼ teaspoon salt

½ cup chopped dried figs

2 tablespoons walnut pieces

1. Preheat oven to 325°F. Lightly coat 8- to 9-inch springform baking pan with nonstick cooking spray.

2. Break up cookies with fingers, then chop by hand with knife or process in food processor until crumbly. Lightly press crust onto bottom and sides of pan. Bake 15 minutes; cool slightly while preparing filling.

3. In large bowl, beat cream cheese with mixer at high speed until smooth. Add pumpkin, SPLENDA®, egg substitute, milk, vanilla, spice mix and salt. Beat until smooth. Spread filling evenly over crust.

4. Place springform pan on baking sheet. Bake 1 hour and 15 minutes or until top begins to crack and center moves very little when pan is jiggled. Cool on wire rack to room temperature; refrigerate 4 to 6 hours or overnight before serving. Just before serving, decorate top with figs and nuts.

Makes 16 slices

Nutrients per Serving (1 slice):
Calories: 157, Calories from Fat: 20%, Total Fat: 3g, Saturated Fat: 2g, Cholesterol: 9mg, Sodium: 310mg, Carbohydrate: 22g, Dietary Fiber: 2g, Protein: 9g

Dietary Exchanges: 1½ Starch, 1 Lean Meat

Pumpkin-Fig Cheesecake

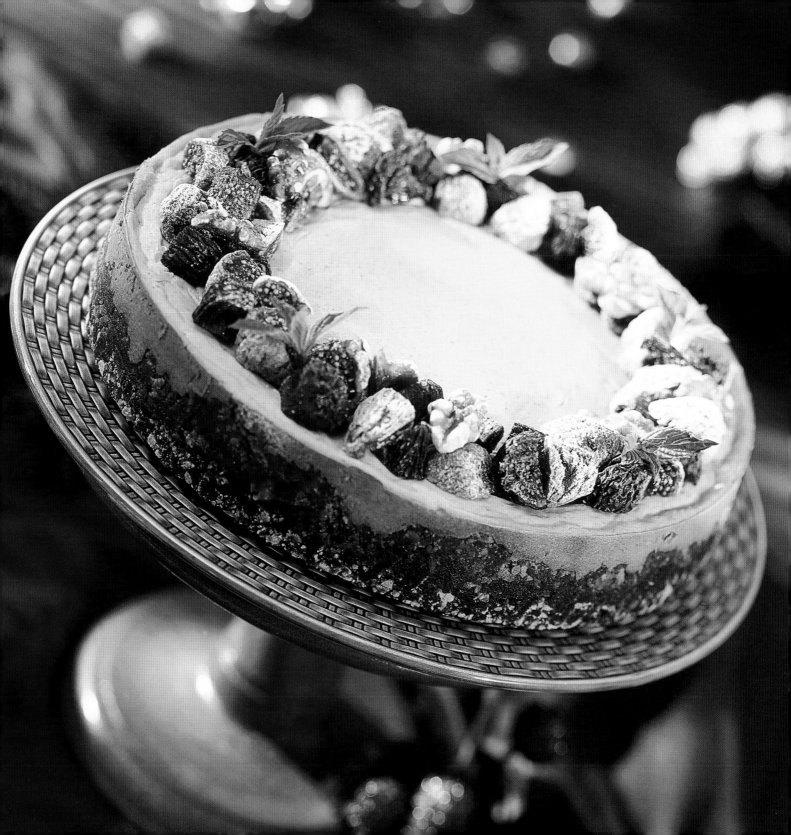

Lemon Meringue Pie

Pastry for single crust 9-inch pie

2¼ cups water

½ cup lemon juice

⅓ cup plus 2 tablespoons cornstarch

10¾ teaspoons EQUAL® FOR RECIPES *or* 36 packets EQUAL® sweetener *or* 1½ cups EQUAL® SPOONFUL™

2 eggs

2 egg whites

1 teaspoon finely grated lemon peel (optional)

2 tablespoons margarine

1 to 2 drops yellow food color (optional)

3 egg whites

¼ teaspoon cream of tartar

3½ teaspoons EQUAL® FOR RECIPES *or* 12 packets EQUAL® sweetener*

Equal® Spoonful™ cannot be used in meringue recipes.

- Roll pastry on lightly floured surface into circle 1 inch larger than inverted 9-inch pie pan. Ease pastry into pan; trim and flute edge. Pierce bottom and side of pastry with fork. Bake in preheated 425°F oven until pastry is browned, 10 to 15 minutes. Cool on wire rack.

- Mix water, lemon juice, cornstarch and 10¾ teaspoons Equal® for Recipes in medium saucepan. Heat to boiling over medium-high heat, stirring constantly; boil and stir 1 minute. Beat eggs, egg whites and lemon peel, if desired, in small bowl; stir in about half of hot cornstarch mixture. Stir egg mixture into remaining cornstarch mixture in saucepan; cook and stir over low heat 1 minute. Remove from heat; add margarine, stirring until melted. Stir in food color, if desired. Pour mixture into baked pie shell.

- Beat 3 egg whites in medium bowl until foamy; add cream of tartar and beat to soft peaks.

continued on page 340

Lemon Meringue Pie

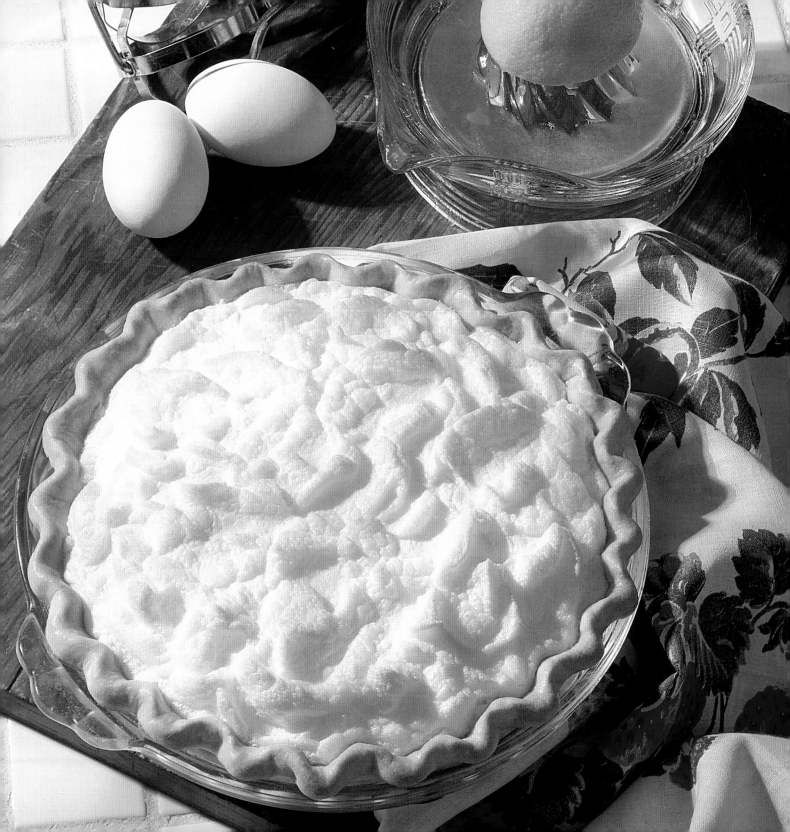

• Gradually beat in 3½ teaspoons Equal® for Recipes, beating to stiff peaks. Spread meringue over hot lemon filling, carefully sealing to edge of crust to prevent shrinking or weeping. Bake pie in preheated 425°F oven until meringue is browned, about 5 minutes. Cool completely on wire rack before cutting.

Makes 8 servings

Nutrients per Serving (⅛ of pie):
Calories: 227, Calories from Fat: 47%, Total Fat: 12g, Saturated Fat: 3g, Cholesterol: 53mg, Sodium: 206mg, Carbohydrate: 24g, Dietary Fiber: 1g, Protein: 5g

Dietary Exchanges: 1½ Starch, 2½ Fat

Strawberry **Cobbler**

1 (10-ounce) package frozen whole strawberries, unsweetened and without juice, chopped
3 packets sugar substitute
1 (8-fluid-ounce) can Vanilla GLUCERNA® Shake
½ cup self-rising flour
4 tablespoons margarine, melted

Preheat oven to 375°F. Grease 9-inch square baking dish. Spread strawberries in baking dish. Sprinkle sugar substitute over strawberries. In medium bowl, combine GLUCERNA® Shake, flour and margarine. Pour over strawberries. Bake 25 to 30 minutes or until golden brown.   *Makes 6 servings*

Nutrients per Serving (⅙ of cobbler):
Calories: 163, Calories from Fat: 54%, Total Fat: 10g, Saturated Fat: 2g, Cholesterol: <1mg, Sodium: 259mg, Carbohydrate: 16g, Dietary Fiber: 2g, Protein: 3g

Dietary Exchanges: 1 Starch, 2 Fat

Chocolate Pudding Cake

Cake

    1 cup all-purpose flour

    ⅓ cup sugar

    10 packets sugar substitute *or* equivalent of 20 teaspoons sugar

    3 tablespoons unsweetened cocoa powder

    2 teaspoons baking powder

    ½ teaspoon salt

    ½ cup warm fat-free (skim) milk

    2 tablespoons canola oil

    2 teaspoons vanilla

Sauce

    ¼ cup sugar

    10 packets sugar substitute *or* equivalent of 20 teaspoons sugar

    3 tablespoons unsweetened cocoa powder

    1¾ cups boiling water

1. Preheat oven to 350°F. Combine all cake ingredients in large bowl; mix well. Pour into ungreased 9-inch square baking pan.

2. To prepare sauce, sprinkle ¼ cup sugar, 10 packets sugar substitute and 3 tablespoons cocoa powder over batter in pan. Pour boiling water over top. *(Do not stir.)*

3. Bake 40 minutes or until cake portion has risen to top of pan and sauce is bubbling underneath. Serve immediately.   *Makes 9 servings*

Nutrients per Serving (⅑ of cake):
Calories: 150, Calories from Fat: 18%, Total Fat: 3g, Saturated Fat: <1g, Cholesterol: <1mg, Sodium: 246mg, Carbohydrate: 26g, Dietary Fiber: <1g, Protein: 4g

Dietary Exchanges: 1½ Starch, ½ Fat

Tropical Fruit Coconut Tart

1 cup cornflakes, crushed

1 can (3½ ounces) sweetened flaked coconut

2 egg whites

1 can (15¼ ounces) pineapple tidbits in juice, undrained

2 teaspoons cornstarch

2 packets sugar substitute *or* equivalent of 4 teaspoons sugar

1 teaspoon coconut extract (optional)

1 mango, peeled and thinly sliced

1 banana, thinly sliced

1. Preheat oven to 425°F. Coat 9-inch springform pan with nonstick cooking spray; set aside.

2. Combine cereal, coconut and egg whites in medium bowl; toss gently to blend. Place coconut mixture in prepared pan; press firmly to coat bottom and ½ inch up side of pan.

3. Bake 8 minutes or until edge begins to brown. Cool completely on wire rack.

4. Drain pineapple, reserving pineapple juice. Combine pineapple juice and cornstarch in small saucepan; stir until cornstarch is dissolved. Bring to a boil over high heat. Continue boiling 1 minute, stirring constantly. Remove from heat; cool completely. Stir in sugar substitute and coconut extract, if desired.

5. Combine pineapple, mango slices and banana slices in medium bowl. Spoon over crust in pan; drizzle with pineapple sauce. Cover with plastic wrap and refrigerate 2 hours. Garnish with pineapple leaves, if desired. *Makes 8 servings*

Nutrients per Serving (⅛ of tart):
Calories: 139, Calories from Fat: 25%, Total Fat: 4g, Saturated Fat: 4g, Cholesterol: 0mg, Sodium: 59mg, Carbohydrate: 25g, Dietary Fiber: 2g, Protein: 2g

Dietary Exchanges: 1 Starch, ½ Fruit, 1 Fat

Tropical Fruit Coconut Tart

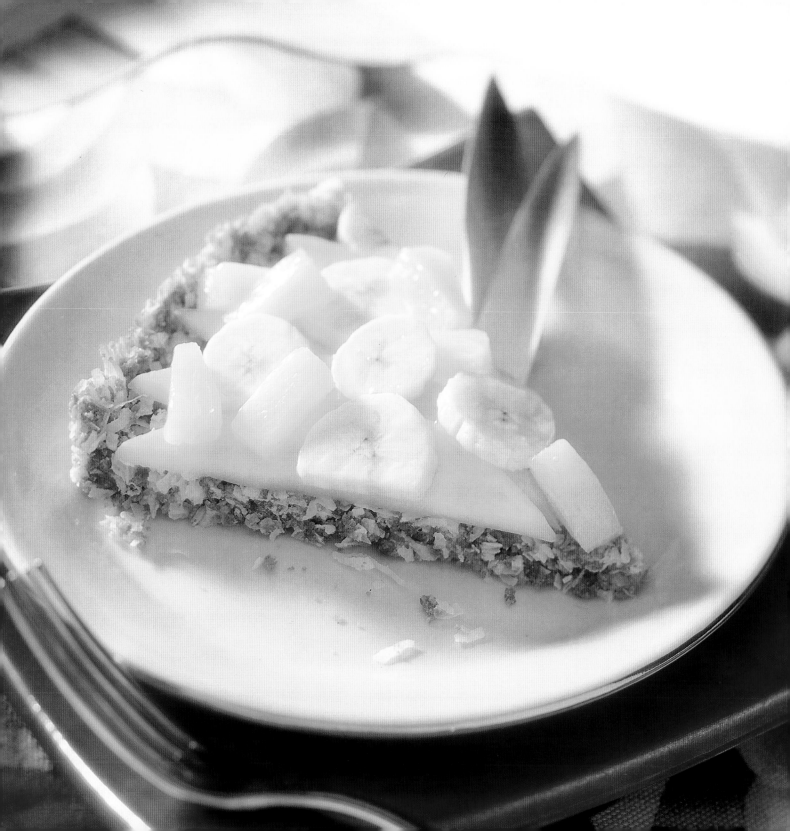

Blueberry Lemon Pudding Cake

¼ cup sugar

¼ cup all-purpose flour

1 cup fat-free (skim) milk

1 egg yolk

2 teaspoons finely grated lemon peel

3 tablespoons fresh lemon juice

2 tablespoons margarine

3 egg whites

2 cups fresh or frozen (not thawed) blueberries

1 cup sugar-free strawberry fruit spread

1. Preheat oven to 350°F. Lightly spray 8-inch square glass or ceramic baking dish with nonstick cooking spray.

2. Combine sugar and flour in small bowl.

3. Combine milk, egg yolk, lemon peel, lemon juice and margarine in large bowl. Add sugar mixture to milk mixture; stir until just blended.

4. Beat egg whites in medium bowl until stiff, but not dry. Gently fold beaten egg whites into milk mixture; spread into bottom of prepared baking dish. Place dish in 13×9-inch baking pan; pour 1 inch hot water into outer pan. Bake 15 minutes.

5. Meanwhile, melt fruit spread. Drop blueberries evenly over top of cake; carefully brush with fruit spread. Bake about 35 minutes or until set and lightly golden. Let cool slightly; serve warm or chilled.

Makes 6 servings

Nutrients per Serving (⅙ of cake):
Calories: 147, Calories from Fat: 29%, Total Fat: 5g, Saturated Fat: 1g, Cholesterol: 36mg, Sodium: 97mg, Carbohydrate: 22g, Dietary Fiber: 2g, Protein: 5g

Dietary Exchanges: 1 Starch, 1½ Fruit, 1 Fat

Blueberry Lemon Pudding Cake

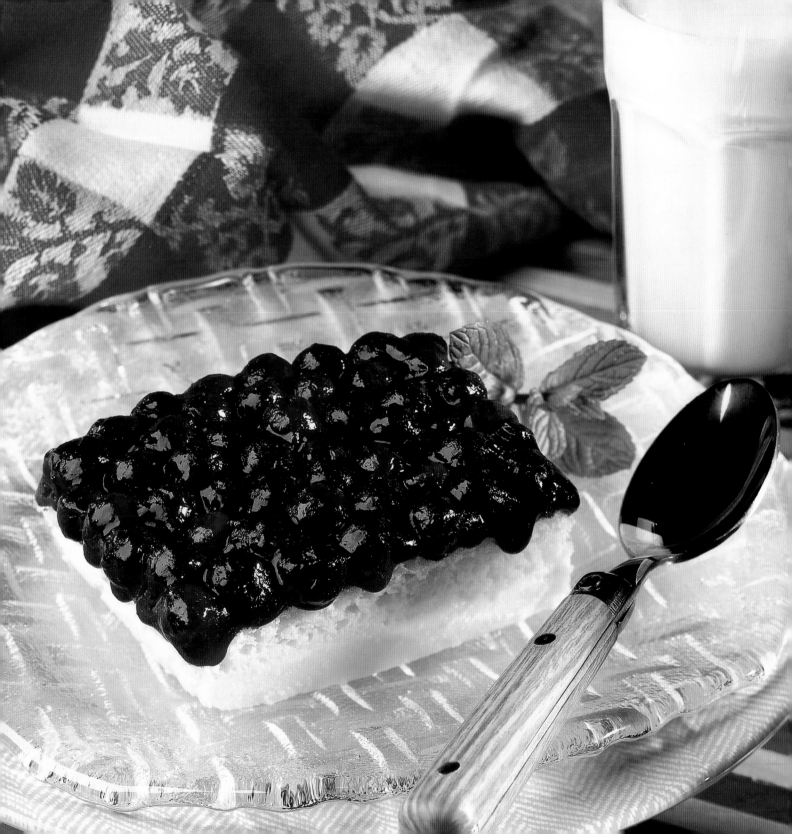

Ginger-Crusted Pumpkin Cheesecake

    12 whole low-fat honey graham crackers, broken into small pieces

     3 tablespoons reduced-fat margarine, melted

    ½ teaspoon ground ginger

     1 can (15 ounces) solid-pack pumpkin

     2 packages (8 ounces each) fat-free cream cheese, softened

     1 package (8 ounces) reduced-fat cream cheese, softened

     1 cup sugar

     1 cup cholesterol-free egg substitute

    ½ cup nonfat evaporated milk

     1 tablespoon vanilla

     1 teaspoon ground cinnamon

    ½ teaspoon ground nutmeg

    ¼ teaspoon salt

     2 cups thawed frozen reduced-fat whipped topping

       Additional ground nutmeg (optional)

1. Preheat oven to 350°F. Coat 9-inch springform baking pan with nonstick cooking spray; set aside.

2. Place graham crackers, margarine and ginger in food processor or blender; pulse until coarse in texture. Gently press crumb mixture onto bottom and ¾ inch up side of pan. Bake 10 minutes or until lightly browned; cool slightly on wire rack.

3. Beat remaining ingredients except whipped topping and additional nutmeg in large bowl with electric mixer at medium-high speed until smooth; pour into pie crust. Bake 1 hour and 15 minutes or until top begins to crack and center moves very little when pan is shaken back and forth. Cool on wire rack to room temperature; refrigerate until ready to serve. Just before serving, spoon 1 tablespoonful whipped topping onto each serving; sprinkle lightly with additional nutmeg, if desired.

Makes 16 servings

Nutrients per Serving (¹⁄₁₆ of cheesecake):
Calories: 187, Calories from Fat: 28%, Total Fat: 6g, Saturated Fat: 4g, Cholesterol: 9mg, Sodium: 338mg, Carbohydrate: 23g, Dietary Fiber: 1g, Protein: 8g

Dietary Exchanges: 1½ Starch, 1 Lean Meat, ½ Fat

Tropical Snack Cake

1½ cups all-purpose flour

1 cup QUAKER® Oats (quick or old fashioned, uncooked)

2 tablespoons fructose

2 teaspoons baking powder

½ teaspoon baking soda

¼ teaspoon salt (optional)

1 can (8 ounces) crushed pineapple in juice, undrained

½ cup fat-free milk

⅓ cup mashed ripe banana

¼ cup egg substitute *or* 2 egg whites

2 tablespoons vegetable oil

2 teaspoons vanilla

Heat oven to 350°F. Grease and flour 8×8-inch square baking pan. Combine first 6 ingredients; mix well. Set aside. Blend pineapple, milk, banana, egg substitute, oil and vanilla until mixed thoroughly. Add to dry ingredients, mixing just until moistened. Pour into prepared pan. Bake 45 to 50 minutes or until golden brown and wooden pick inserted in center comes out clean. Cool slightly before serving.

Makes 12 servings

Nutrients per Serving (¹⁄₁₂ of cake):
Calories: 150, Calories from Fat: 18%, Total Fat: 3g, Saturated Fat: 0g, Cholesterol: 0mg, Sodium: 110mg, Carbohydrate: 26g, Dietary Fiber: 1g, Protein: 4g

Dietary Exchanges: 1 Starch, ½ Fruit, ½ Fat

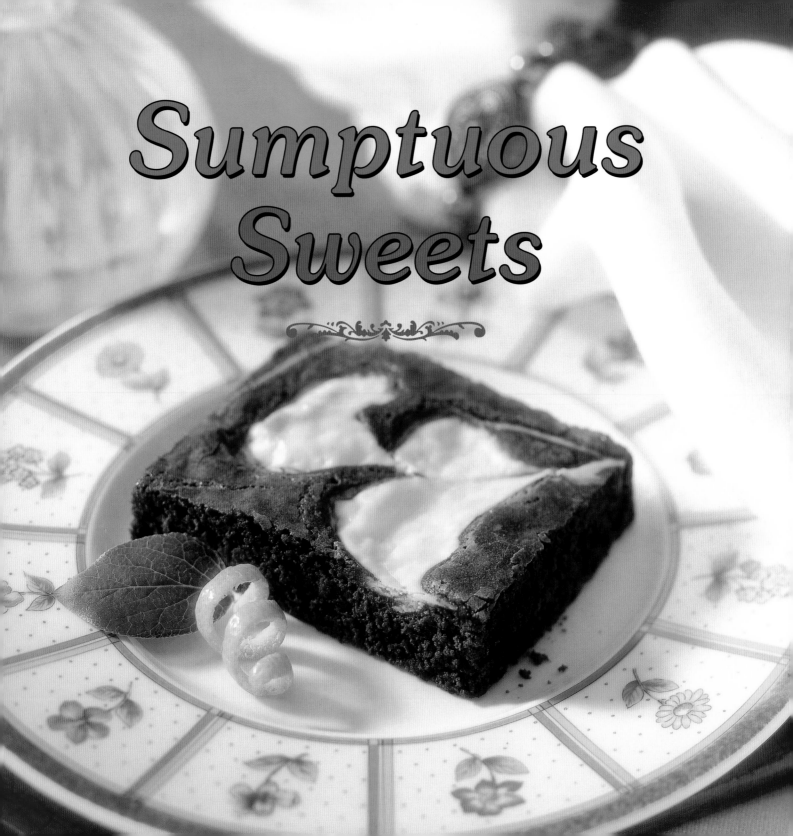

Sumptuous
Sweets

Cream Cheese Brownie Royale

1 package (about 15 ounces) low-fat brownie mix
⅔ cup cold coffee or water
1 package (8 ounces) reduced-fat cream cheese, softened
¼ cup fat-free (skim) milk
5 packets sugar substitute *or* equivalent of 10 teaspoons sugar
½ teaspoon vanilla

1. Preheat oven to 350°F. Coat 13×9-inch nonstick baking pan with nonstick cooking spray.

2. Combine brownie mix and coffee in large bowl; stir until blended. Pour brownie mixture into prepared pan.

3. Beat cream cheese, milk, sugar substitute and vanilla in medium bowl with electric mixer at medium speed until smooth. Spoon cream cheese mixture in dollops over brownie mixture. Swirl cream cheese mixture into brownie mixture with tip of knife.

4. Bake 30 to 35 minutes or until toothpick inserted in center comes out clean. Cool completely in pan on wire rack.

5. Cover with foil and refrigerate 8 hours or until ready to serve. Garnish as desired.

Makes 16 servings

Nutrients per Serving (¹⁄₁₆ of total recipe):
Calories: 167, Calories from Fat: 25%, Total Fat: 5g, Saturated Fat: 2g, Cholesterol: 7mg, Sodium: 181mg, Carbohydrate: 28g, Dietary Fiber: 1g, Protein: 4g

Dietary Exchanges: 2 Starch, ½ Fat

Cream Cheese Brownie Royale

Blackberry Sorbet

1 (8-fluid-ounce) can chilled Vanilla GLUCERNA® Shake

1 cup frozen whole blackberries, unsweetened

¼ teaspoon nutmeg

½ teaspoon cinnamon

    Sugar substitute to taste

1. In blender, combine all ingredients. Blend until thick.

2. Serve immediately or freeze 10 to 15 minutes. Garnish as desired. *Makes 2 servings*

Nutrients per Serving (¾ cup):
Calories: 161, Calories from Fat: 31%, Total Fat: 6g, Saturated Fat: 1g, Cholesterol: 1mg, Sodium: 106mg, Carbohydrate: 23g, Dietary Fiber: 5g, Protein: 6g

Dietary Exchanges: 1 Starch, 1 Fruit, 1 Fat

recipe tip

Glucerna® Shakes were specially designed to serve as an occasional meal replacement or a snack for people with diabetes. You can find them in pharmacies and in most large supermarkets.

Blackberry Sorbet

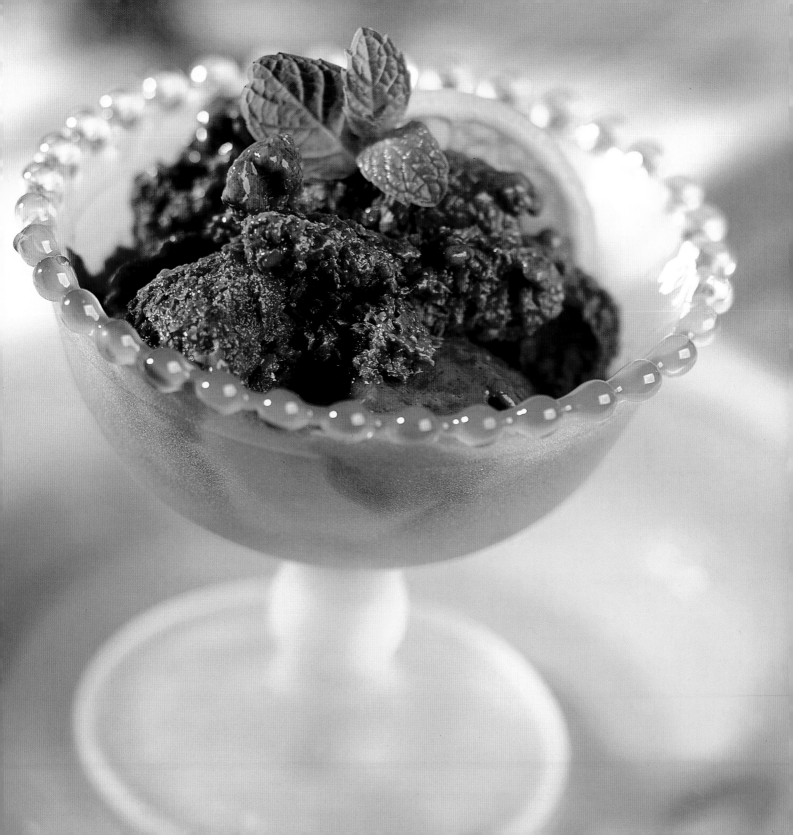

Grandma's Apple Crisp

¾ cup apple juice

3½ teaspoons EQUAL® FOR RECIPES *or* 12 packets EQUAL® sweetener *or* ½ cup EQUAL® SPOONFUL™

1 tablespoon cornstarch

1 teaspoon grated lemon peel

4 cups sliced peeled apples

¼ cup all-purpose flour

2½ teaspoons EQUAL® FOR RECIPES *or* 8 packets EQUAL® sweetener *or* ⅓ cup EQUAL® SPOONFUL™

1 teaspoon ground cinnamon

½ teaspoon ground nutmeg

3 dashes ground allspice

4 tablespoons cold margarine, cut into pieces

¼ cup each quick-cooking oats and unsweetened flaked coconut*

Unsweetened coconut can be purchased in health food stores.

Combine juice, Equal®, cornstarch and lemon peel in medium saucepan. Add apples; heat to boiling. Reduce heat; simmer, uncovered, until thickened and apples begin to lose crispness, about 5 minutes. Arrange apples in 8-inch square baking pan. Combine flour, Equal® and spices in small bowl; cut in margarine with pastry blender until mixture resembles coarse crumbs. Stir in oats and coconut. Bake in preheated 400°F oven until topping is browned and apples are tender, about 25 minutes. Serve warm.

Makes 6 servings

Nutrients per Serving (⅙ of Apple Crisp):
Calories: 165, Calories from Fat: 33%, Total Fat: 6g, Saturated Fat: 2g, Cholesterol: 0mg, Sodium: 91mg, Carbohydrate: 28g, Dietary Fiber: 3g, Protein: 2g

Dietary Exchanges: 2 Fruit, 1 Fat

Grandma's Apple Crisp

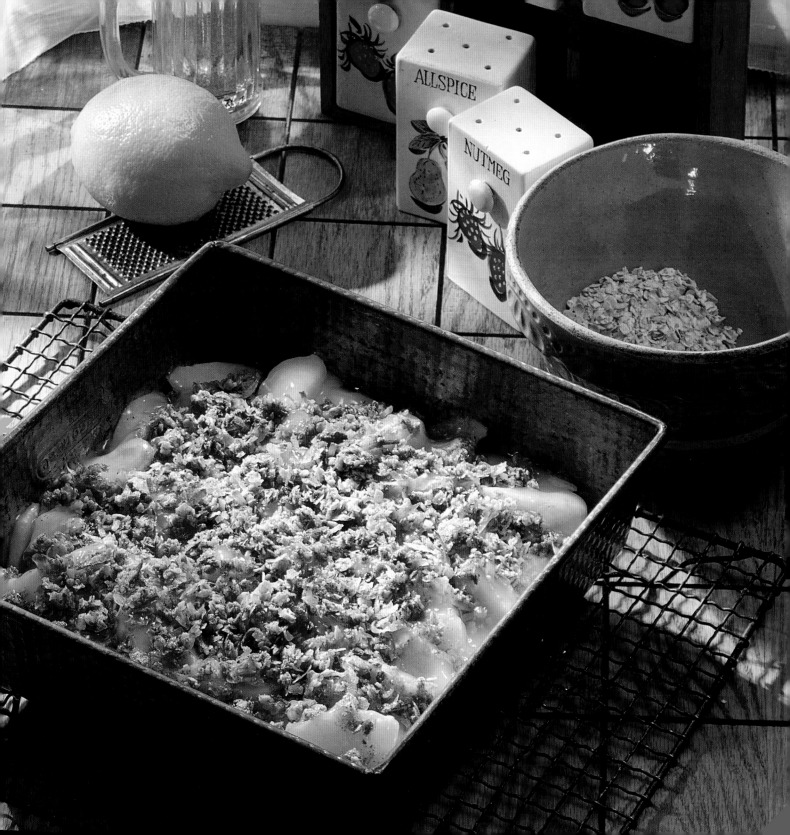

Apricot and Toasted Almond Phyllo Cups

Butter-flavored nonstick cooking spray

½ **cup (1%) low-fat cottage cheese**

4 **ounces reduced-fat cream cheese**

2 **packets sugar substitute** *or* **equivalent of 4 teaspoons sugar**

1 **tablespoon fat-free (skim) milk**

¼ **teaspoon vanilla**

4 **sheets phyllo dough**

3 **tablespoons apricot or blackberry preserves**

¼ **cup sliced almonds, toasted**

1. Preheat oven to 350°F. Coat 8 (2½-inch) muffin cups with cooking spray; set aside.

2. Beat cottage cheese, cream cheese, sugar substitute, milk and vanilla in large bowl with electric mixer at high speed until completely smooth; refrigerate until needed.

3. Place 1 sheet phyllo dough on work surface. Keep remaining sheets covered with plastic wrap and damp kitchen towel. Lightly spray phyllo sheet with cooking spray; top with another sheet; spray with cooking spray. Repeat with remaining sheets of phyllo.

4. Cut stack of phyllo into 8 pieces, using sharp knife or kitchen scissors. Gently fit each stacked square into prepared muffin cup. Bake 5 minutes or until lightly browned; cool on wire rack.

5. Place preserves in small microwavable bowl. Microwave at HIGH 20 seconds or until just melted. Spoon 2 tablespoons cream cheese mixture into each phyllo cup; drizzle 1 teaspoon melted preserves on top of cheese mixture. Top with 1½ teaspoons almonds. *Makes 8 servings*

Nutrients per Serving (1 filled Phyllo Cup):
Calories: 109, Calories from Fat: 41%, Total Fat: 5g, Saturated Fat: 2g, Cholesterol: 8mg, Sodium: 174mg, Carbohydrate: 12g, Dietary Fiber: 1g, Protein: 5g

Dietary Exchanges: 1 Starch, 1 Fat

Strawberry Lime Dessert

2 cups boiling water
1 package (4-serving size) JELL-O® Brand Lime Flavor Sugar Free Low Calorie
    Gelatin Dessert
½ cup cold water
1 container (8 ounces) BREYERS® Vanilla Lowfat Yogurt
1 package (4-serving size) JELL-O® Brand Strawberry Flavor Sugar Free Low
    Calorie Gelatin Dessert
1 package (10 ounces) frozen strawberries in lite syrup, unthawed

STIR 1 cup of the boiling water into lime gelatin in medium bowl at least 2 minutes until completely dissolved. Stir in cold water. Refrigerate about 45 minutes or until slightly thickened (consistency of unbeaten egg whites). Stir in yogurt with wire whisk until smooth. Pour into 2-quart serving bowl. Refrigerate about 15 minutes or until set but not firm (gelatin should stick to finger when touched and should mound).

STIR remaining 1 cup boiling water into strawberry gelatin in medium bowl at least 2 minutes until completely dissolved. Stir in frozen berries until berries are separated and gelatin is thickened (spoon drawn through leaves definite impression). Spoon over lime gelatin mixture.

REFRIGERATE 2 hours or until firm. Garnish as desired.   *Makes 10 servings*

Preparation Time: 15 minutes
Refrigerating Time: 3 hours

Nutrients per Serving (using JELL-O® Brand Strawberry and Lime Flavors Sugar Free Low Calorie Gelatin Dessert):
Calories: 37, Calories from Fat: 12%, Total Fat: <1g, Saturated Fat: <1g, Cholesterol: 1mg, Sodium: 60mg, Carbohydrate: 6g, Dietary Fiber: <1g, Protein: 2g

Dietary Exchanges: ½ Milk

Chocolate Fudge Cheesecake Parfaits

1½ cups nonfat cottage cheese

4 packets sugar substitute *or* equivalent of 8 teaspoons sugar

2 teaspoons packed brown sugar

1½ teaspoons vanilla

2 tablespoons semisweet mini chocolate chips, divided

2 cups fat-free chocolate ice cream or fat-free frozen yogurt

3 tablespoons graham cracker crumbs

1. Combine cottage cheese, sugar substitute, brown sugar and vanilla in food processor or blender; process until smooth. Stir in 1 tablespoon mini chips with wooden spoon.

2. Spoon about ¼ cup ice cream into each stemmed glass. Top with heaping tablespoon cheese mixture; sprinkle with 2 teaspoons graham cracker crumbs. Repeat layers. Freeze parfaits 15 to 30 minutes to firm slightly.

3. Garnish each parfait with remaining 1 tablespoon mini chips and remaining cracker crumbs.

Makes 4 servings

Nutrients per Serving (1 parfait):
Calories: 199, Calories from Fat: 9%, Total Fat: 2g, Saturated Fat: 1g, Cholesterol: 0mg, Sodium: 419mg, Carbohydrate: 28g, Dietary Fiber: 1g, Protein: 17g

Dietary Exchanges: 1½ Starch, 1½ Lean Meat

Chocolate Fudge Cheesecake Parfaits

Sumptuous Sweets

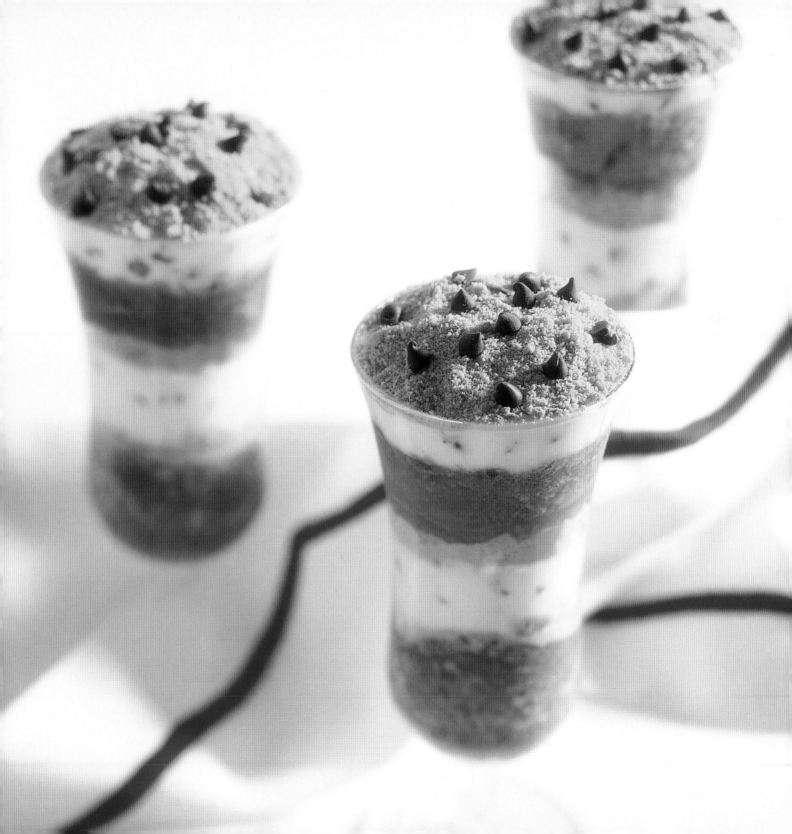

Lemon Mousse Squares

1 cup graham cracker crumbs
2 tablespoons reduced-fat margarine, melted
1 packet sugar substitute *or* equivalent of 2 teaspoons sugar
⅓ cup cold water
1 packet unflavored gelatin
2 eggs, well beaten
½ cup lemon juice
¼ cup sugar
2 teaspoons grated lemon peel
2 cups thawed frozen fat-free nondairy whipped topping
1 container (8 ounces) lemon-flavored nonfat yogurt with sugar substitute

1. Spray 9-inch square baking pan with nonstick cooking spray. Stir together graham cracker crumbs, margarine and sugar substitute in small bowl. Press into bottom of pan with fork; set aside.

2. Combine cold water and gelatin in small microwavable bowl; let stand 2 minutes. Microwave at HIGH 40 seconds to dissolve gelatin; set aside.

3. Combine eggs, lemon juice, sugar and lemon peel in top of double boiler. Cook, stirring constantly, over boiling water, about 4 minutes or until thickened. Remove from heat; stir in gelatin mixture. Refrigerate about 25 minutes or until mixture is thoroughly cooled and begins to set.

4. Gently combine lemon-gelatin mixture, whipped topping and lemon yogurt. Pour into prepared crust. Refrigerate 1 hour or until firm. Cut evenly into 9 squares. *Makes 9 servings*

Nutrients per Serving (1 square):
Calories: 154, Calories from Fat: 29%, Total Fat: 5g, Saturated Fat: 1g, Cholesterol: 47mg, Sodium: 124mg, Carbohydrate: 24g, Dietary Fiber: 1g, Protein: 3g

Dietary Exchanges: 1½ Starch, 1 Fat

Lemon Mousse Squares

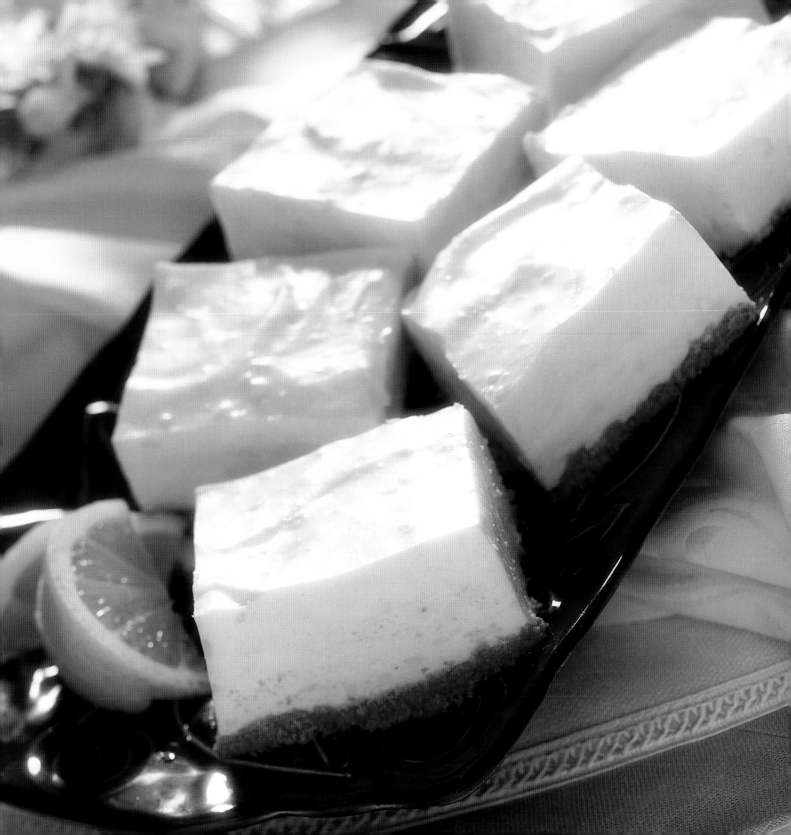

Sinfully Slim Crêpes Suzette

Crêpes
>   1 cup fat-free (skim) milk
>   3 egg whites
>   ¼ cup plus 2 tablespoons all-purpose flour

Filling
>   2½ tablespoons reduced-fat margarine
>   2 tablespoons sugar

Orange Sauce
>   1 cup fresh orange juice
>   2 tablespoons sugar
>   Peel of 1 orange, cut into ⅛-inch julienne strips
>   2 tablespoons orange-flavored liqueur

1. To prepare crêpes, combine milk, egg whites and flour in food processor or blender; process until smooth. Refrigerate at least 1 hour.

2. Heat 6- or 7-inch nonstick skillet over medium-high heat. Spray lightly with nonstick cooking spray. Pour 2 tablespoons crêpe batter into hot skillet; quickly rotate pan to distribute batter evenly. Cook 1 to 2 minutes or until nicely browned. Flip crêpe and cook on other side about 30 seconds. Stack crêpes on clean kitchen towel. Repeat with remaining batter, spraying skillet with cooking spray before each crêpe.

3. To prepare filling, combine margarine and 2 tablespoons sugar in small bowl; set aside.

4. To prepare sauce, combine orange juice and 2 tablespoons sugar in small saucepan. Bring to a boil over high heat; reduce heat to medium-high and continue cooking until reduced by half. Add orange peel; set aside. Pour liqueur into separate small saucepan; heat over medium-high heat until warm. Light with match and immediately stop flame with lid. Combine liqueur and orange sauce; keep warm. Set aside.

5. To serve, spread each crêpe with about ½ teaspoon filling mixture. Fold crêpes in half, then in half again to form a triangle. Arrange 2 crêpes on each dessert plate; repeat with remaining crêpes. Top each serving with about 1 tablespoon orange sauce; serve warm.   *Makes 6 servings (12 crêpes)*

Nutrients per Serving [2 crêpes plus 1 teaspoon filling mixture (½ teaspoon per crêpe) plus 1 tablespoon orange sauce]:
Calories: 139, Calories from Fat: 16%, Total Fat: 3g, Saturated Fat: <1g, Cholesterol: 1mg, Sodium: 106mg, Carbohydrate: 23g, Dietary Fiber: <1g, Protein: 4g

Dietary Exchanges: 1½ Starch, ½ Fat

Lighter Than Air Chocolate Delight

2 envelopes unflavored gelatin
½ cup cold water
1 cup boiling water
1⅓ cups nonfat dry milk powder
⅓ cup HERSHEY'S Cocoa or HERSHEY'S Dutch Processed Cocoa
1 tablespoon vanilla extract
Dash salt
Granulated sugar substitute to equal 14 teaspoons sugar
8 large ice cubes

1. Sprinkle gelatin over cold water in blender container; let stand 4 minutes to soften. Gently stir with rubber spatula, scraping gelatin particles off sides; add boiling water to gelatin mixture. Cover; blend until gelatin dissolves. Add milk powder, cocoa, vanilla and salt; blend on medium speed until well mixed. Add sugar substitute and ice cubes; blend on high speed until ice is crushed and mixture is smooth and fluffy.

2. Immediately pour into 4-cup mold. Cover; refrigerate until firm. Unmold onto serving plate.

Makes 8 servings

Note: Eight individual dessert dishes may be used in place of 4-cup mold, if desired.

Nutrients per Serving (⅛ of total recipe):
Calories: 72, Calories from Fat: 5%, Total Fat: <1g, Saturated Fat: <1g, Cholesterol: 2mg, Sodium: 67mg, Carbohydrate: 10g, Dietary Fiber: 1g, Protein: 6g

Dietary Exchanges: 1 Starch

Creamy Tapioca Pudding

2 cups skim milk
3 tablespoons quick-cooking tapioca
1 egg
⅛ teaspoon salt
3½ teaspoons EQUAL® FOR RECIPES *or* 12 packets EQUAL® sweetener *or* ½ cup
    EQUAL® SPOONFUL™
1 to 2 teaspoons vanilla
    Ground cinnamon and nutmeg

• Combine milk, tapioca, egg and salt in medium saucepan. Let stand 5 minutes. Cook over medium-high heat, stirring constantly, until boiling. Remove from heat; stir in Equal® and vanilla.

• Spoon mixture evenly into serving dishes; sprinkle lightly with cinnamon and nutmeg. Serve warm, or refrigerate and serve chilled. Garnish as desired.

Makes 4 servings

Nutrients per Serving (⅔ cup):
Calories: 105, Calories from Fat: 13%, Total Fat: 1g, Saturated Fat: 1g, Cholesterol: 56mg, Sodium: 152mg, Carbohydrate: 16g, Dietary Fiber: 0g, Protein: 6g

Dietary Exchanges: ½ Starch, ½ Milk, ½ Fat

recipe tip
Uncooked tapioca will keep for long periods of time if it's stored in a cool, dark place.

Creamy Tapioca Pudding

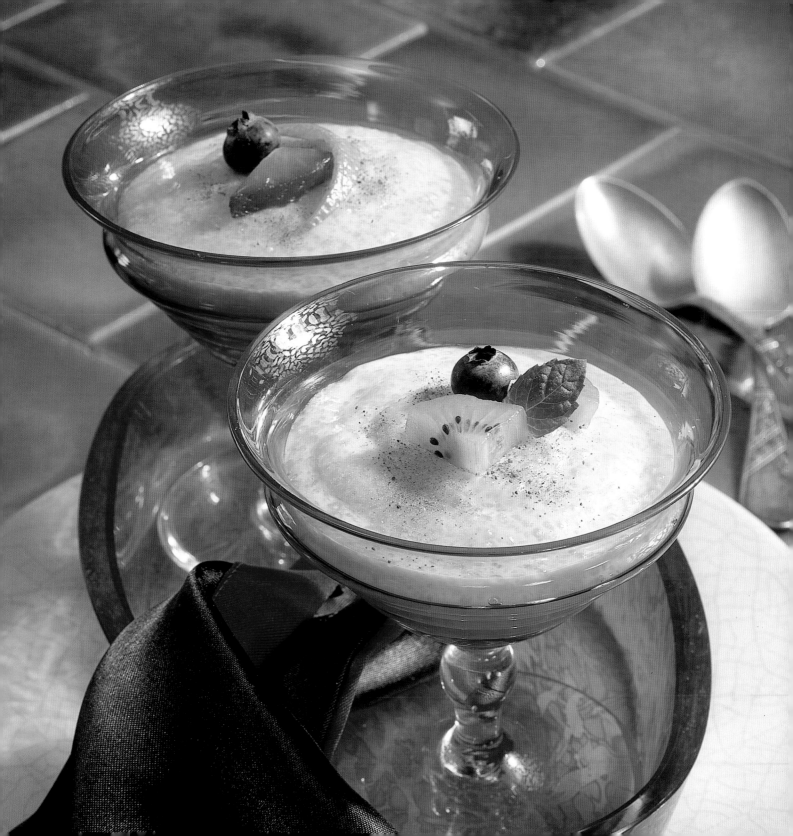

Chocolate-Strawberry Crêpes

Crêpes

⅔ cup all-purpose flour

2 tablespoons unsweetened cocoa powder

6 packages sugar substitute *or* equivalent of ¼ cup sugar

¼ teaspoon salt

1¼ cups fat-free (skim) milk

½ cup cholesterol-free egg substitute

1 tablespoon margarine, melted

1 teaspoon vanilla

Nonstick cooking spray

Filling and Topping

4 ounces fat-free cream cheese, softened

1 package (1.3 ounces) chocolate-fudge-flavored sugar-free instant pudding mix

1½ cups fat-free (skim) milk

¼ cup all-fruit strawberry preserves

2 tablespoons water

2 cups fresh hulled and quartered strawberries

1. To prepare crêpes, combine flour, cocoa, sugar substitute and salt in food processor; process to blend. Add milk, egg substitute, margarine and vanilla; process until smooth. Let stand at room temperature 30 minutes.

2. Spray 7-inch nonstick skillet with cooking spray; heat over medium-high heat. Pour 2 tablespoons crêpe batter into hot pan. Immediately rotate pan back and forth to swirl batter over entire surface of pan. Cook 1 to 2 minutes or until crêpe is brown around edge and top is dry. Carefully turn crêpe with spatula and cook 30 seconds more. Transfer crêpe to waxed paper to cool. Repeat with remaining batter, spraying pan with cooking spray as needed. Separate crêpes with sheets of waxed paper.

continued on page 366

Chocolate-Strawberry Crêpes

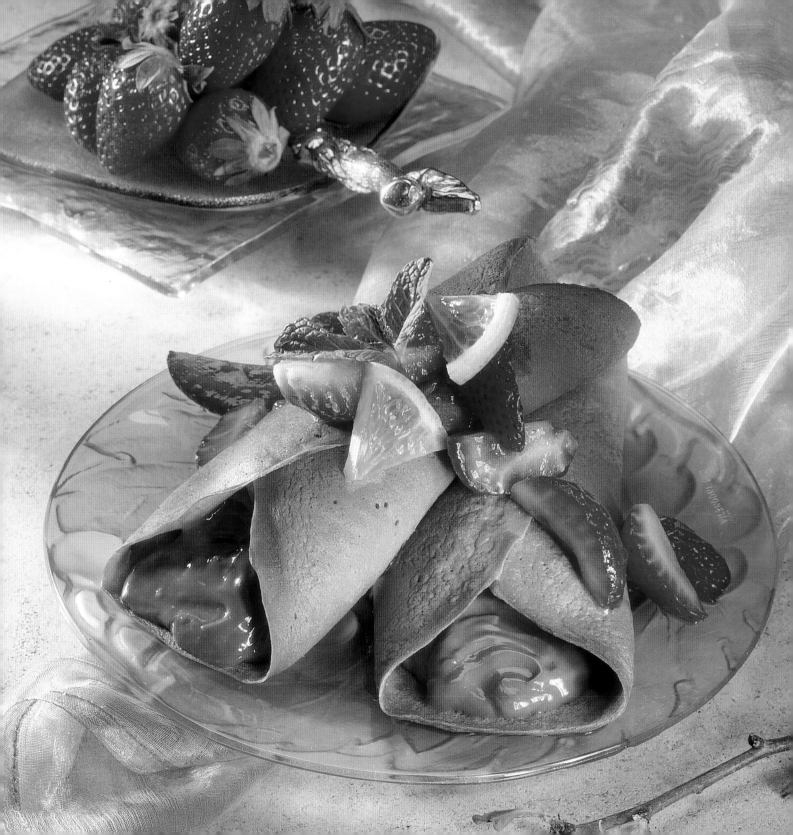

3. To prepare chocolate filling, beat cream cheese in medium bowl with electric mixer at high speed until smooth; set aside. Prepare chocolate pudding with skim milk according to package directions. Gradually add pudding to cream cheese; beat at high speed 3 minutes. To prepare strawberry topping, combine preserves and water in large bowl until smooth. Add strawberries; toss to coat.

4. Spread 2 tablespoons chocolate filling evenly over surface of each crêpe; roll tightly. Repeat with remaining crêpes. Place 2 crêpes on each plate. Spoon ¼ cup strawberry topping over each serving. Serve immediately. *Makes 8 servings*

Nutrients per Serving (2 filled crêpes plus ¼ cup strawberry topping):
Calories: 161, Calories from Fat: 13%, Total Fat: 2g, Saturated Fat: <1g, Cholesterol: 1mg, Sodium: 374mg, Carbohydrate: 27g, Dietary Fiber: 1g, Protein: 8g

Dietary Exchanges: 2 Fruit

Summer Melon Soup

1 medium-size ripe cantaloupe, cut into cubes
⅓ cup orange juice
¼ cup plain nonfat yogurt
3 tablespoons lime juice
2 tablespoons honey
6 thin slices lime, for garnish
Dash ground nutmeg

Combine cantaloupe, orange juice, yogurt, lime juice and honey in food processor or blender; process until smooth. Refrigerate, covered, 1 to 2 hours or until chilled. Serve soup in chilled bowls. Garnish with lime slices; sprinkle with nutmeg. *Makes 6 servings*

Nutrients per Serving (⅙ of total recipe):
Calories: 74, Calories from Fat: 4%, Total Fat: <1g, Saturated Fat: <1g, Cholesterol: <1mg, Sodium: 17mg, Carbohydrate: 18g, Dietary Fiber: 1g, Protein: 2g

Dietary Exchanges: 1 Fruit

Pumpkin Mousse Cups

1 can (15 ounces) solid pack pumpkin
½ cup low-fat sweetened condensed milk
4 packets sugar substitute *or* equivalent of 8 teaspoons sugar
1 teaspoon ground cinnamon
¼ teaspoon ground ginger
¼ teaspoon salt
1 packet unflavored gelatin
2 tablespoons water
2 cups thawed frozen low-fat nondairy whipped topping

1. Combine pumpkin, milk, sugar substitute, cinnamon, ginger and salt in medium bowl; set aside.

2. Combine gelatin and water in small microwavable bowl; let stand 2 minutes. Microwave at HIGH 40 seconds to dissolve gelatin. Stir into pumpkin mixture. Gently fold whipped topping into pumpkin mixture until well combined.

3. Spoon into 8 to 10 small dessert dishes. Refrigerate 1 hour or until slightly firm.

Makes 8 servings

Nutrients per Serving (⅛ of total recipe):
Calories: 113, Calories from Fat: 16%, Total Fat: 2g, Saturated Fat: <1g, Cholesterol: 5mg, Sodium: 112mg, Carbohydrate: 22g, Dietary Fiber: 2g, Protein: 3g

Dietary Exchanges: 1½ Starch

Spun Sugar Berries with Yogurt Crème

2 cups fresh raspberries*
1 container (8 ounces) lemon-flavored nonfat sugar-free yogurt
1 cup thawed frozen fat-free nondairy whipped topping
3 tablespoons sugar

*You may substitute your favorite fresh berry for the fresh raspberries.

1. Arrange berries in 4 glass dessert dishes.

2. Combine yogurt and whipped topping in medium bowl. (If not using immediately, cover and refrigerate.) Top berries with yogurt mixture.

3. To prepare spun sugar, pour sugar into heavy medium saucepan. Cook over medium-high heat until sugar melts, shaking pan occasionally. *Do not stir.* As sugar begins to melt, reduce heat to low and cook about 10 minutes or until sugar is completely melted and has turned light golden brown.

4. Remove from heat; let stand 1 minute. Coat metal fork with sugar mixture. Drizzle sugar over berries with circular or back and forth motion. Ropes of spun sugar will harden quickly. Garnish as desired. Serve immediately. *Makes 4 servings*

Nutrients per Serving (¼ of total recipe):
Calories: 119, Calories from Fat: 2%, Total Fat: <1g, Saturated Fat: <1g, Cholesterol: 0mg, Sodium: 45mg, Carbohydrate: 26g, Dietary Fiber: 4g, Protein: 3g

Dietary Exchanges: 2 Fruit

Spun Sugar Berries with Yogurt Crème

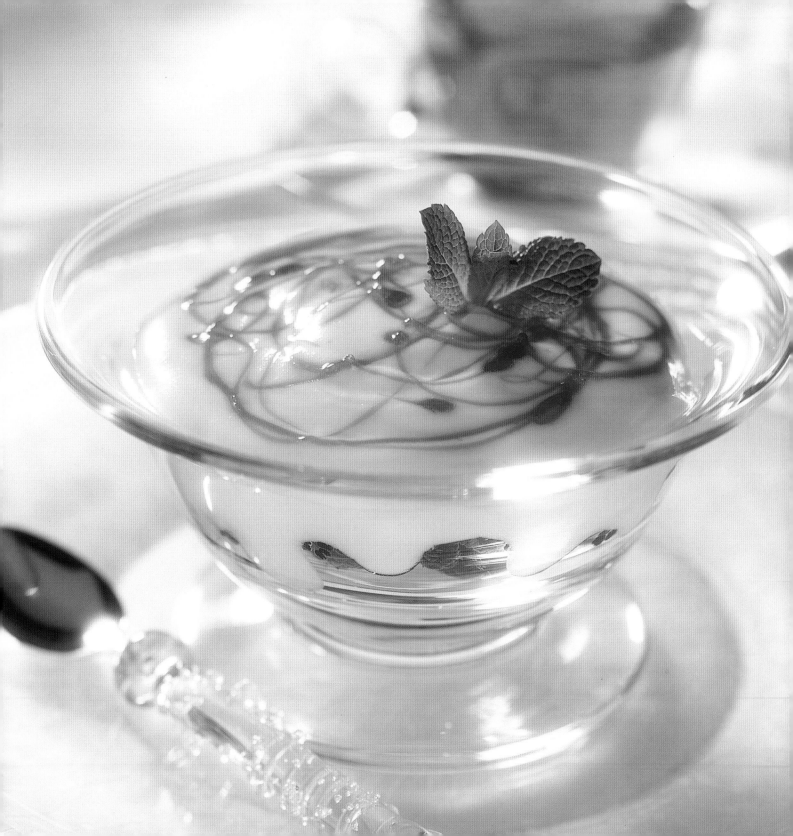

Crispy Rice Squares

3 tablespoons Dried Plum Purée (recipe follows) or prepared dried plum butter
1 tablespoon butter or margarine
1 package (10 ounces) marshmallows
6 cups crisp rice cereal
   Colored nonpareils

Coat 13×9-inch baking pan with vegetable cooking spray. Heat dried plum purée and butter in Dutch oven or large saucepan over low heat, stirring until butter is melted. Add marshmallows; stir until completely melted. Remove from heat. Stir in cereal until well coated. Spray back of wooden spoon with vegetable cooking spray and pat mixture evenly into prepared pan. Sprinkle with nonpareils. Cool until set. Cut evenly into squares. *Makes 24 squares*

Dried Plum Purée: Combine 1⅓ cups (8 ounces) pitted dried plums and 6 tablespoons hot water in container of food processor or blender. Pulse on and off until dried plums are finely chopped and smooth. Store leftovers in a covered container in the refrigerator for up to two months. Makes 1 cup.

Favorite recipe from **California Dried Plum Board**

Nutrients per Serving (1 square):
Calories: 74, Calories from Fat: 7%, Total Fat: 1g, Saturated Fat: <1g, Cholesterol: 1mg, Sodium: 62mg, Carbohydrate: 17g, Dietary Fiber: <1g, Protein: 1g

Dietary Exchanges: 1 Starch

Crispy Rice Squares

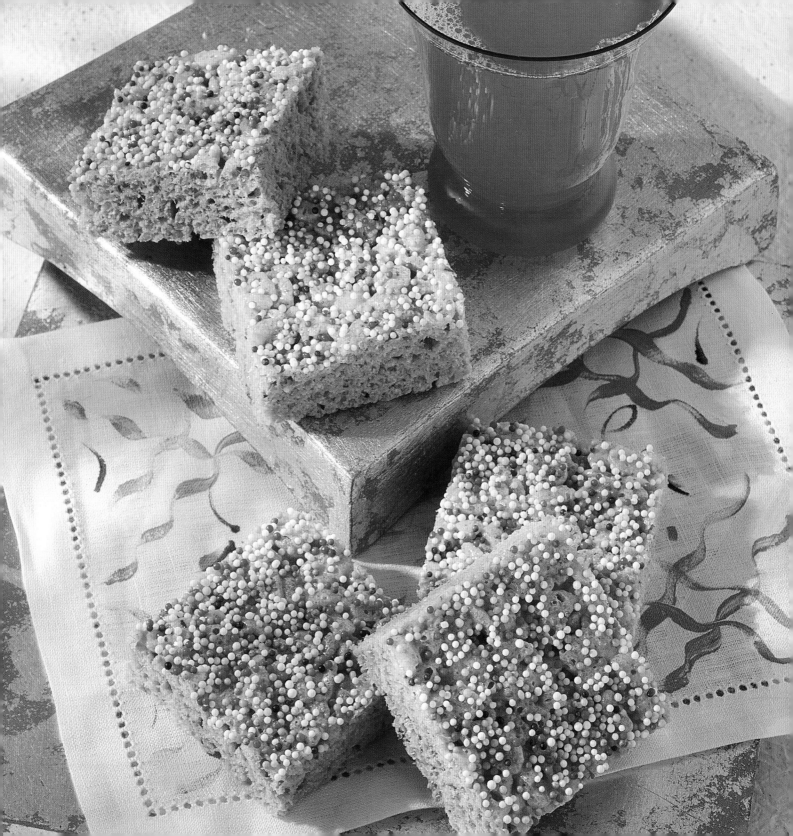

Yogurt Fluff

¾ cup boiling water

1 package (4-serving size) JELL-O® Brand Sugar Free Low Calorie Gelatin
   Dessert or JELL-O® Brand Gelatin Dessert, any flavor

½ cup cold water or fruit juice

   Ice cubes

1 container (8 ounces) BREYERS® Vanilla Lowfat Yogurt

½ teaspoon vanilla (optional)

5 tablespoons thawed COOL WHIP FREE® or COOL WHIP LITE® Whipped
   Topping

STIR boiling water into gelatin in large bowl at least 2 minutes until completely dissolved.

MIX cold water and ice cubes to make 1 cup. Add to gelatin, stirring until slightly thickened. Remove any remaining ice. Stir in yogurt and vanilla. Pour evenly into 5 dessert dishes.

REFRIGERATE 1½ hours or until firm. Top each with 1 tablespoon whipped topping.

Makes 5 servings

Preparation Time: 10 minutes
Refrigerating Time: 1½ hours

Nutrients per Serving (⅕ of total recipe, using JELL-O® Brand Sugar Free Low Calorie Gelatin Dessert, water and COOL WHIP FREE®):
Calories: 61, Calories from Fat: 13%, Total Fat: 1g, Saturated Fat: <1g, Cholesterol: 3mg, Sodium: 92mg, Carbohydrate: 9g, Dietary Fiber: 0g, Protein: 3g

Dietary Exchanges: 1 Starch

Yogurt Fluff

Sumptuous Sweets

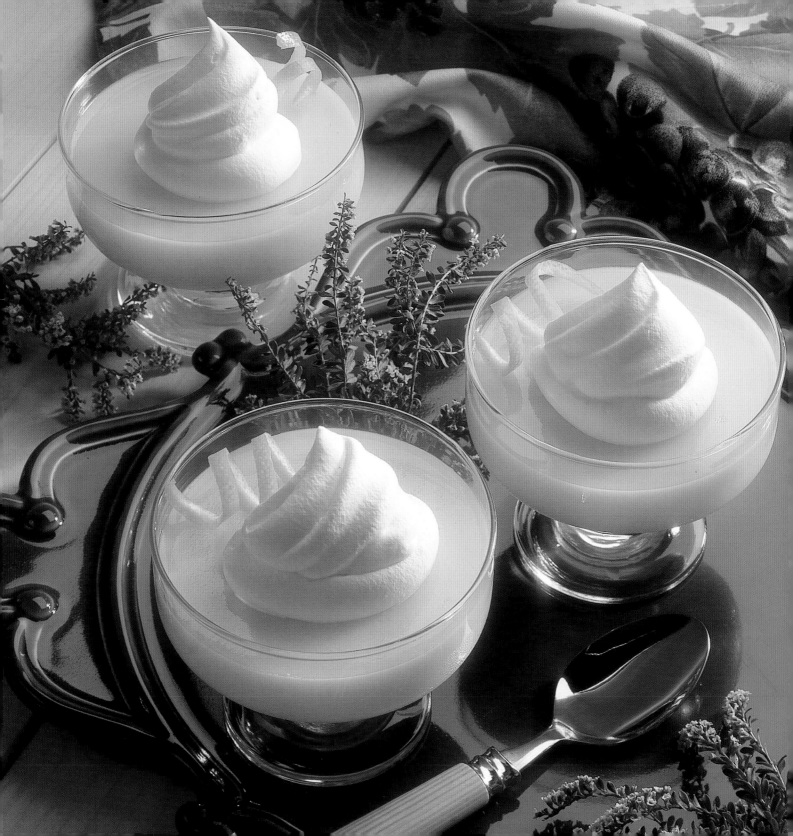

Acknowledgments

The publisher would like to thank the companies and organizations listed below for the use of their recipes and photographs in this publication.

A.1.® Steak Sauce

Barilla America, Inc.

Birds Eye®

Butterball® Turkey Company

California Dried Plum Board

California Poultry Federation

Del Monte Corporation

Dole Food Company, Inc.

Egg Beaters®

Equal® sweetener

Filippo Berio® Olive Oil

Glucerna® is a registered trademark of Abbott Laboratories

The Golden Grain Company®

Guiltless Gourmet®

Hershey Foods Corporation

Holland House® is a registered trademark of Mott's, Inc.

Kikkoman International Inc.

The Kingsford Products Company

Kraft Foods Holdings

Lawry's® Foods, Inc.

Mushroom Council

National Chicken Council/US Poultry & Egg Association

National Fisheries Institute

National Pork Board

National Turkey Federation

North Dakota Wheat Commission

Peanut Advisory Board

Perdue Farms Incorporated

The Quaker® Oatmeal Kitchens

Reckitt Benckiser Inc.

Riviana Foods Inc.

The J.M. Smucker Company

Splenda® is a registered trademark of McNeil Specialty Products Company

StarKist® Seafood Company

Property of © 2003 Sunkist Growers, Inc. All rights reserved.

Texas Peanut Producers Board

Tyson Foods, Inc.

Uncle Ben's Inc.

Walnut Marketing Board

Wisconsin Milk Marketing Board

Index

METRIC CONVERSION CHART

VOLUME MEASUREMENTS (dry)

1/8 teaspoon = 0.5 mL
1/4 teaspoon = 1 mL
1/2 teaspoon = 2 mL
3/4 teaspoon = 4 mL
1 teaspoon = 5 mL
1 tablespoon = 15 mL
2 tablespoons = 30 mL
1/4 cup = 60 mL
1/3 cup = 75 mL
1/2 cup = 125 mL
2/3 cup = 150 mL
3/4 cup = 175 mL
1 cup = 250 mL
2 cups = 1 pint = 500 mL
3 cups = 750 mL
4 cups = 1 quart = 1 L

VOLUME MEASUREMENTS (fluid)

1 fluid ounce (2 tablespoons) = 30 mL
4 fluid ounces (1/2 cup) = 125 mL
8 fluid ounces (1 cup) = 250 mL
12 fluid ounces (1 1/2 cups) = 375 mL
16 fluid ounces (2 cups) = 500 mL

WEIGHTS (mass)

1/2 ounce = 15 g
1 ounce = 30 g
3 ounces = 90 g
4 ounces = 120 g
8 ounces = 225 g
10 ounces = 285 g
12 ounces = 360 g
16 ounces = 1 pound = 450 g

DIMENSIONS

1/16 inch = 2 mm
1/8 inch = 3 mm
1/4 inch = 6 mm
1/2 inch = 1.5 cm
3/4 inch = 2 cm
1 inch = 2.5 cm

OVEN TEMPERATURES

250°F = 120°C
275°F = 140°C
300°F = 150°C
325°F = 160°C
350°F = 180°C
375°F = 190°C
400°F = 200°C
425°F = 220°C
450°F = 230°C

BAKING PAN SIZES

Utensil	Size in Inches/Quarts	Metric Volume	Size in Centimeters
Baking or Cake Pan (square or rectangular)	8×8×2	2 L	20×20×5
	9×9×2	2.5 L	23×23×5
	12×8×2	3 L	30×20×5
	13×9×2	3.5 L	33×23×5
Loaf Pan	8×4×3	1.5 L	20×10×7
	9×5×3	2 L	23×13×7
Round Layer Cake Pan	8×1½	1.2 L	20×4
	9×1½	1.5 L	23×4
Pie Plate	8×1¼	750 mL	20×3
	9×1¼	1 L	23×3
Baking Dish or Casserole	1 quart	1 L	—
	1½ quart	1.5 L	—
	2 quart	2 L	—